THE CLINICAL MANAGEMENT

OF

BASIC MAXILLOFACIAL ORTHOPEDIC APPLIANCES

VOLUME III: TEMPOROMANDIBULAR JOINT

Terrance J. Spahl, D.D.S.

*in collaboration with
and presenting the case studies of*

John W. Witzig, D.D.S.

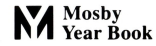
Mosby
Year Book

St. Louis   Baltimore   Boston   Chicago   London   Philadelphia   Sydney   Toronto

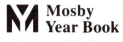

**Mosby
Year Book**

Dedicated to Publishing Excellence

Sponsoring Editor: Robert Reinhardt
Associate Managing Editor, Manuscript Services: Deborah Thorp
Production Project Coordinator: Carol A. Reynolds
Proofroom Manager: Barbara Kelly

Library of Congress Cataloging-in-Publication Data
(Revised for volume 3)
Spahl, Terrance J.
    The clinical management of basic maxillofacial
orthopedic appliances.
    Vol. 3-Temporomandibular joint—by John
Witzig and Terrance J. Spahl.
    Vol. 3-   has imprint: Chicago : Mosby-Year
Book, Inc.
    Includes bibliographies and indexes.
    Contents: v. 1. Mechanics—
v. 2. Diagnostics—
v. 3. Temporomandibular joint–
    1. Orthodontic appliances. I. Witzig, John W.
[DNLM: 1. Orthodontic Appliances. WU 400
S733c]
RK527.S63 1987   617.6'43   86-91476
ISBN 0-8841-6558-2 (v. 1)
ISBN 0-8841-6559-0 (v. 2)

Printed in Hong Kong

To those who were there
when needed.

ABOUT THE AUTHORS

Terrance J. Spahl, D.D.S., has been in private practice in St. Paul, Minnesota since 1971. He is a dental products consultant for the 3M Company and Ohlendorf Company Orthodontic Laboratory, and a clinical consultant for Ortho-Diagnostics Ltd.

Dr. Spahl has lectured widely to dental and medical groups on the subject of the temporomandibular joint and co-developed the Witzig-Spahl Analysis, the first computerized method for analyzing TMJ X-rays.

A clinician with extensive orthodontic experience, Dr. Spahl has studied under noted experts in the United States and abroad. He is a member of the American Equilibration Society, the American Endodontic Society, the American Dental Association, the American Academy of General Dentistry, and the American Association of Functional Orthodontics.

John W. Witzig, D.D.S., maintains a private practice devoted exclusively to orthodontics and TMJ pain patients, in Minneapolis, Minnesota. He is regional editor of *The Journal of Cranio-Mandibular Practice* and contributing editor to *The Functional Orthodontist*.

Dr. Witzig is author of *Orthodontic and Orthopedic Appliances* and co-author of *Orthodontics and Its Effect on the TMJ and Clinical Management of TMJ Pain*. He developed and patented the Orthopedic Corrector I Appliance and the Orthopedic Corrector II Appliance and is co-holder of the U.S. patent on the Sagittal III Appliance. Dr. Witzig is a member of the American Equilibration Society, the American Association of Functional Orthodontics, the European Orthodontic Society, the International Association of Orthodontics, and the American Dental Association.

An experienced clinician who has studied in the United States and Europe, he was honored as "Man of the Year" in 1984 by the American Association of Functional Orthodontics. Since 1972, Dr. Witzig has conducted dental education courses for more than 15,000 doctors in North America.

CONTENTS

v

FOREWORD

It has been estimated there may be as many as 45 million Americans who suffer from temporomandibular joint disorders. For those people and the dentists who treat them, Drs. Witzig and Spahl have written this book. The answers to their perplexing pains are to be found in this concise, informational, and entertaining treatise.

The dental profession has long awaited just such a book as this. For the first time, all the important elements have been combined to give the student of temporomandibular disorders the tools necessary to diagnose and treat those disorders. Literally thousands of hours have gone into the production of this text. Hundreds of cases have been reviewed and many of the leading authorities in the treatment of temporomandibular disorders have contributed to the pages of this book. It gives the best overview of joint anatomy available today. A careful study of that section will give the reader a true understanding of joint function and an appreciation of dysfunction.

The authors have painstakingly detailed the major symptoms of temporomandibular disorders with explanations of those symptoms and their relationship with other anatomical structures and sites of referred pain. This information is invaluable in understanding the progression of TM disorders and in explaining it to the patient.

The careful delineation of diagnostic techniques with their description and interpretation is most enlightening at a time when so many new materials, modalities, and methods are flooding the marketplace. The authors offer some very practical advice in this section for the selection and use of diagnostic procedures in the everyday practice of dentistry by those treating TM disorders. In particular, the chapter on radiography is a valuable tool for understanding the often complicated area of joint imaging. Here the reader is taken from simple transcranial or transparietal films all the way through nuclear magnetic resonance imaging with a clear explanation of each type of image.

After a detailed discussion of diagnostics, the topic of treatment is undertaken. Once again, the thoroughness of the authors is manifest. Many of the authors' cases, as well as those from other contributors, are shown and explained in detail. This information is most useful in helping the reader relate to his own patients and understand treatment modalities that can be employed in difficult situations.

We are indebted to the authors for their untiring efforts in bringing forth this book. This is the third in a series that has enlightened us all. Some will praise and some will find fault. However, most of us would do nothing if we waited until we could do it so well that no one could find fault with what we had done. We often discover what will do by finding out what will not do; and probably he who never made a mistake never made a discovery. Dr. Samuel Johnson is reported to have said, "knowledge always desires increase; it is like fire, which must first be kindled by some external agent, but which will afterwards propagate itself." We express our gratitude to Dr. Witzig and Dr. Spahl for expanding our knowledge and understanding in the area of temporomandibular joint disorders. You have kindled a fire within us.

James S. Colt, D.D.S., M.D.
Director, TMJ Clinic
University of Colorado Health Sciences Center
Denver, Colorado

PREFACE

We meet again. And this third time it is on the highly contested terrain of the diagnosis and treatment of temporomandibular joint pain and dysfunction. It is a jousting field littered with the broken lances of failed therapeutic regimens, bits of the battered armor of pedantic opinion, and—of course—the vestiges of crumpled and wounded ego. But beyond this din there are also the victories, the champions; those who have faced the test and have endured. Their work and contributions herald the true progress in this discipline, and the greatest victory to date, so far as the application of practical and effective therapeutics is concerned, has been registered by those leading clinicians who have determined the method of applying the principles of functional jaw orthopedics to the treatment of functionally induced TMJ problems. What makes this approach so important is the incredible number of patients to which it applies.

In a field as highly controversial as TMJ, one of the major problems both the dental and medical professions have had to confront is not one of etiology, but rather one of epidemiology. It is true that there are many varied etiologic agents that cause pain and dysfunction in the TMJs. Many agents may also cause the headaches (cephalalgia) and neckaches (cervicalgia) that are so intimately associated with the TMJ pain-dysfunction patient on such a consistent basis. However, all but one basic etiologic agent have been observed clinically to be quite rare. What has emerged over the decades to surprise even those most closely associated with treatment of TMJ disorders is the relationship of the series of TMJ pain-dysfunction-headache-neckache signs and symptoms to the status of the functional occlusion. Put simply, too many patients are suffering from functional malocclusions that force the mandible to bite too far back. When this happens on a consistent enough basis, and with a sufficient enough level of intensity, the TM joints become disarticulated and physical breakdown begins. This in turn initiates a whole raft of TMJ pain, dysfunction, headache, and neckache problems. Imbalanced, improper dysfunction is the problem, rebalanced proper normal function is the solution. Other conditions can and do exist, of course. That is why there will always be a need for the true specialist and the avant garde technique. But the incidence of TMJ problems of a functionally induced nature account for 99% of those patients who suffer classic TMJ pains, joint sounds, headache, facial pains, and neckaches.

Differential diagnosis is not only essential in determining the true nature of the patient's TMJ problems, but also in determining if a true TMJ problem even exists. Yet once that diagnostic process has been properly understood and executed, the clinician will be amazed at the repetitive nature of the signs, symptoms, cause, and resultant treatments indicated. Each patient varies somewhat as to symptomatic details and clinical findings. Yet they will be observed to generally fall into a repetitive pattern with alarming constancy. Something in the functional occlusion drives the mandible/condyle unit too far superiorly and posteriorly during full force occlusion for Nature to find it acceptable. A deranged occlusion will often be seen as the true cause of the patient's particular symptomatic picture. A rearranged occlusion will often be seen as the means of resolving the case and relieving the pains. Effecting this is not the problem. The problem lies in the reticence of both the medical and dental professions to realize the cause-and-effect relationship of the malocclusion/TMJ pain-dysfunction/headache neckache scenario. Its occurence is ubiquitous in the general population of patients. It can be caused by a naturally occurring malocclusion or it may result from, or be worsened by, certain types of "traditional" dental treatments and/or trauma. Unusual cases with rare or unusual etiological agents can and do exist. There are even cases that defy diagnosis and resolution by means of conventional technology. Fortunately, as previously stated, such cases are relatively rare and for them the team approach of sophisticated institutional settings are appropriate.

Because of the self-consciousness of the lack of a true understanding of the nature of the TMJ pain-dysfunction problem, the health care professions have approached the establishment of universally acceptable diagnostic and treatment planning regimens with the greatest of trepidation. The wide range of rare types of TMJ problems no doubt intensifies this caution. There has not even been a generally accepted method developed to date as to how to categorize the problem or what to even call it. Yet one fact remains: the average functionally induced TMJ problem follows a predictable pattern of etiology and treatment response and the incidence of occurence of these common types of TMJ conditions, when compared to the less common types, is so great that they dominate the field in an overwhelming fashion. Hence, although the TMJ clinician must keep a "diagnostic eye" out for the rare or the exotic, these common types of TMJ pain-dysfunction problems command the most direct attention. One should not be led to assume the 99% are like the 1%. Conversely, one should be careful not to assume the 1% are like the other 99%. Yet unless the medical and dental disciplines are prepared to accept that the basic principles of functional jaw orthopedics are the appropriate method of resolution of functionally induced TMJ pain-dysfunction problems, and these types of problems are by far and away the most prevalent variety, there is a great danger the 99% will be figuratively dumped into the "live-with-it" clump of the 1%.

Another unnecessary conflict is the clash between the scientific method and the human method. The former has no innate power to negate the latter. The clinically observed evidence over the past few decades has been such that inertia on the acknowledgement of the significance of the relationship of functional jaw orthopedics to functionally induced TMJ problems is totally unjustified and intolerable. The condescending criticisms and resistance to change of those who feel threatened by such a revolutionary concept contributes nothing to the advancement of the cause of helping clinicians help their patients. Rather, such only serves to brace the academic narcissism with which these resisters adorn themselves. Some forget to whom they own their allegiance. The patient's need for proper care commands the foremost position on our list of priorities.

Instead of controversy, rejection, and self-serving "turf protection," what is needed is an open-minded willingness to search out the truth, whatever it may turn out to be and whereever its source may be. This must be done for the sake of the patient. Just such a search has been going on quietly and steadily and it is now bearing fruit. Its source has been private clinical practice. One cannot deny that a common consensus among common practitioners is what will eventually set the standards of care. And when the good and honest people of this profession are given the facts and the truth, the great body of common practitioners will be found to seldom make a mistake. This text represents a step in the direction of reaching that consensus. It is designed, therefore, to be an introductory medium to the most basic aspects of the TMJ problem and concentrates mainly on the singular most prevalent variety. Such a concentration is effected in an effort to deliver the greatest amount of assistance to the greatest number of clinicians and, in turn, to eventually benefit the greatest number of patients. There will always be other texts, other methods, new techniques, and new scientific findings. There is so much we must yet learn. But one must always begin with the basics. From there, advancement of individual skills may take whatever course necessary. It should also be an undertaking performed in the proper spirit. The needs of the patient demand that for their sakes we professionals of the healing arts stand shoulder to shoulder against disease, not nose to nose against each other.

Terrance J. Spahl, D.D.S.

"What we have beaten in Nature we cannot conquer in ourselves"

Adlai E. Stevenson
American Statesman

ACKNOWLEDGMENTS

John Donne was right, "No man is an island." This is especially true in the book-writing business. When this author was approached with the proposition of writing a series of texts for Dr. John Witzig that would not only chronicle his particular message but would also expound upon the ancillary aspects supportive of that message, neither side envisioned that the project would stretch out over a decade. Yet in these troubled times, with respect to the controversial and revolutionary movements in both orthodontic and temporomandibular joint therapeutics, an important statement had to be made and properly supported. The welfare of not only the patients but also the clinicians who care for them was at stake.

The breakthroughs in knowledge of functional orthodontics and current TMJ treatment techniques not only showed us the superiority of certain aspects of the new ways but also showed us the error of certain aspects of our old ways. This set the stage for enormous changes in the ways in which we deliver orthodontic and TMJ health care. Dr. John Witzig has been responsible for being one of the first to bring this message to the dental profession through his lectures and teaching. It has been this author's responsibility to bring this message to the profession through this series of texts. As a team, we have endeavored to put these new ideas and techniques in their proper perspective relative to the overall scheme of things through the spoken word of John Witzig's teachings and the written word of this author's endeavors. Neither of us did it alone. To fail to acknowledge the many fine people that have not only assisted me with the details of the production of this text, but also the entire series as well, would be unthinkable. It would also fail to acknowledge how interdependent we all are.

As usual, I would first like to begin with the Germans. This time a debt of gratitude is owed to the publishing firm of Urban and Schwarzenberg of Munich for their cooperation in allowing us to reproduce some of the exquisite anatomical artwork from Eduard Pernhopf's *Atlas of Applied Head and Neck Anatomy*. This publishing firm has always been most helpful over the years and their cooperation is deeply appreciated. We have also received assistance on this particular volume from our British colleagues. I would like to thank Dr. R.M.H. McMinn of the Royal College of Surgeons of England, R.J. Hutchings, former Chief Medical Laboratory Scientific Officer, Royal College of Surgeons of England, and B.M. Logan of the Department of Anatomy, Royal College of Surgeons of England, for their assistance in providing some of the anatomical photography used in this text. Special thanks is also due to Michael Manson, Managing Director of Wolfe Publishing Ltd. of London. To round out our "European tour" we also received help from our colleagues in France. We are enormously grateful to Dr. Richard Marguelles-Bonnet, Professor of Prosthodontics at the Faculté de Chirurgie Dentaire, Paris, and Professor Jean-Pierre Yung, Attaché de Consultation for the Department of Basic Dental Services, Faculté de Chirurgie Dentaire, Laboratoire de Recherches Orthopediques—CRNS, Paris, for providing us with a truly spectacular series of stained anatomical, microscopic serial section slides of the temporomandibular joint.

On the American side, again, many fine people answered the call for assistance. First and foremost among these is Dr. James Colt, Director of the TMJ Disorder Clinic at the University of Colorado. The technical assistance and the vast number of illustrations and technical photography provided by this kind and patient man have been of the greatest importance to the production of this text. I will always be grateful for his personal help and remember the wonderful times we spent working together. He is truly one of the great TMJ practitioners and clinical instructors of our time. We are also grateful to Dr. R. Edward Hendrick, Ph.D., Department of Radiology, University of Colorado Health Science Center, Denver, and to Anne G. Osborn, M.D., Department of Radiology, University of Utah School of Medicine, for their contributions of illustrative materials. Another leading TMJ pioneer and nationally known authority in the field is "the grand old man of TMJ" himself, Dr. Harold Gelb of New York. His enthusiastic support for this project and the technical assistance he provided were rendered in a fashion consistent with the personality of this great man. We are honored that he chose to assist us by providing a tremendous series of illustrations of pretreatment and posttreatment transcranial radiographs of the temporomandibular joint. A debt of gratitude is also owed to Dr. Steve Messing of Albany, NY, for his photographic contributions. We would also like to acknowledge the assistance of Dr. Janet Travell, whose contributions of the superb anatomical drawings of Barbara D. Cummings were a great addition to the text. Additional illustrative material was also provided through courtesy of Dr. William K. Solberg, and Dr. Glen T. Clark, both of the Section of Gnathology and Occlusion and the Temporomandibular and Facial Pain Clinic of the School of Dentistry, University of California at Los Angeles, and Quintessence Publishing Co, Chicago. We also gratefully acknowledge the contributions of Dr. Riley Lunn, Editor of the Journal of Craniomandibular Practice, and Ruby K. Napier, Assistant Editor.

Once again an enormous debt of gratitude is owed to Mr. Mark Ohlendorf, President of Ohlendorf Co., St. Louis. The willingness to assist in all the ways asked of this extremely knowledgeable and generous man will always be remembered with great fondness. The profession is fortunate that such honorable men and women occupy the ranks of its supportive services. Thanks are also due to Mr. Donald Neuschwander of John's Dental Laboratory, Terre Haute, and to Mr. Russ Reichel, of Hermanson Dental Laboratory, St. Paul.

Special assistance with the research for this project was expertly provided, as always, by Jolene Vicchiollo and the staff of the Biomedical Library at the University of Minnesota. We are also grateful to Linda Pierpoint for her help with the procurement of illustrative materials from foreign publishers. Without the assistance of this gracious lady, such procurements would have been near impossible. And once again the contributions of the splendid original artwork of Jan Bilek is gratefully acknowledged. Her work provided some of the most important original art produced for this text. I would also like to thank Judy Cloutier who patiently deciphered endless sheets of illegible hand written script and some how turned it into readable manuscript. She has typed every page of this entire series of texts.

I would also like to thank my personal staff of Dr. Peter Hill, Jackie Blossom, Nancy Elert, Marilyn Wiedell, Mary Jo Cichy, Bonnie Westphal, Lisa Vono, and Heidi Jeanson. Personal support was also rendered through this entire project by Mr. Jerome L. Testa, Dr. Steven P. Kulenkamp and Dr. James M. Gayes. The wise counsel of Dr. Joe Dunlap of Clearwater, Fla, is also deeply appreciated. A special thanks is due to Stan and Nancy Weaver of Big Sandy, Montana. The nurturing of body and heart that they and their children Kelly Ann, David, and Daniel so freely rendered truly helped brace a weathered mind.

And of course I cannot fail to thank my friend and colleague Dr. John Witzig for allowing me the privilege of designing and writing this series of texts. His steady hand and gentle ways were always a source of inspiration and support. I only hope these writings prove worthy to stand as his testament. Finally, and most important, I must thank my wife Susan and our children EmmaLee, Teddy, and Joey. Their strength and sacrifice over the nearly ten years it took to produce this trilogy displayed a true lesson in quiet heroism as they somehow managed to endure the unendurable.

Many people contributed in many ways over many years. The time has now come for all to take a long slow walk by the River Peace.

Terrance J. Spahl, D.D.S.

"Salus populi suprema lex esto!"
"Let the welfare of the people be the
supreme law."
(Missouri State Motto)

"DeLegibus"
Cicero
Roman orator 129-43 B.C.

CHAPTER 1
The Temporomandibular Joint: Wind Tunnel for Change

OVERVIEW

Until only recently, for clinicians who dreamed of an orderly, concise, accurate, and manageable way of advancing themselves by means of their own self-initiated continuing education in the various fields of dentistry, the pursuit of the discipline of the diagnosis and treatment of temporomandibular joint (TMJ) problems has represented an academic nightmare. Fortunately, however, clarity and understanding have now emerged to make addressing this problem on a daily basis practical for rank-and-file practitioners. Until recently, individuals wishing to master the discipline and bring relief to their suffering patients were at the mercy of a vast horde of pedantic authorities, all of whom professed empirically derived treatment modalities that drew from an incredibly wide variety of disciplines. Diagnostic nomenclature was vague, poorly defined, overlapping in its terminology, and therefore in its very essence, confusing. Many of the forms of treatment that were recommended were supportive, but only ancillary to the main etiological agents that remained hidden. Some of the treatment approaches that were at one time in vogue even worsened the condition. This, however, we see from the safety of the fortress of hindsight. Yet at the time, all were practiced in good faith in an effort to gradually tighten the ring of knowledge around the essence of the TMJ pain-dysfunction problem. The end result of these somewhat uncoordinated empirical efforts was a sort of diagnostic and therapeutic "smorgasbord" from which individual practitioners were burdened with the responsibilities of selecting what they thought to be most helpful and

1

applicable to their own patients. But due to the overlap and lack of complete understanding of the role of the various approaches to the pain-dysfunction problems of the joint, the amount of confusion, controversy, and even disenchantment associated with these approaches sometimes increased faster than did the actual knowledge in these fields themselves. This left practitioners not quite well enough prepared to understand the full scope of the problems that patients with TMJ pain-dysfunction presented to them and as a result prevented them from fully resolving many of their patient's needs in these types of situations. Their knowledge was incomplete, and therefore by necessity some of the treatments of their cases were incomplete. Things are better now.

The reasons for the history of this near academic pandemonium are many. Two that might be cited, however, as being major contributors are first, the assumed multiplicity of etiologies, and second, the definite multiplicity of treatment techniques. To a certain extent it is true that the etiological agents responsible for the onset of the pain-dysfunction symptoms are indeed multifactorial, that is, many different medical situations might lead to the appearance of similar symptoms. Thus the important process of differential diagnosis becomes critical in deciphering which patients have true TMJ pain-dysfunction resulting from a maxillomandibular imbalance as opposed to those who have similar symptoms and possibly even similar dysfunction as a result of a more distantly related systemic disease. A general or localized systemic problem might coincide with a true TMJ pain-dysfunction problem, either masking or, most likely, intensifying it. Conversely, a chronic, functionally induced, degenerative arthritis of the joint under certain conditions may secondarily result in pain and even some forms of dysfunction in related structures of the head, neck, or other more distant parts of the body. It used to be said that syphilis was the "great imitator" by virtue of that disease's penchant for presenting a confusing set of signs and symptoms to diagnosing physicians, leading them to believe other conditions were possibly present when in fact they were not. Chronic TMJ arthrosis also may produce secondary signs and symptoms to a limited degree so that the patient presents a varied and multicolored diagnostic picture. This multiplicity of signs and symptoms associated with the patient's joint pain-dysfunction circumstance led many different individuals to select various components of the complex problem as their theoretical prime etiological agent. Diagnosis involved expanding one's knowledge into the various tissue changes observed, the psychological condition of the patient, evaluation of the patient's resistance levels to stress, the frequency and intensity of bruxism, etc., in addition to a general medical evaluation to rule out systemic problems that might be contributing factors. And as might be imagined, each individual clinician placed emphasis on that particular component of the "etiological jigsaw puzzle" that he felt was most appropriate, usually a result of viewing the problem from the outlook from which he felt most comfortable.

Our current understanding (which is by no means complete) of the interplay between secondary intensifying etiological agents with what has now been observed to be a prime overriding etiological agent (in most cases) presently allows us to better understand why for so long the TMJ pain-dysfunction problem has oft been viewed as a ferocious multiheaded hydra of cause and effect. Considering how each of the secondary etiological "heads" manifests itself with respect to TMJ signs and symptoms, it is no wonder many a concerned clinician felt that a given head must be the subject of direct therapeutic combat when all along the heart of the beast actually lay deeper. Although severing a head may have superficially seemed a success, often two more heads representing confusion and inconclusive results appeared in its place. Striking at the core of the problem, as we now see it to often be, is what is actually needed to put the monster to rest and secure a true victory.

For example, after years of only marginally acceptable function of a mandible/condyle unit that is inappropriately driven too far distally by the occlusion, the condyle/disc/bilaminar zone assembly has certainly been given more than its fair share of abuse. The joint structure as a whole may have become so physiologically and biomechanically "threadbare" that a singular traumatic blow to the chin, as in a motor vehicle accident or contact during active sports, may be enough to "push the joints over the edge" and result in the occurrence of TMJ-type symptomatology. The combination of a contusion of the bilaminar area, an enhanced elongation of already compromised collateral and accessory TMJ ligaments, and a traumatic wrenching of highly innervated TMJ musculature may easily produce acute TMJ signs and symptoms in such circumstances. Such circumstance may even add up to produce a temporary acute malocclusion or possibly even a severe limitation of opening. And such symptoms of the acute type may progress to the headache, neck ache, and myofascial pains of the chronic variety due to the fact that the initially, functionally compromised joint is always in use and never has quite enough of an opportunity to "catch up" as far as complete recovery is concerned due to the ever-present noxious stimuli represented by the original compromising agent, the distal-driving malocclusion. Such patients would most likely eventually succumb to the chronic trauma of such malocclusion anyway. The incident of acute trauma merely hastens the occurrence of symptoms. Such people have been referred to by one nationally prominent TMJ expert as "Mount Vesuviuses waiting to erupt." This has led some to feel that trauma is a chief source of TMJ troubles. The etiological agent in such cases (the trauma) is not the question; rather it is the time span qualifying it that becomes deceiving.

A certain small portion of patients with functionally induced TMJ problems appear to suffer from classic signs of clicking and headache pains for a period of time, and then the symptoms seem to disappear after awhile. In severely involved cases, this "silent stage" may be a precursor to more serious joint degeneration to follow. However, occasionally it masks a true end to the major symptomatology due to the fact that the joint structures and even the temporal bone itself have either become worn or resorbed or have otherwise adapted to the point where the entire joint-occlusion complex may operate at a satisfactory, albeit borderline level. Nature has an incredible ability to adapt if given the chance.

Conversely, others have observed (due to the wonders of modern high technology) that once a condyle starts to suffer erosion, resorption, or other forms of osseous breakdown such changes may be observed to alter even the deeper marrow structures of the condyle. Disc displacement, degeneration, and perforation may now be routinely detected, as may be joint effusion and other arthritic breakdown processes. Once such full-scale breakdown begins, it often paves the way for further osseous condylar degeneration and even articular eminential breakdown that can result in skeletal "acute" malocclusions of the seemingly anterior open-bite variety (which under such circumstances actually represent a posterior skeletally closed vertical bite). This causes the entire mandible to teeter on the last molars in the arches, which become a fulcrum point, as the mandible tips up in back with the bite correspondingly opening in the front. The resemblance of such processes as these to the well-known phenomena of osteoarthritis led some to think that advanced TMJ conditions were essentially osteoarthritic in nature and were somehow metabolically influenced, irrespective of any other factor.

The muscle abuse required to effect the level of mandibular/condylar retrusion necessary to elongate the restrictive TMJ ligaments, displace articular discs anteriorly and medially, and cause the condyle to impinge on sensitive retrodiscal bilaminar tissues superiorly and posteriorly in order to satisfy the occlusion demands of some forms of malocclusion resulted in a series of muscle signs and symptoms that led others to feel that the "TMJ syndrome" was primarily myogenic in origin. As a result, many obscure muscle conditions and pathologies were thought of as lying at the base of the TMJ problem. Muscles are most often not the true villains but rather are merely the victims.

In a closely related field of endeavor, the ability of muscles that have been abused to refer pain to secondary sites, thus compounding the headache–myofascial pain picture, along with the observed relationship of headaches to increased periods of stress logically led some investigators to believe that a strong psychological component was the most guilty etiological agent.

The association of hypertension with exacerbation of headache symptoms and the occurrence of certain signs and symptoms indicative of blood vessel wall exhaustion and distension coupled with the observed temporary relief provided by medications concerned with blood vessel constriction led some to feel there was a strong vascular component to the chronic headache problem.

Neurological-type pain patterns that camouflaged actual structurally oriented TMJ pain-dysfunction problems influenced the TMJ symptomatic picture, especially those symptoms concerned with headache. Often practitioners of both medicine and dentistry who are unfamiliar with the true nature of the TMJ pain-dysfunction problem refer chronic headache patients to a neurologist for evaluation.

The entire field of dietary control was also implicated as a means of quelling the storms of TMJ pain-dysfunction problems. Since it was known that simple hypoglycemia could cause headaches and that certain foodstuffs could cause urticaria and other allergic reactions in sensitive individuals, nutritional deficiencies and/or excesses of various types were felt to be an important factor in exacerbating headache symptoms or even causing them totally on their own.

And, of course, when high spots on the occlusal table or balancing side interferences were eliminated in certain circumstances, the relief afforded to overworked muscles and battered joints led a great many to believe that occlusal equilibration alone was the answer. It was in fact of some limited assistance, but only for prematurities that resulted in the mandible being deflected distally. The concept of "long centric" was evidence of things done almost right for reasons that were unrelated to the true needs of the case. The indictment of occlusal prematurities as prime offenders in the TMJ etiological puzzle was fortified by the introduction of the intraoral acrylic occlusal splint to TMJ therapeutics. The wonders these little devices sometimes seemed to effect, if constructed properly and used in the proper types of cases, convinced many that the heart of the problem must lie in equilibration. The occlusal prematurity had to be the villain regardless of how discreet it was. The contradicting significance of the observance of heavy occlusal wear of amalgam or gold restorations in non–TMJ pain-dysfunction patients was somehow ignored by this school of thought.

The myriad of available answers in the TMJ multiple-choice quiz left many a dismayed clinician groping for an answer when in actuality the main factor for the functionally induced–type TMJ problem hadn't even been proposed. Had it been, it would have been in the form of "all of the above," but only as secondary modifying, enhancing, or exacerbating factors to the true, main etiologic agent, i.e., posteriorly displaced condyles.

As previously noted, this multiplicity of contributing factors also allowed for a multiplicity of therapeutic approaches to be developed, and not without a certain noteworthy degree of success, it might be added. Thus there were those who delved off into the fields of dietary control and occlusal balancing through equilibration or coronoplasty, and biofeedback and tension relief principles were employed, as was the use of muscle exercises, physical therapy, and electronic and thermal stimulations. In addition to these other types of therapy, a great boon to the field was felt with the discovery and concerted employment of intraoral removable acrylic splints of every conceivable variety. Some splints made an effort to capture the bite but at a different vertical or horizontal level of occlusion. Others were flat on their occlusal surface in an effort to allow the occlusion to seek its own level of horizontal positioning. Splints were made for both upper and lower arches. Some were worn 24 hours per day, others at night only, while others were recommended for periodic use during times when the patient felt under undue stress of one kind or another. At the more radical end of the therapeutic spectrum, surgery was also employed in various forms. Nerves were cut, intra-articular discs were removed, condyles were reshaped and recontoured,[1-6] mandibles were sectioned and repositioned, and implants of an endless variety were inserted.

The scene of TMJ analysis and treatment has been dominated over the last half century by many players. The time from Costen's first attempts at describing the condition[7, 8] until the present is divided into various phases of development as the pendulum of therapeutic thought has swung from one philosophical approach to another. The mere fact that such wide oscillations in approach have occurred in the past bears mute testimony to the fact that both the dental and medical professions never really grasped the essence of the problem in its entirety to begin with but rather focused in uncertain and faltering fashion on singular portions of it.[9-11] As often happens when things are ill understood, the entire issue was cloaked in a veil of mystery and "considered opinion" that was no doubt a product of the intimidation spawned by a lack of true certainty. The condition took on the aegis of an extremely sophisticated multiplicity of etiologies, symptomatic significances, and diagnostic processes, not to mention a variety of proposed treatment methodologies. The uncertainty inherent in such a process caused many to view TMJ treatment as a diagnostic and therapeutic "no man's land" in which practitioners were forced to size up the situation as best they could and empirically fend for themselves as far as constructing a viable treatment plan was concerned. A lack of a vertical dimension was one of the first etiological culprits to be singled out. Thus certain treatment approaches took on the aspect of "bite raising." But some clinicians disagreed with this approach and said that the lack of a vertical dimension of occlusion was not the chief offender but that the aforementioned occlusal interferences were the cause.[12, 13] This debate began in the decade of the 1940s and has persisted in some form or other to the present day. Yet at the beginning, the first pioneers in the field of TMJ therapeutics actually were closer to the truth than they realized. TMJ "syndrome" became defined in the 1950s as a type of degenerative arthritis caused by a lack of a vertical dimension of occlusion and/or mandibular condylar displacement. However, the displacement was never clearly or firmly defined as to its *direction*. So near and yet so far!

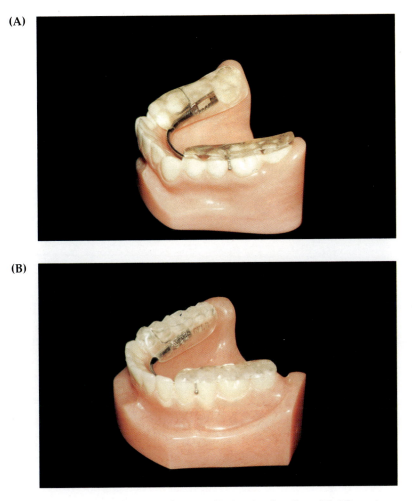

Figure 1–1 **(A)** Flat-plane "occlusion-eliminating" splint. **(B)** "Occusion-grabbing" splint. (Courtesy of Ohlendorf Co, St Louis.)

(A)

(B)

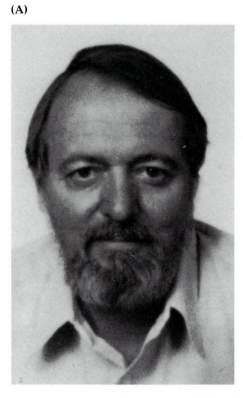

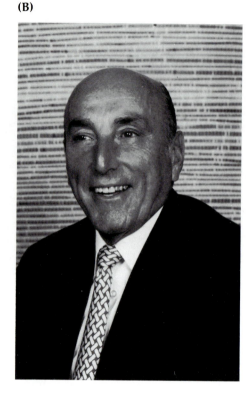

Figure 1–2   (A) Dr. William B. Farrar. **(B)** Dr. Harold Gelb.

The decade of the 1960s saw the first appearance of the term "TMJ pain-dysfunction syndrome" as coined by Dr. Laszlo Schwartz.[14] Somewhat later the more psychologically oriented "myofascial pain-dysfunction (MPD) syndrome" of Laskin[15] appeared and was defined as a closely related but separate entity. This temporarily shifted the spotlight from the theater of the equilibrationists (those concerned with occlusal interferences and biomechanics) to the theater of relaxing the muscles (and the patient) by the use of intraoral acrylic splints. But one of the major strides forward with respect to the TMJ problem was made in the early 1970s by Dr. W.B. Farrar.[16] He was the first to clearly and accurately describe the phenomenon of reciprocal clicking as he demonstrated how the condyle hops on and off the disc during opening and closing movements. On the heels of this revelation, the eloquent and energetic Dr. Harold Gelb of New York City demonstrated the clinical importance of repositioning posteriorly displaced mandibles down and forward to effect TMJ pain relief with his famous mandibular orthopedic repositioning appliance (MORA), or Gelb splint.[17]

Yet, through all this maze of diagnostic differentiation and therapeutic variety, although the ring around the TMJ pain-dysfunction problem tightened and knowledge and skills advanced, the key issue remained yet unresolved. The workers were busily buzzing around the hive in preparation and anticipation, but the "etiological queen bee" had not yet emerged.

Although successful cases inspired practitioners to redouble their efforts at understanding the problems of TMJ pain-dysfunction conditions on an ever more complete and accurate level, unfortunately the failure of certain patients to respond or the recurrence of signs and symptoms after an interim of what at first appeared to be initial success threw a disconcerting light on the advancement of the science that led even the most prestigious and articulate leaders in the field to inwardly and sometimes outwardly second-guess both their treatment approaches and themselves. As a result, some became all the more adamant and dogmatic as to the particular portion of their practice of the discipline with which they were most sure. In the meantime the main body of clinicians became steadily more confused and disillusioned. The entire picture simply had not yet been made complete.

And then there transpired an event that seems to occur only once in a lifetime. A concept was proposed that, like all great and revolutionary scientific theories, seemed at once both inspired and yet at the same time incredibly simple. The concept was that of the correction orthodontically of TMJ pain-dysfunction problems by means of mandibular advancement with functional appliances such as the Bionator to bring the condyles down and forward in the glenoid fossae, increase the vertical dimension of the occlusion, and retrain the Class II neuromuscular sling with resultant decompression of the highly vascular and neurologically sensitive bilaminar zone of the joint in the process, and one of this theory's first great proponents was none other than my colleague, the man with whom this author has written and produced this series of texts, Dr. John Witzig of Minneapolis, Minn. If for no other reason than this alone, Dr. Witzig shall be recognized by history as having been the individual who most singularly represents the change in both the treatment and diagnostic philosophy of American orthodontics. Relative to the efforts of the professional community to wrestle with the problems of the TMJ series of disorders and its stinted efforts at true resolution, Dr. Witzig almost single-handedly effected a coup of truly stunning proportions by means of the promulgation of his ideas to the clinical orthodontic world. The answer had always been there. It was a vital component of the very foundations upon which the functional jaw orthopedics (FJO) philosophy was built. All it merely needed was redirection to its ultimate conclusions. These newly appreciated concepts cut like a saber through the confusion surrounding TMJ problems of a functional nature and have proved to be unequivocally the most important aspects of a correct and complete approach to treatment of this type. They are treatment concepts that already

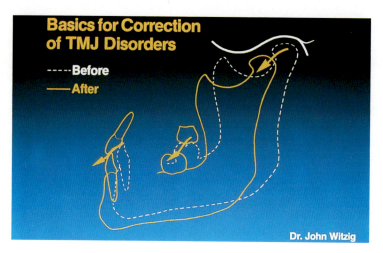

Figure 1–3   Dr. John Witzig's basic concept of the correction of functionally induced TMJ problems by using FJO and orthodontic techniques to deliver the mandible-condyle unit down and forward. (Courtesy of Dr. John Witzig.)

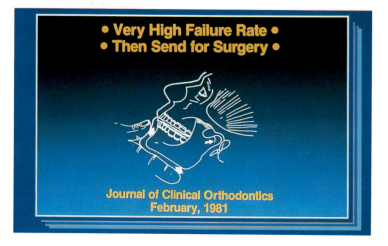

Figure 1–4   Erroneous concepts of mandibular condyle positioning.

lie at the very heart of the FJO philosophy.

As may be surmised from even the most cursory review of the material presented so far in this entire series of texts, the "gauntlet is down" with respect to the position the FJO philosophy takes relative to the importance of a properly balanced, condyle-disc-fossa relationship and decompressed bilaminar zone under any circumstances, let alone those in which the patient is already suffering from signs and symptoms of TMJ arthrosis. Although the many other supportive and ancillary techniques and treatments for TMJ problems are important, the contribution that the FJO methodology is capable of making to the field of common, functionally related TMJ disorders is nothing short of monumental. In the area of treatment for the TMJ patient, there are many instances when the FJO methodology represents not only a correct and workable treatment solution to the patient's problem but is the *only* treatment solution if the exacerbation and intensification of the condition or eventual surrender to the surgeon is to be avoided.

CHANGES IN APPROACH IN DEALING
WITH THE TEMPOROMANDIBULAR JOINT

The amount of information that has recently become available concerning the diagnosis and treatment of TMJ problems is voluminous. The last decade or so has seen an explosion of popularity for the subject crop up throughout the rank and file of the general dental community. Various schools of thought have sprung up concerning methods of treatment, and a wide variety of techniques, along with experts who support and promote their use, now command a major portion of the spotlight of methods available for addressing the subject. Being that it is extremely difficult to perform carefully controlled experiments in this field, the profession has evolved many of its techniques in this area as a result of trial and error on the general populace of patients themselves. As a result, the evolution of this specific discipline has taken a meandering and somewhat disorganized path to its present "state of the art." It would be impossible to present a comprehensive review of all the techniques and philosophical approaches used to confront TMJ problems, yet we would be remiss not to discuss the scope of research and development on the subject and the most general of terms prior to our discussion of the place FJO methodology occupies in the field. This better enables our understanding of that position to be well founded in an overall view of the scene.

Without a doubt, the single most important step in the evolution of the diagnosis and treatment of TMJ arthrosis has been at its most basic and fundamental level, that of the definition of the ideal relationship of the lower jaw to the rest of the skull. Regardless of how sophisticated, well planned, and accurately implemented any treatment technique may be, until this most elemental physiological position of the maxillomandibular relationship is correctly secured, only a compromised result at the completion of that treatment plan would be obtainable at best.

There was a time, and not too long ago, when students learning to make dentures or taking wax bite registrations for removable partials or fixed crowns and bridgework were trained that the ideal position for the mandible (one chosen simply because it could be consistently reproduced) was for the condyle of the mandible to be in its most superior and retruded position during maximum full contact, molar-to-molar interdigitated occlusion. Great efforts were taken to ensure that this position was being attained, especially during denture construction bite registration. Students were taught to place their thumbs and forefingers on the patient's chin in order to apply a firm but gentle pressure posteriorly to ensure that the mandible was being closed forcibly in its most retruded position during registration of the wax bite. What effect this might have on the status of the joint and muscles themselves or whether or not this was *actually* a physiologically correct position ubiquitously occurring in Nature was never thought of as being a point to consider. The position so obtained merely had the attribute of consistent reproducibility and a theoretically induced sense of logic, and that was all that was sought after. Yet for decades it sounded like a reasonable thing to do. (Eventually that highly touted reproducibility proved to be only an illusion.) Meticulous attention to detail in the accurate transferral of this relationship to any one of a variety of mechanical articulators was surpassed only by the level of complexity of design engineered into the building of these articulators so as to attempt to reproduce the naturally occurring movements of the mandible in this retruded position as nearly as possible. Seminars, study clubs, and even great national-level societies were founded and governed by men of true genius whose devotion and efforts to the perfection of the techniques involved in this approach were to be justifiably commended by the rest of the dental community. Their prime focus of attention was the development and perfection in balance and function of the occlusion in this reproducible, theoretically "stable," albeit retruded mandibular position. The high level of advancement of their technique has greatly contributed to our present level of understanding. Like others before them in other areas, theirs was a standard for the world! But what about that founding premise? What would Nature have to say about all this? How many "dental authorities" actually went to anatomy laboratories, looked at cadaver joints, and studied what was actually behind those condyles? If they would have, they would have seen that the discs were on the front side of those condyles, but only nerves and blood vessels were on the back side!

It was common knowledge that if the occlusion was imbalanced, if prematurities existed, if inclined-plane action interfered with normal occlusal function, or if occlusal "slides" existed in one direction or another, the patient might potentially suffer from some sort of symptoms of the TMJ. This was found to be especially true if the case were reconstructed to be of such an occlusion as to permit only the most superior retruded position of the condyle in the glenoid fossa to be obtained upon full interdigitation of the teeth. The maximum superior retruded position of the mandible was given the term "centric relation," whereas situations where the teeth brought the mandible upon full, naturally occurring interdigitation were called "centric occlusion." The goal seemed to be to make both one and the same. In such close quarters as that represented by an occlusion built to the myth of centric relation, occlusal imbalances or interferences could not be tolerated. Everything had better work smoothly! It was partially to this end that the science of occlusal equilibration was developed. The tooth-to-tooth contact had to be a tripodal cusp/fossa relationship, with every effort to keep working and balancing sides in complete harmony during anterior and lateral excursive movements. This, along with an adequate vertical dimension anteriorly, was theorized to be all that was required to give patients the ideal in function and comfort for the jaw-to-jaw relationship more posteriorly, always using the aforementioned superior, most retruded position as a standardized frame of reference and always attempting to resolve the discrepancies between centric occlusion and centric relation. It was a noble end, but alas, it all only represented a pipe dream!

Due to the problems of its founding premise, the entire thrust of clinical effort of this philosophy was crusading off in the wrong direction. The campaign resolved itself to the level of the pursuit of a "holy grail-like" therapeutic goal that in the end actually proved to be physiologically and biomechanically compromised. Although some helpful techniques resulted from this effort over the years, the true clinical solution at the most basic foundations of the whole TMJ problem still remained hidden, waiting to be discovered. The path of discovery was gradual and arduous. Yet its most formidable obstacles presented themselves, surprisingly, not in the form of the physical difficulties and problems of technique but rather in the form of the metaphysical problems of faith.

Gradually and in areas totally independent of each other came a new field of endeavor in handling TMJ discomfort, that of occlusal splint therapy. Removable acrylic intraoral splints were found to make dramatic improvements in patient comfort, although at first the mechanisms by which they achieved relief of symptoms were ill understood. But the relief of muscle and joint pain or attending chronic headaches was so welcomed by both patient and doctor that in spite of a lack of a thorough understanding of its mechanisms, splint therapy was embraced by the profession with open arms. But some clinicians carried their dependence on the use of occlusal splints to extremes only to be disappointed to find that the patient was sometimes worse off after prolonged splint usage than before.

Other disciplines that evolved as ancillary components to this strug-gling field were those of dental kinesiology, diet control, electronic stim-ulation, biofeedback, and a whole raft of other disciplines associated with another very important component of TMJ therapy—stress control.

Yet all of these newer disciplines are devoted to alleviation of symp-toms—praiseworthy in their own right—but nevertheless still only symptomatic in essence. What was also needed in addition to the above was a discipline designated to address correcting the primary *causes* of temporomandibular pain-dysfunction problems. It is now sincerely felt by many that such a discipline exists in the form of the proper use of FJO technique. The where, when, why, and how of that technique is predi-cated upon a broad, general background knowledge of the TMJ "syn-drome" and what the major thoughts on its etiology and treatment are today.

It would be improper to presume to be able to present any form of survey of TMJ treatment that would do justice to every aspect of this enormous field. Entire textbooks are devoted to the discussion of singular aspects of it. Yet we may present a categorized summary of major points of interest that will help the reader decipher the important and specific position FJO techniques occupy; these will serve as a springboard from which the clinician may launch into more detailed pursuits of individual areas. What will be presented here is no doubt colored by empirical clini-cal observations for which it is hoped the reader will be graciously indul-gent.

EVOLUTION OF A "SYNDROME"

A clearer understanding of the reasons for the confusion, despera-tion, and overlapping of both the disciplines and terminologies of TMJ pain-dysfunction conditions may be derived from a brief survey of the history of the evolution of the profession's view of the problem. The rec-ognition of joint problems, or more generally the relationship between the occlusion and headaches, is nothing new to the organized healing arts but surprisingly goes as far back as the time of the Egyptians and was even described by the "father of medicine" himself, Hippocrates. In mod-ern times, one of the first and for the longest time the only description of the problem to be generally accepted by the medical community was that of the otolaryngologist J.B. Costen in the form of his famous "Costen's syndrome." In 1934 Costen described a group of symptoms including ear and sinus problems that he attributed to improper functioning of the TMJs. This he observed primarily in edentulous patients with severe loss of vertical. To this day the only knowledge many physicians have of TMJ problems of a functional nature is through knowledge of the syndrome bearing Costen's name. But Costen's descriptions of otic symptoms were based on the then-radical theory of pressure being placed on extracapsular areas behind the TMJ area by the condyles. In the late 1940s extremely important contributions were made to the field by H. Sicher, J.P. Weinmann, J.R. Thompson, and A.A. Zimmerman. It was Sicher who first refuted Costen's theories on biomechanical grounds and would later describe more correctly some of the facets of the complex TMJ problem.[18, 19] In the meantime, it was L.L. Schwartz who, after treating a number of patients with TMJ pain-dysfunction, noted that Costen's set of otic symptoms were not the ones primarily observed by Schwartz but rather pain and dysfunction were the chief clinical characteristics of the condition.[20] Schwartz was also one of the first to note the now famous 4:1 ratio of females to males presenting with the problem. British dental surgeon J. Campbell, one of the "founding fathers" of splint therapy, did a monumental study over a 10-year period whereby he noted that the pain associated with the "syndrome" was localized to origins and insertions of muscles of mastication and also to the joint itself! He was also instrumental in developing the concepts of a "sister science" to FJO-type treatment, i.e., full-mouth occlusal reconstruction after a period of palliative and diagnostic splint therapy. The idea of optimal maxillomandibular skeletal and muscular relationships had finally come of age. Yet at that time only occlusal rehabilitative techniques were seen as an answer. Another phenomenon was also being noted. It was that of the painful involvement of areas quite removed from the immediate locale of the joint itself such as the head, neck, and shoulders. It was gradually seen that a great many problems of a myofunctional and even systemic nature could be directly related to imbalances in the occlusion. The science of the "trigger point" phenomenon and referred pain was going through its embryonic stages.

Yet it was Sicher who made the critical analysis that the pain, joint sounds, and other observed dysfunctions were the result of the joint being in a state of traumatic degenerative arthritis, i.e., a joint and surrounding musculature mechanically stressed beyond their ability to adapt and compensate. Noting also the importance of the vertical dimension of occlusion and the problems represented by posterior and/or superior condylar displacement, Sicher was also one of the first to propose that muscle spasms could cause many of the observed problems, even in the ear, and also proposed the just now generally recognized and all-important concept of the pain of the joint and surrounding areas arising from condylar impingement in the bilaminar zone! He stated that this condylar impingement process into retrodiscal tissues could manifest itself in the form of associated muscular pain. What Sicher told the profession of dentistry in the 1950s has proved correct. In an ocean of theories and conjecture on TMJ, his perceptive genius went almost unnoticed. Years later students at universities throughout the country were still being taught to obtain bite registrations for dentures, partials, and bridges in the most superior and posterior relationship of the condyle to the fossa that was clinically possible for them to produce through posteriorly directed, manual

(A)

(B)

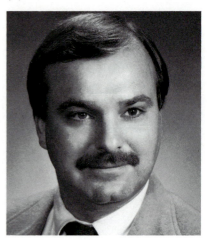

Figure 1–5   **(A)** Dr. J. Cambell, British dental surgeon and "father of splint therapy." **(B)** Dr. Ronald Levandoski, prosthodontist extraordinaire.

manipulation of the mandible! Later, others besides Sicher would also make major contributions to the understanding of TMJ problems.

For the sake of organizing the various approaches to the TMJ problem into a clearer picture, it might be safe to think of the various theories of TMJ diagnosis and treatment as falling into three major camps. The first is that of the occlusionists (or more correctly, "equilibrationists"). This camp feels that occlusal irregularities in the form of interferences and/or prematurities are responsible for TMJ-type pains and dysfunction. All sorts of intricate theories of occlusion of the most fastidious nature may be found to reside in this group. For them, precisely mounted models in the most elaborate and sophisticated of articulators, the finest of articulating papers, and little blue and red marks on the cusps of teeth are the order of the day. None of this is ever related to the position of the condyle in the joint at full occlusion, however. Although some modicum of success is occasionally observed with this approach (usually only enough to keep this group inspired), the failures are far too many. Nor can this theoretical basis account for the commonly observed fact that many patients have all sorts of interferences, irregularities, prematurities, and imbalances to their occlusions; yet since condyles are not forced too far up and back during function because of the same, no TMJ signs or symptoms whatsoever may be observed if the condyles are correctly positioned smack dab in the middle of the disc with plenty of room posteriorly for each bilaminar zone to "breathe freely" during function. How can an occlusal prematurity of 1/100th of an inch be of any significance to one of Nature's best-designed shock absorbers? The second school of thought believed that psychological and emotional stress were key elements to the TMJ circumstance, and one of their chief proponents was D.M. Laskin. In

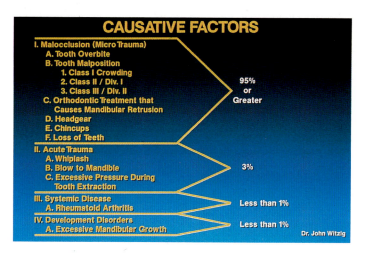

Figure 1–6 Causes of TMJ pain and dysfunction.

spite of the attention given to stress by this camp, the cardinal signs and symptoms they listed as prime indicators of a TMJ problem were head, neck, joint, and facial pains; reciprocal clicking; associated muscle tenderness; and a limited range of mandibular motion. Again, condylar position, its relation to the guidance (or misguidance) of the occlusion, and the relationship of the degree of superior and posterior displacement of the condyle to the severity of the patient's signs and symptoms continued to remain unrecognized and unappreciated in an amorphic state of diagnostic apogee. Yet Laskin still stressed a strong psychological aspect to the TMJ problem and proposed that spasm caused by muscle fatigue due to persistent, psychologically motivated, tension-relieving oral habits such as bruxism were a prime etiological factor to consider. He placed such importance on the muscular aspects of the problem that he suggested the use of the now famous term "myofascial pain-dysfunction syndrome." The third and most current school of thought is the approach represented by the discipline of FJO. This represents the first time a method was developed that addressed all three components of the maxillofacial triangle, i.e., the teeth, bones, and muscles, and related the location of the condyle to all of these components as well as to the overall condition of the patient. It also looked at the variety of symptoms observed in various patients as different levels of involvement of the same condition. This outlook, however, is not yet generally accepted by the majority of the main body of academicians but appears to be more popular among those involved in clinical practice.

One of the vestigial carryovers from these early formative years of the discipline is the somewhat misleading terminology used to describe it. The term *TMJ syndrome* is ubiquitous throughout the literature, yet it is actually a misnomer. A syndrome is defined as "a number of signs and symptoms occurring together and characterizing a specific disease." Yet signs and symptoms may be observed in great variety in TMJ patients. Some have headaches and myofascial pains, with or without clicking. Some have the clicking only. Some have crepitus or no joint sounds at all. For some the signs and symptoms are bilateral, for others they are only unilateral. Some have regular, frequent myofascial pains, cephalgia (headaches), and cervicalgia (neck aches) of a very predictable and well-defined nature. Others have only periodic episodes of headache or clicking that seem only to be associated with periods of intensified stress, bruxism, or even something as innocuous as gum chewing. Some people are "borderline" individuals with mild, sporadic symptoms and well-shaped condyles that do not appear displaced too far superiorly and posteriorly within the confines of the TMJ fossa. Yet others exhibit the most untoward series of intense chronic head and facial pains with attending hypomobility of the jaw; superior and posterior joint spaces that are all but obliterated by overwhelming condylar intrusion; condyles that are lipped, flattened, eroded, and grotesquely misshapen; and discs and posterior attachments that are torn, severed, or otherwise shredded and mangled. Pains may be localized, generalized, lancinating, or dull. They can even cause referred pain to other areas that results in the most confusing of diagnostic pictures when observed by the treating clinician. Therefore, the multiplicity of signs and symptoms varying from individual to individual makes the term *TMJ syndrome* rather suspect, likewise the terms *disease* and *pathology*. These terms are strongly associated with an invasive agent of some sort such as a bacterium or virus. Actually, this phenomenon, more than anything else, truly represents a "condition" just as a sprained ankle, obesity, or common physical fatigue are conditions. The TMJ condition, at least the condition we are concerned with in this text, is functional in nature and is a result of overstressing at the joint by means of something in the occlusion that forces the condyle to a final position that is too far up and back in the fossa or otherwise out of its normal position (such as in posterior crossbite situations) during full occlusion to be considered acceptable by Nature. The symptomatic picture presented by the patient with TMJ pain-dysfunction is really nothing more than the sum total of factors such as the severity of the malocclusion, the severity of the condylar displacement superiorly and posteriorly, the chronicity of that particular state, the amount of use (or abuse) the entire mechanism is given, as well as the all-important factor of host resistance (or more correctly, durability). That particular aspect is in turn a product of sex, age, general homeostasis, general medical health, as well as emotional and psychological makeup. However, at its most basic of levels, TMJ arthrosis should be thought of as primarily a problem of an overly retruded mandibular arc of final closure that causes superior, posterior condylar displacement up past the back edge of the disc into the bilaminar zone. Once this is corrected via FJO techniques, the clinician will observe a sort of biological "domino effect" that will clear up a whole raft of head, neck, and back pains as well as numerous other vague and intractable complaints patients have. Put the condyle in the right place, keep it there during both function and rest, and one will be amazed at how many patients will simply thrive.

Many other individual contributions were made by many fine gentlemen over the years, but when one stands back and looks at the entire spectrum of events, one may then begin to visualize the central truths such men as Costen, Sicher, Schwartz, Campbell, Laskin, and many others were "homing in" on. There are three major components to be addressed in treating the triad of problems of TMJ pain and dysfunction. They are the joint itself, its supportive musculature, and the occlusion. Mild occlusal imbalances with slight muscular discomfort and negligible joint involvement all the way to major chronic functional degenerative arthritic inflammatory involvement with associated muscle pain, spasm, osteolytic changes, and irreparable intracapsular damage are all manifestations of the various levels of severity of the exact same condition! It is often merely a matter of degree, a matter of how far the patients have traveled down the path of TMJ involvement that induces them to present the signs and symptoms peculiar to their individual state. Their particular position on the "pathological pathway" from the most mild to the most severe manifestations of this condition is a cumulative product of the degree of involvement (or imbalance) of the occlusion, the musculature, and the joint. Barring extraneous overriding and complicating systemic medical conditions such as the previously mentioned arthritides, trauma, infection, collagen diseases, neoplasms, etc., these three aspects of TMJ problems—*the occlusion, the musculature, and the joint*—will always be present and together combine to make up the overall structural status of a given individual. The teeth-bone-muscle triangle must always be before the minds of the clinician in both diagnosis and treatment planning. What does each side of the triangle mean? What role does each side of the triangle play in the overall picture of the patient's condition? What are the needs of each component of the triangle that must be addressed therapeutically to effect a permanent correction? Since the TMJ pain-dysfunction pathological path is contiguous from mild to severe, there can be as many positions along its course as there are individuals who present with problems. Classification of all the various varieties and levels of intensity and of signs, symptoms, and conditions by whatever form of nomenclature is regionally popular at the time is not as important as the understanding of what these signs and symptoms mean and what they are telling the clinician about the three things he is most capable of addressing in the patient, i.e., the occlusion, the muscles, and the joint. Questions then traverse the mind of the clinician concerning the patient with TMJ pain or dysfunction. How far along the path has the patient progressed (or more correctly, degenerated)? Is he stable at a given point or slowly worsening, slowly sliding farther down the path? What will be required to bring the patient back? What must be done to relieve the patient's pain? What must be done to treat the occlusion orthodontically or even restoratively? What must be done to treat the bones orthopedically to provide normal joint relationships. What must be done myofunctionally to retrain the Class II neuromuscular sling? If the functional occlusion is cramped, restricted, and causing the whole complex to work incorrectly, how does everything have to be rearranged and realigned to make everything work right?

CHANGES IN PERSPECTIVE ON OCCLUSION

Some of the early practitioners of over a century and a half ago found that they could increase the stability of the artificial dentures they constructed in those days by setting the teeth in what they confusingly called "balanced occlusion." They developed extremely primitive articulators to assist them in setting the artificial teeth in the dentures so as to ensure balancing side contacts during mastication. No thought whatsoever was ever given to what effect this might have on the joints or muscles. Dentures always moved slightly during function anyway. The concept of balancing side contacts during function or similar ideas of multiple contacts to aid in denture stability were embraced by the general dental community and unthinkingly transferred from the realm of artificial occlusions to that of natural occlusions! Thus two gigantic theories developed that have remained unquestioned ever since: first, that multiple and simultaneous occlusal contacts during mastication are necessary and desirable, and second, that in order to create and control all this multiplicity of occlusal contact within the mouth, various types of mechanical articulators could be engineered and would prove of service for the construction of either fixed or removable prostheses outside the mouth for use in a treatment plan involving occlusal therapeutics. Well, maybe these notions are at least partially right! Yet to this day the design and construction of mechanical articulators have persistently been perfected and elaborated upon so as to be able to provide a guiding mechanism that would produce an occlusion that possessed another generally accepted, yet unproven offshoot attribute of early occlusal mechanics that is well entrenched in the profession, i.e., that of having the angulation of the cuspal inclined planes of the posterior teeth as near as possible to the same angulation of the slope of the eminential pathway of the tuberculum of the joint. To this arena of theoretical, somewhat incomplete, and ill-founded "dogma" also came two other totally apocryphal concepts, one of which, with the benefit of hindsight, has been shown to be the singular most detrimental obstacle to the overall elucidation of the truths of occlusion. In the early 1920s McCollum proposed two theories that have haunted the world of occlusal therapeutics to this day. First, he suggested that a most superior, retruded position of the mandible could be established as a baseline for constructing occlusions simply because he observed that it was a universally reproducible stereoscopic point of refer-

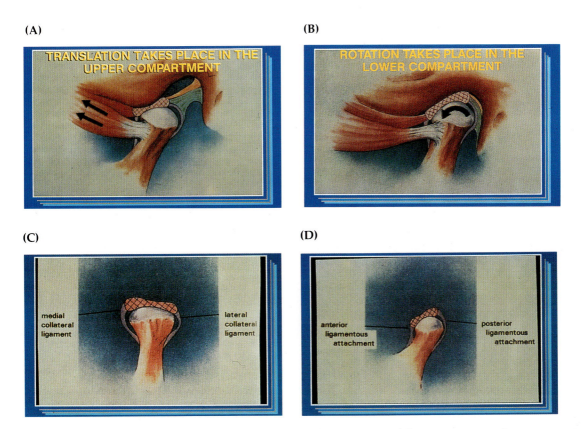

Figure 1–7 **(A)** Condylar translation; **(B)** condylar rotation; **(C)** anterior view of the condyle with medial and lateral collateral ligaments; **(D)** lateral view of the condyle with anterior and posterior ligament attachments. Note that the posterior attachment represented here is actually one of two. The inferior ligament or lamina attaches the disk to the posterior condylar neck as shown. The superior lamina (not shown) is not a true ligament because it is highly elastic and runs from the posterior edge of the disc to the back of the fossa. The area in between these two lamina or connective tissue attachments is referred to as the bilaminar zone. It is filled with highly sensitive nerves and blood vessels.

ence for positioning the mandible. Second, although he was correct in noting the two types of condylar movement within the TMJ capsule, rotational and translatory, the questionable concept arose that the rotational or "hinge axis" position is indeed a truly functioning position, which we now see may not necessarily be the case. This most superior, retruded hinge-axis position of the head of the condyle within the glenoid fossa was given the name "centric relation" to denote that it was a condyle-fossa relationship irrespective of how the teeth occluded when that most superior retruded relationship existed within the joint. The term *centric occlusion* or *habitual occlusion* was the term coined to describe the counterpart to the above, i.e., the fully interdigitated occlusion of the posterior teeth in their most stable mechanical relationship to one another irrespective of what that might do to the condyle-fossa relationship further back. As previously stated, the main thrust of the rehabilitative efforts of the profession over the years seems to have been to make the two relationships somehow coincide as one and the same. These principles were professed with an almost religious fervor. The profession was bristling with the rush of its fascination with mechanical articulators and the search for the true hinge axis and centric relation. Few seemed interested in listening to what Nature had to say about all this. Common logic was looked upon with a great deal of suspicion in spite of the fact that very few patients could be found who walked around with their thumbs on their chins.

Yet sooner or later there always appears on the scene that type of individual whose incisive and truly scientific perception is capable of penetrating such areas of commonly accepted truisms and deciphering deeper hidden truths. There are just some people who seem to have the uncanny knack of being able to eat sacred cows for lunch! Such was bound to occur in the field of occlusion, and one of the prime examples of just such an individual was Dr. Bernard Jankelson[21] of Seattle. Jankelson was one of the first to chart a new path through the complex theories of occlusion. He and others like him have contributed greatly to the redirection of thinking (sometimes in a totally opposite direction) as to what actually is "normal" and natural in properly balanced and functional occlusion. Some of his particular contributions to new ideas on occlusion are the critical concepts that the most superior/retruded condyle-fossa relationship, referred to as centric relation, is in fact not a true naturally occurring functional position, with the important exception being, as we now know, the state of forced positioning of the condyle into that relationship by the improperly directing forces of a malocclusion. Jankelson believed that, barring such extenuating circumstances as a malocclusion, the normal structurally balanced individual neither chews at that position nor braces his teeth at that position during swallowing. He correctly theorized that they perform these functions at the most biomechanically stable position their particular structural and occlusal status will allow, i.e., centric or habitual occlusion! He also has shown that teeth actually make minimal contact during mastication and, theorizing another dynamic concept, that true hinge-axis rotational movement seldom if ever occurs in nature, but rather the mandible engages in combined rotational and immediate translatory motion during all its functional movements. The occlusion determines where the condyle will reside within the discal confines of the joint, not vice versa. Therefore, centric relation as we have seen it defined by early clinicians is all but physiologically useless as a reference point for constructing occlusion. Not only that, we have now come to know that such a position can actually be detrimental to the patient. The paths of thought have come full cycle, and not without a great deal of rejection and resistance along the way as is common to all revolutionary ideas.

The coup de grace to traditional concepts on what constitutes a normal occlusion was delivered by Dr. Ronald Levandoski, whose revolutionary ideas on the TMJ and its relationship to dentition have changed forever not only the way we look at TMJ therapeutics but also the way we look at articulators. He was the first to resurrect a nearly century-old concept that as the mandible advances, the posterior vertical dimension of occlusion (due to the rotation or hinge axis phase of motion within the joint during translation) actually increases faster than does the anterior vertical dimension of occlusion. He even designed and built the first truly anatomically correctable articulator capable of compensating for this phenomenon that, when coordinated with proper transcranial radiographic findings, is able to allow the practitioner to adjust the articulator; mount study models; and construct splints, orthodontic appliances, full dentures, or other dental prostheses that will position the condyle perfectly within the fossa during function or as near perfect as the available data of a given case will allow. The notion of building such an articulator that allows the clinician to forcibly and precisely reposition a disfavorably displaced condyle represents the single most revolutionary concept of this century with respect to the relationship of mechanical articulators and their ability to relate the occlusion to the functional balance of the condyle-disc-fossa relationship.

In the decade of the 1980s, the maturation of the Witzig-type techniques of FJO for patients with full dentitions, staunchly fortified by the Levandoski approach of prosthetic methodologies for patients with less than full dentitions, has combined to make sound, sensible, effective, and humanly practical TMJ treatments readily available to both patient and practitioner alike. The concept of restructuring the dysfunctional occlusion to change it from driving the condyle up and back to one that delivers it down and forward against the disc and eminence if possible, but at least not against sensitive retrodiscal bilaminar tissues, is a therapeutic approach that has stood the test of time and is now fully coming of age. Yet, what is most incredible in all this, is the amazing amount of difficulty some individuals exhibit as to their willingness to accept the significance of these great clinical discoveries. Although opponents to this movement are vociferous, even among some of the ranks of the upper echelon of leadership of this profession, common human observation will divulge that their resistance to change may be founded on ignorance and/or arrogance, but definitely not on science. For the thousands of clinicians in this new FJO/TMJ camp and the hundreds of thousands of patients who have been successfully treated by them, the truth behind the basic premise of the movement has been witnessed regardless of the obstacles represented by doddering academic institutions, manipulative third-party carriers, or intellectually myopic professional associations. The levels of advancement and success have come too far for too long. The truth simply cannot be beaten down with a hammer. From this point forward it might temporarily resolve itself to a matter of will, but the ultimate resolution is ensured. Nature has seen to it.

"If this were played
upon a stage now, I could
condemn it as improbable
fiction."

William Shakespeare
Twelfth Night, *Act III; scene iv*

References

1. Kiehn CL: Meniscectomy for internal derangement of the temporomandibular joint. *Am J Surg* 1952; 83:364–373.
2. Morgan DH: Temporomandibular joint surgery, correction of pain, tinnitus and vertigo. *Dent Radiol Photogr* 1973; 46:27–39.
3. Henny FA, Baldridge OL: Condylectomy for the persistently painful temporomandibular joint. *J Oral Surg* 1957; 15:24–31.
4. Kameros J, Himmelfarb R: Treatment of temporomandibular joint ankylosis with methyl methacrylate interpositional arthroplasty. *J Oral Surg* 1975; 33:282–287.
5. Ward TG, Smith DG, Sommar M: Condylotomy for mandibular joint. *Br Dent J* 1957; 103:147–148.
6. Dingman RO, Morrman WC: Meniscectomy in the treatment of the temporomandibular joint. *J Oral Surg* 1951; 9:214–224.
7. Costen JB: Syndrome of ear and sinus symptoms dependent upon disturbed function of the temporomandibular-joint. *Ann Otol Rhinol Laryngol* 1934; 43:1–15.
8. Costen JB: Some features of the mandibular articulation as it pertains to medical diagnosis, especially otolaryngology. *J Am Dent Assoc* 1937; 24:1507–1511.
9. Schultz LW: A curative treatment for subluxation of the temporomandibular joint, or of any joint. *J Am Dent Assoc* 1937; 24:1947–1950.
10. Goodfriend DJ: Symptomatology and treatment of abnormalities of the mandibular articulation. *Dent Cosmos* 1933 1106; 75:844, 947.
11. Goodfriend DJ: Dysarthrosis and subarthrosis of the mandibular articulation. *Dent Cosmos* 1932; 74:523–535.
12. Schuyler CH: Fundamental principles in the correction of occlusal disharmony, natural and artificial. *J Am Dent Assoc* 1935; 22:1193–1202.
13. Gottlieb B: Traumatic occlusion and the rest position of the mandible. *J Periodontol* 1947; 18:7–21.

14. Schwartz LL: A temporomandibular joint pain-dysfunction syndrome. *J Chronic Dis* 1956; 3:284–293.
15. Laskin DM: Etiology of the pain-dysfunction syndrome. *J Am Dent Assoc* 1969; 79:147–153.
16. Farrar WB, McCarty WL: Diagnosis and treatment of anterior dislocation of the articular disc. *NYJ Dent* 1971; 41:348–351.
17. Gelb H (ed): *Clinical Management of Head, Neck and TMJ Pain and Dysfunction.* Philadelphia, WB Saunders Co, 1977.
18. Sicher H: *Oral Anatomy.* St Louis, CV Mosby Co, 1949.
19. Sicher H: Problems of pain in dentistry. *Oral Surg* 1954; 7:149–160.
20. Schwartz L et al (eds): Disorders of the Temporomandibular Joint; Diagnosis, Management, Relation to Occlusion of Tooth. Philadelphia, WB Saunders Co, 1959.
21. Jankelson B, Hoffman GM, Hendron JA: Physiology of the stomatognathic system. *J Am Dent Assoc* 1953; 46:375–386.

CHAPTER 2
The Pillars of Hercules

ANATOMY

The temporomandibular joint (TMJ), on its most basic of levels, represents a sort of anatomical isthmus between what might conceptually be thought of as the two great bones of the head: the craniomaxillary bone above and the mandibular bone below.[1-4] As such, it also acts as a major channeling mechanism for absorbing its fair share of the "thousand natural shocks that flesh is heir to" Hence the intervening mediation of a resilient fibrocartilagenous disc since when it comes to considerable degrees of chronic biomechanical loading Nature doesn't like bare bone rubbing against bare stone.[5-7] The TMJ is an exquisite example of natural engineering and architectural design. Like all joints in the body, it permits movement of adjacent parts by means of simple rotation. However, in addition, it also allows for something almost unique to modern man, the phenomenon of translation. The entire condyle-disc assembly is capable of moving en masse from an original starting location in the glenoid fossa in such a fashion that the entire lower jaw may move in a coordinated fashion not only up and down but also back and forth while continually maintaining its excellent shock-absorbing abilities of condyle on disc on eminence during the entire process! This enables our species to perform precise functional activities such as eating corn on the cob, tearing open cellophane bags, or biting off pieces of monofilament fishing line. It also facilitates the more entirely human attributes of speech, song, and even whistling! The Almighty thinks of everything.

Long cloaked in mystery and viewed from a respectful distance with the greatest of trepidation by the early pioneering clinicians in this field, the human TMJ as we have now come to know it in modern times is pli-

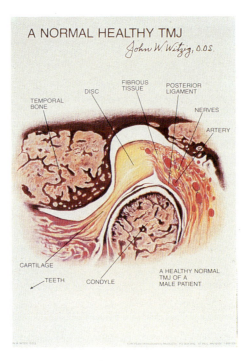

Figure 2–1   Artist's rendition of a sagittal view of a normal healthy TMJ.

able, functionally adaptable, symptomatically culpable, and even reasonably understandable. It has an enormous capacity for abuse. However, when it is abused chronically beyond its ability to adapt or recover from such common things as occlusal misguidance, it can become a source of a great many localized and even generalized problems of pain and dysfunction for its host. Fortunately, because of our relatively new found knowledge of functional jaw orthopedic (FJO) techniques, such problems are easy to remedy!

OSSEOUS ANATOMY

There are various types of joints in the body when considered from a biomechanical standpoint. The broadest general division is into two types: the synarthrodial (fibrous) joints and the diarthrodial (synovial) joints. Synarthrodial joints are limited in nature and may be thought of more in terms of unions or connections rather than joints. The most common example of a synarthrodial joint would be the sutures of the calvarium. Motion, at least to any appreciable extent, is not the object of these joints. Therefore, they are usually approximated by continuous fibrous connective tissue, hence the term *fibrous joint*. The diarthrodial joint on the other hand is primarily designed for motion in one or any number of all three planes of space. They commonly are enclosed by synovial membranes, which is where the alternative term comes from. They may be composed only of two opposing articular surfaces (simple synovial joints) or three or more opposing articular surfaces (compound synovial joints). Joints that permit only hinge-type movement, such as the finger joints (phalangeal), are referred to as ginglymoid joints. Those that permit a sliding motion are dubbed arthrodial joints. Therefore, the human TMJ, by virtue of its ability to both simultaneously rotate and translate, in semantic white tie and tails may be addressed as a compound synovial ginglymoarthrodial articulation. In colloquial sneakers and blue jeans, it's a sliding ball-and-socket–type affair.[8] Although the mandible is one bone in humans, it phylogenetically originated as two. In humans it is fused at the midline, or the symphysis menti, although in most all other mammalian species the two halves remain paired. Movement of one condyle, therefore, automatically implies movement of the other, although not necessarily to the same extent. The mandible does all the moving, hinge type and translating type, against the stationary temporal bones. Both have special features to assist in attainment of Nature's design objective.

The Condyle

The mandibular condyle represents the articulating portion of the mandible with the temporal bone and, other than the teeth, also represents the only place where the forces of occlusion may be absorbed by the mandible. It also represents a key component in understanding TMJ problems because its excessively superior posterior stereoscopic location within the confines of the glenoid fossa upon full occlusion is all but pathognomonic for classic functionally induced TMJ arthrosis. From a gross anatomical aspect, the condyle is shaped like an oversized kidney bean and is wider mediolaterally than it is anteroposteriorly or superoinferiorly. It's perched atop the condylar neck at about a 90-degree angle to the plane of the main body of the ramus. There is a slight concavity or notch at the point where the anteromedial surface of the condylar head meets the condylar neck that represents a small fossa for the insertion of the tendon of the inferior head of the lateral pterygoid. The mediolateral width of the condyle, about 15 to 20 mm, causes an axis to exist from the more prominent medial pole to the more diminutive lateral pole. This condylar polar axis angulation may vary from 0 degrees to an extreme 45 degrees to the midsagittal plane. However, about 20 degrees is average. An important biomechanical distinction that should be noted is that the

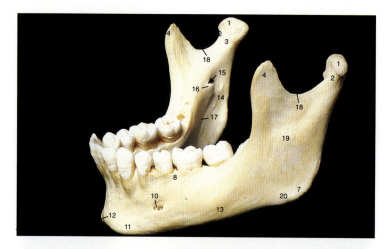

Figure 2–2(A)

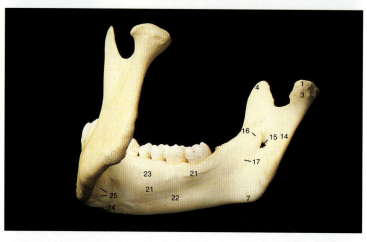

(B)

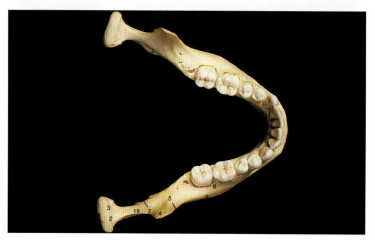

(C)

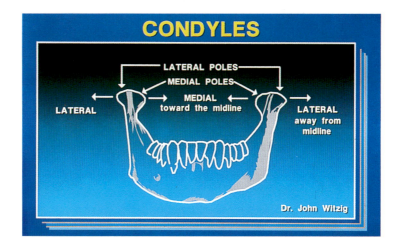

(D)

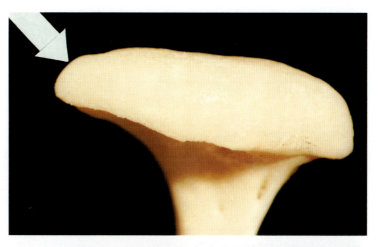

(E)

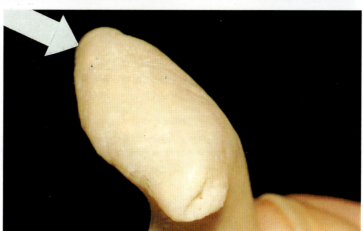

(F)

articular surfaces of the condyle are the anterior and superior surfaces. It should also be kept in mind that the articular facet of the condylar head is more robust in the superior posterior portion of its generally convex outline. This, as we shall see later, comes into play to worsen the situation when superior posterior displacement into the ever-sensitive bilaminar zone takes place.

On a histological level, the unique aspects of the condylar head stand out. The articular substance that covers the osseous surfaces of most bones in synovial joints is hyaline cartilage. It is also referred to as *articular cartilage*. This is quite different from growth cartilage. The two are almost always separated by an intervening layer of bone as in the epiphyseal areas of the long bones. The purpose of the articular hyaline cartilage is load bearing. The purpose of the growth or epiphyseal cartilage is endochondral-type bony proliferation. From basic principles of embryology, it must be remembered that endochondral bone growth (as in the bones of the appendicular skeleton), with the exception of certain hormonal and nutritional influences, is primarily governed by genetic control. Endochondral bones always arise from an embryonic cartilagenous precursor. Dermal or membrane bones, on the other hand, have no cartilagenous precursors but merely arise from primitive dermal tissues and oddly are *not* under genetic control. Nearly all of the bones of the skull are dermal in origin. Another distinction to bear in mind is that endochondral bone growth cannot be influenced by external mechanical or hydraulic inhibitory forces, whereas membrane bones are subject to tensile, mechanical, and/or hydraulic forces, which would tend to stimulate proliferation. Now as surprising as it seems for all the mechanical loading it is expected to bear, the cartilagenous covering of the head of the condyle is *not* hyaline or articular cartilage. It is *growth cartilage*,[9–12] and as such it sits right on top of the bony surface of the condylar head and is covered itself by a

---

Figure 2–2 The mandible. **(A)** left superior oblique view; **(B)** left inferior oblique view; **(C)** superior view; **(D)** the condylar poles; **(E)** condylar head, frontal view: note lipping of the anterior rim; **(F)** lateral superior oblique view. *White arrows* in **E** and **F** represent the medial pole of the condyle. 1 = head (capitulum); 2 = neck; 3 = pterygoid fovea; 4 = coronoid process; 5 = anterior border of the ramus; 6 = oblique line; 7 = angle; 8 = alveolar part; 9 = body; 10 = mental foramen; 11 = mental tubercle; 12 = mental protuberance; 13 = base; 14 = posterior border of ramus; 15 = mandibular foramen; 16 = lingula; 17 = myohyoid groove; 18 = mandibular notch; 19 = ramus; 20 = inferior border of ramus; 21 = mylohyoid line; 22 = submandibular fossa; 23 = sublingual fossa; 24 = digastric fossa; 25 = superior and inferior mental spines. In this mandible the third molar teeth are unerupted. (From McMinn RMH, Hutchings RT, Logan BM: *Color Atlas of Head and Neck Anatomy.* Chicago, Year Book Medical Publishers, Inc, 1985, p 34–35. Used by permission.)

thin but articular surface covering that is essentially a dense fibrous articular tissue.[13] In the long bones the articular cartilage is separated from the
growth (epiphyseal) cartilage by an intervening layer of bone in the epi-
physis. However, in the condyle it is as if there is no separating or intervening layer of bone between the condylar (growth) cartilage and the articulating layer that covers it. And in this case the topmost articular portion of this arrangement is not the normal hyaline or articular cartilage
but rather a dense fibrous articular tissue cap. Also of membranous origins embryonically, the condylar cartilage is not primarily under genetic
control but rather is more sensitive to tensile stimulations. The condylar
neck is another situation, but the condylar head is a base of bone covered
by growth-type cartilage capped off by a helmetlike covering of fibrous
articulator tissue, and the whole thing is sensitive to tensile forces and
has an ability to adapt to a certain degree to the particular biomechanical
demands of its loading. This simple fact is the reason that the discipline
of FJO exists. Although the condylar cartilage will obligingly adapt to tensile forces, especially in the growing child, compressive forces of the
wrong amount or in the wrong direction can be devastating.

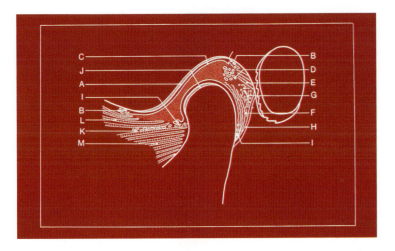

Figure 2–3 Normal TMJ anatomy (sagittal view, left TMJ). A = articular surface
of temporal bone; B = synovial membrane of superior cavity; C = superior
cavity; D = vascular knee; E = superior stratum of bilaminar zone; F = inferior
stratum of bilaminar zone; G = loose areolar connective tissue; H = posterior
capsule; I = inferior cavity synovial membrane; J = articular surface of condyle;
K = blood vessels; L = superior belly of lateral pterygoid; M = inferior belly of
lateral pterygoid muscle. (From Solberg WK, Clark GT: *Temporomandibular Joint
Problems, Biologic Diagnosis and Treatment*. Chicago, Quintessence Publishing Co,
1980, p 34. Used by permission.)

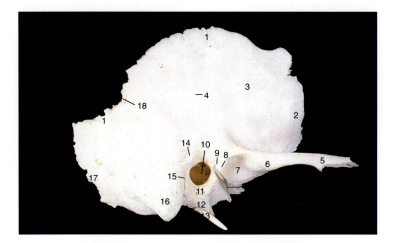

(A)

(B)

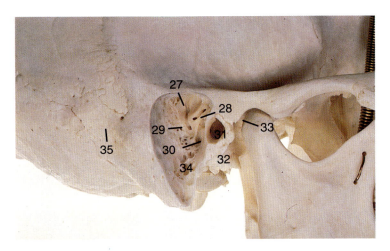

(C)

Figure 2–4 **(A)** The temporal bone (lateral view). 1 = parietal margin; 2 = sphenoidal margin; 3 = temporal surface of squamous part; 4 = groove for middle temporal artery; 5 = zygomatic process; 6 = articular tubercle (tuberculum); 7 = mandibular fossa; 8 = postglenoid tubercle; 9 = squamotympanic fissure; 10 = external acoustic meatus; 11 = tympanic part; 12 = sheath of styloid process; 13 = styloid process; 14 = suprameatal pit and spine (suprameatal triangle); 15 = tympanomastoid fissure; 16 = mastoid process; 17 = occipital margin; 18 = parietal notch. **(B)** Articular eminence of the temporal bone in relation to the external base of the skull (inferior view). 1 = musculus uvulae; 2 = palatopharyngeus; 3 = superior constrictor of pharynx; 4 = pterygoideus lateralis (deep head); 5 = pterygoideus lateralis (superficial head); 6 = pterygoideus lateralis (upper head); 7 = masseter; 8 = styloglossus; 9 = stylohyoid; 10 = stylopharyngeus; 11 = pharyngeal raphe; 12 = longus capitis; 13 = rectus capitis anterior; 14 = rectus capitis lateralis; 15 = posterior belly of digastric; 16 = longissimus capitis; 17 = splenius capitis; 18 = sternocleidomastoideus; 19 = occipital belly of occipitofrontalis; 20 = trapezius; 21 = semispinalis capitis; 22 = superior oblique; 23 = rectus capitis posterior minor; 24 = rectus capitis posterior major; 25 = capsule of atlanto-occipital joint; 26 = levator veli palatini; 27 = tensor veli palatini; 28 = articular eminence of temporal bone. **(C)** Condyle and glenoid fossa in relation to the mastoid process. 27 = anterior; 28 = lateral semicircular; 29 = posterior canal; 30 = canal for facial nerve; 31 = external acoustic meatus; 32 = tympanic part of temporal bone; 33 = postglenoid tubercle; 34 = mastoid air cells; 35 = mastoid foramen. (From McMinn RMH, Hutchings RT, Logan BM: *Color Atlas of Head and Neck Anatomy.* Chicago, Year Book Medical Publishers, Inc, 1985, pp 24, 50, 148. Used by permission.)

The Temporal Bone

Compared with its opponent in the masticatory process (the condylar head), the temporal bone is somewhat more complex. Yet its anatomy is a simple matter of utility and a good example of the principle that form follows function. The temporal bone serves as the base against which the condyle of the mandible articulates, but it started out embryonically as three bones.[14] They are the squamous portion, the tympanic portion, and the petrous portion. They are fused into one bone during the first year of life, and only the squamous and tympanic portions are dermal (membrane) in origin. The petrous portion is chondral in origin. The famous facial nerve (cranial nerve VII) courses through the bone at the stylomastoid foramen, an important communicating branch of which is the auriculotemporal nerve, which passes through the retrocondylar area in the bilaminar zone. The petrous portion contains the mastoid process and internal mastoid air cells. The tympanic portion contains, of course, the external auditory meatus and hearing apparatus. But it is the squamous portion that contains the glenoid fossa and the articular eminence against which the condylar head and disc assembly articulate. Sometimes referred to as the tuberculum of the fossa, the temporal articular facet of the glenoid fossa, which serves as functional stress-bearing opposition to the mandible's disc-condyle assembly, courses from the anterolateral portion of the fossa down over the whole of the articular eminence and even slightly anterior to the eminence. The facet area beyond the base of the eminence inclines slightly upward. Confluent with the slope of the bony eminence and slightly obstructing it from a strictly lateral view is the base of the supra-articular crest, which courses out and forward to form the zygomatic arch. The base of the supra-articular crest often appears as the superior surface of the articular facet of the slope of the eminence when viewed on a transcranial radiograph, when in fact the actual slope of the eminence is somewhat obscured by this structure. It usually lies deeper and at less of an angle than is revealed by the outline of the base of the supra-articular crest. However, the difference is not great. The actual location of the surface of the eminence, which lies slightly superior to the outline of the base of the supra-articular crest, can only be visualized by sequential-slice images of tomographic techniques. Interestingly, the roof of the fossa is a very thin noncancellous bony plate averaging only about 1.0 mm in thickness or less! It separates the glenoid fossa from the temporal lobes of the brain and was obviously not intended by Nature to absorb shock from the mandibular condyle. However, the articular facet of the anterior portion of the roof of the fossa and the slope of the articular eminence or tuberculum are designed for load bearing and have ample amounts of cancellous bone backing them up to prove it. The articular surfaces of the facet area are covered by a layer of dense fibrous tissue that, like the condylar head, is *not* hyaline cartilage (as with other joints of the body) but rather is this dense stress-absorbing articular tissue, which has occasional cartilagenous-type cells present, indicative of remodeling potential. This fibrous articular tissue is (like the bone it covers) thinnest at the roof of the fossa and quickly becomes much thicker down over the eminential slope. The articular tissue has bundles of fibers arranged in layers, with an outer layer running parallel to the bony surface (sliding forces) and an inner layer running perpendicular to the bony surface (loading). The biomechanical inferences of the bony trabecular patterns and articular surface tissue densities of both the articular surface of the temporal bone and the condylar head of the TMJ indicate that the general direction of the absorbed vectors of stress during functional loading is in a combined upward and forward direction. One thing is certain: there is definitely no stress-absorbing–type tissue anywhere in the posterior portions of the glenoid fossa. All that can be found there are the superior and inferior retrodiscal ligaments, the huge auriculotemporal neurovascular bundle, and loose connective tissues of the bilaminar zone.

CONNECTIVE TISSUE ANATOMY

To the student of anatomy, the words "connective tissue" mean many things. But for the sake of our little discussion here they mean two things: the intra-articular disc and the associated TMJ ligaments. The intra-articular disc of the TMJ is an important component in the overall workings of the joint mechanism. It is important because it allows for rotational movement of the condyle against its lower surface. It is important because it allows for translation of the entire condyle-disc assembly against the articular facet of the fossa via its upper surface. It is important because it allows two convex surfaces, the head of the condyle (capitulum) and the articular eminence (tuberculum), to be juxtaposed against one another in a state of totally compatible biomechanical stability. But it is most important to the clinician when things in the maxillofacial complex are functionally awry. For when the condyle is forced out of its normal, intimate, cradled relationship with the disc at full occlusion, forcing it to be displaced down and forward as the condyle is forced too far up and back, the signs that appear as a result of that forward discal displacement lend tremendous support to the accumulation of symptoms to give the clinician a clearer picture of what is going on and what needs to be done treatment-wise with respect to the joint. But for all its importance to the patient for its ability to facilitate complex joint movements, the intra-articular disk is most important to the clinician for the role it plays in the form of a "biological tattletale" revealing the effects of the status of the present occlusion on the overall functional integrity of the TMJ. The disc is also referred to as the meniscus, which comes from the Greek root *meniskos* which means crescent, a bit of a misnomer. The disc is not actu-

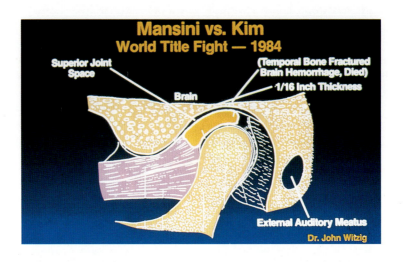

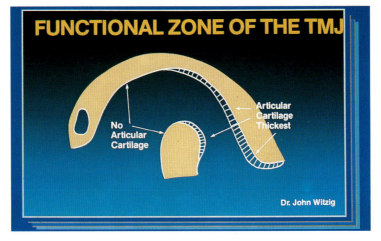

Figure 2–5   **(A)** Boxing fracture. **(B)** TMJ functional zone.

ally crescent shaped (as the fluid meniscus in a small graduated cylinder) but is shaped more like a common red blood cell. Discs that have been completely dissected free during surgical procedures have been observed to resemble dried apricot halves. It is ovoid in surface area, thick on the edges, and thinner in the middle. The posterior portion, sometimes referred to as the posterior band or heel of the disc, is usually much thicker than the anterior portion, also called the anterior band or toe of the disc. It is composed of a dense fibrous tissue that is essentially fibrocartilaginous in nature. It is shaped so as to snugly fit the corresponding articulating surface of the condylar head, which rotates against its bottom surface, and it is also contoured on its upper surface so as to closely adapt to the articular surfaces of the superior portion of the fossa and the slope of the articular eminence. The upper surface is what allows for the translation of the entire disc-condyle assembly across the surface of the articular eminence. The disc is attached to the condylar head by ligaments to the medial and lateral poles. It is indirectly attached to the roof or superior head of the lateral pterygoid anteriorly via the anterior capsular wall. Posteriorly, it has two ligaments. One elastic lamina attaches to the posterior wall of the fossa or tympanic plate, and the other attaches to the back edge of the condylar neck. The connective tissue enclosed between these two lamina is what is referred to as the bilaminar tissue or bilaminar zone. The superior lamina is elastic in nature but only exerts tension on the disc in the more forward ranges of the translatory motion.[15] The superior lamina does not exert any tension on the disc in the closed position. Hence the location of the disc in the close position is determined by the tension of the superior head of the lateral pterygoid and the amount of space present between the condylar head and the contours of the roof of the fossa and articular eminence. The inferior lamina is not elastic in nature but is more like a true ligament in that it serves to stabilize the disc and prevents excessive forward rotation of the disc over the front of the condylar head. The bilaminar tissues in between consist of highly vascularized and highly innervated loose connective tissue. The volumetric amount of connective tissue present that represents the retrodiscal tissues between the superior and inferior laminae is what is responsible for the height of the dome or roof of the fossa, for this is where most of this tissue goes when the condyle assumes its *proper* relationship in the fossa at full occlusion. Only the most anterior portion of the roof of the fossa is occupied by the thickened heel of the disc. The rest of the dome is filled with these sensitive connective tissues of the bilaminar area and are pulled down behind the heel of the disc as the condyle translates inferiorly down and forward along the path of the eminence. As the condyle returns to its "home" position, these retrodiscal tissues get shoved by the condylar head into the superior and posterior portions of the dome of the fossa. There should be plenty of clearance back there for them so they don't become bludgeoned by excessive, occlusion-misguided, full-force

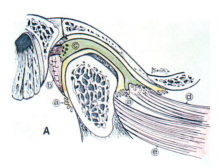

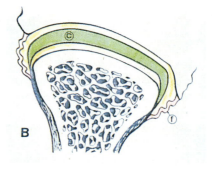

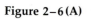

Figure 2–6 (A)

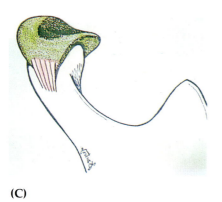

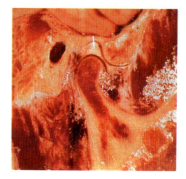

(C)

(D)

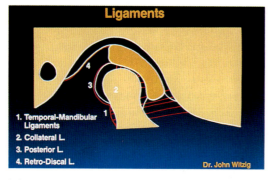

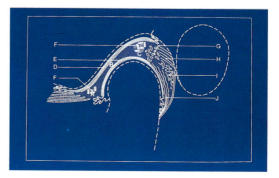

(E)

(F)

condylar intrusion. Again, this area is for vascular circulation and nervous innervation, *not* functional articulation.

The articular ligaments of the TMJ serve a variety of functions, but their general purpose is to act as a set of restraints to excessive movements of the various components of the joint in specific directions. They do not contract, nor do they stretch, at least not on purpose. Therefore, they do not assume an active part in joint function but merely act as confining agents, biomechanical policemen if you will, that limit the amount of linear movement possible during function. They are bundles, sheets, or cablelike structures composed of collagenous connective tissue that remind one often of the way plastic bags are gathered and pursed together at the twist tie. Not being elastic or contractile, as a muscle for instance, they do not cause a tension to be created at the articular surfaces when muscles are at rest; only when the joint is extended to its maximum ranges of movement do they exert their limiting forces. (The elasticity of the posterior discal attachments, specifically the superior lamina, is due to specialty tissues that *are* elastic.) Because of their lack of elasticity, chronic trauma of the stretching (hyperextension and/or hyperflexion) variety can loosen or, more correctly, *elongate* ligaments, which once so damaged tend to remain so. Ligaments are very poorly vascularized and as a result have very poor healing potential once elongated, damaged, or torn. However, they are often very well innervated by two main types of nerves; nociceptors, or pain nerves, and proprioceptors. Chronic abuse in the form of the type of microtrauma that can come from the phenomenon of neuromuscular reflexive displacement of the mandible causing superior

---

Figure 2–6 **(A)** Articular disc in relation to the condylar head and articular eminence of the temporal bone (sagittal view: a = synovial membrane; b = posterior capsular wall; c = thickened posterior band or heel of disc; d = superior head lateral pterygoid; e = inferior head lateral pterygoid). **(B)** Articular disc (anteroposterior view: c = heel of disc; f = medial collateral ligament). **(C)** Biconcave shape of the disc in relation to the condylar head; note the lateral collateral ligament. **(D)** Cryosection of a normal TMJ with a biconcave appearance of the disc and thickened heel *(white arrow)*. **(E)** Schematic view of the relation of various TMJ ligaments. **(F)** Details of the articular disc and bilaminar zone anatomy (A = foot or toe of meniscus [pes]; B = thin, avascular part [pars gracilis]; C = pars posterior; D = sheet of parallel collagen fibers on superior surface; E = sheet of parallel collagen fibers on inferior surface; F = zones of collagen fibers oriented in all three directions; G = vascular knee; H = superior stratum of bilaminar zone; I = loose areolar connective tissue, vessels, and nerves; J = inferior stratum of bilaminar zone). (Parts A to D courtesy of Dr. James Colt, Denver. Part E courtesy of Dr. John Witzig. Part F from Solberg WK, Clark GT: *Temporomandibular Joint Problems, Biologic Diagnosis and Treatment.* Chicago, Quintessence Publishing Co, 1980, p 35. Used by permission.)

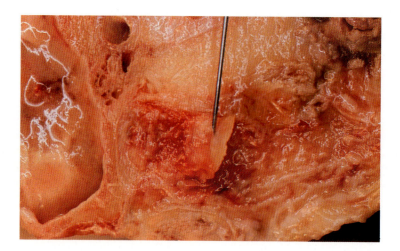

Figure 2–7   Coronal section showing the back edge of the condyle reflected to expose soft tissues, nerves, and blood vessels of the bilaminar zone. (Courtesy of Dr. James Colt, Denver.)

posterior displacement of the condyle (NRDM/SPDC) can cause a low-grade inflammation, which would place the nociceptors in a state of hyperexcitability. This in turn can make the normally quiet ligaments "bark" with pain in direct proportion to the amount of force placed on the ligaments during the outer ranges of functional movements.[16] Proprioceptors on the other hand tell the brain just where things are. This input in combination with similar types of proprioceptive input that comes from the muscles themselves provides a central nervous system (CNS)-controlled

Figure 2–8   **(A)** Gross anatomy of the TMJ area. **(B)** Detailed anatomy of the TMJ area (masseter muscle reflected). Note the direction of pull of the masseter muscle. 1 = inferior temporal line; 2 = temporalis muscle; 3 = temporalis tendon; 4 = zygomatic arch; 5 = middle layer; 6 = superficial layer; 7 = submandibular gland; 8 = neck of mandible; 9 = temporomandibular ligament; 10 = styloid process; 11 = posterior belly of digastric; 12 = sternocleidomastoid; 13 = cartilage of external acoustic meatus; 14 = temporalis fascia; 15 = superior temporal line; 16 = coronoid process; 17 = ramus; 18 = medial pterygoid; 19 = cut edge of mucous membrane of mouth. (From McMinn RMH, Hutchings RT, Logan BM: *Color Atlas of Head and Neck Anatomy*. Chicago, Year Book Medical Publishers, Inc, 1985, pp 114–115. Used by permission.)

Figure 2–9   **(A)** Temporomandibular ligaments, horizontal and oblique fibers *(black arrows)*. **(B)** Schematic representation of the insertions of the temporomandibular ligament. (Part A courtesy of Dr. James Colt, Denver; part B courtesy of Dr. John Witzig.)

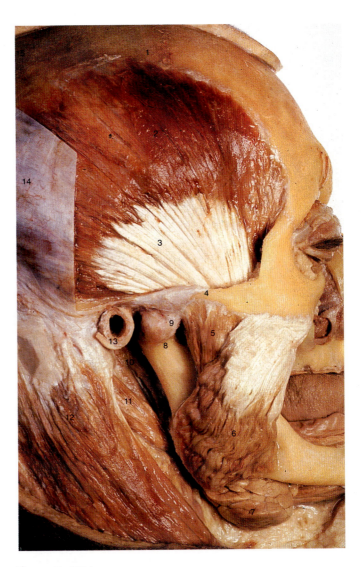

Figure 2–8(A)

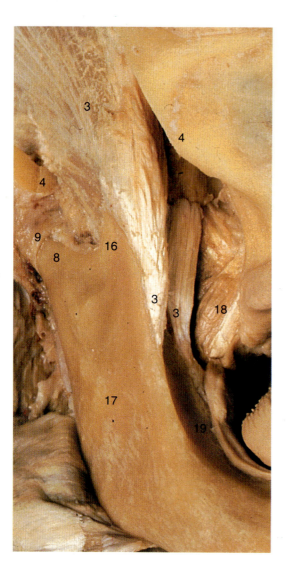

(B)

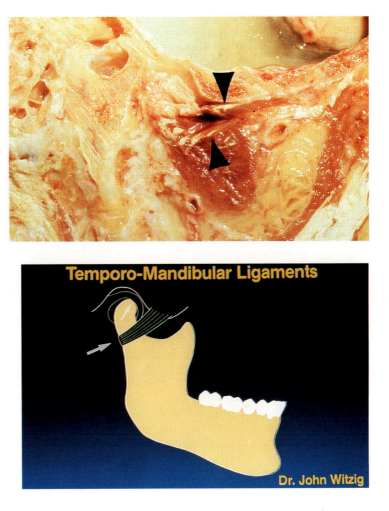

Figure 2–9(A)

(B)

neuromuscular circuit that both monitors and protects the function of the entire TMJ mechanism. Nature likes to continually know not only what it's doing but also how well things are going.

The first specific TMJ ligament we shall discuss resembles not so much a ligament as it does a connective tissue veil. It is a tough, fibrous connective tissue cocoon that envelops the entire temporomandibular articulation, the capsular ligament. More of an enclosure and less of a source of limitation of movement, although it can provide some limitation of movement of the condyle at the most extreme ranges of forward translation, the fibrous capsular ligament of the TMJ attaches to the temporal bone at the articular borders of the eminence and roof of the glenoid fossa superiorly and to the squamotympanic fissure in the posterior areas of the fossa. It attaches inferiorly to the neck of the condyle. Its lateral wall over the condyle-disc assembly area is relatively thin and is theorized by some to be more concerned with assisting in the circulation of synovial fluid during functional movements because its inner surface is lined with synovial membrane tissue. Although the fibrous capsular ligament is relatively loose so as to permit free translation of the condyle-disc assembly back and forth, it does offer a modicum of resistance to inferior and lateral movement of the condyle that would act to pull the joint apart. It is also highly innervated with both nociceptive pain fibers and proprioceptive fibers.

The second main ligament of the TMJ is actually two ligaments that are referred to by the single name of temporomandibular ligament. It is a suspensory ligament meant to limit inferior and posterior displacement of the condylar head and neck. In overall arrangement, this ligament runs from the outer edge of the articular tubercle and supra-articular crest downward and backward at about a 45-degree angle to attach to the condylar neck at its inferior posterior border. The outer oblique portion is the larger of the two sections of this ligament and runs from the supra-articular crest and tubercle to the condyle in the fashion just described; however, the smaller inner horizontal portion of the ligament arises from the same place but runs almost horizontally to attach to the lateral pole of the condylar head and even has a few fibers extending as far back as the posterior portion of the disc. The outer oblique ligament prevents inferior and posterior mandibular displacement. The inner horizontal ligament is designed to limit the extent to which the condyle may be displaced posteriorly. This is one of the ligaments that becomes elongated when the occlusion is such that occlusal misguidance of the NRDM/SPDC-type phenomenon forces the condyle too far superiorly and posteriorly up off the back edge of the disc. Because chronic abuse progressively elongates all the associated ligaments, it becomes progressively easier for the condyle to be displaced superiorly and posteriorly where the full forces of occlusion may be directed to the helpless bilaminar zone. The entire temporomandibular ligament also courses across the fibrous capsule and fortifies it over its lateral aspect where the capsular ligament is thinnest.

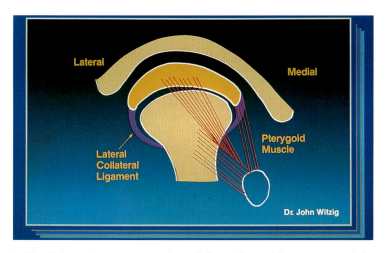

Figure 2–10   Schematic representation of the collateral ligaments and direction of the pterygoid muscle (anteroposterior view). (Courtesy of Dr. John Witzig.)

The final set of ligaments to consider are the collateral ligaments that firmly keep the intra-articular disc attached to the condylar head. There are two, the medial collateral ligament, which is the more stout of the two and attaches the medial surface of the disc to the medial pole of the condyle, and the finer lateral collateral ligament, which attaches the lateral surface of the disc to the lateral pole of the condyle. These collateral ligaments keep the disc in close approximation to the condylar head but do not prevent rotation of the condylar head against the underside of the disc. They do keep the disc moving with the condylar head during sliding or translation-type movements of the joint. These ligaments also serve as the final components needed to separate the two synovial compartments of the joint into superior and inferior synovial joint spaces. These ligaments must also elongate (along with the aforementioned inner horizontal portion of the temporomandibular ligament) in order to permit the undesired condylar intrusion up and back off the disc into the bilaminar zone. This entire process of condylar displacement up and back makes for a very unstable joint status, and since ligaments have good nervous innervation but poor vascular supply, damaged or elongated ligaments require greatly lengthened healing times. Some authorities feel that it is not uncommon for "optimal healing" in severely involved joints to take as long as 2 years after completion of treatment, i.e., correction of the malocclusion, removal of the misguidance of the teeth, increasing of the vertical, and full-scale mandibular advancement with attending posterior and superior joint space decompression.

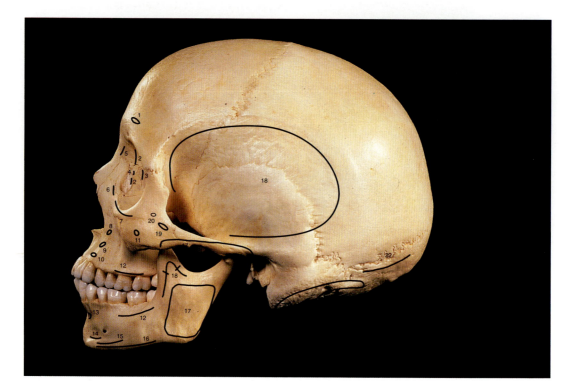

Figure 2–11   Attachment sites of the muscles of the head and neck. **(A)** Left lateral view: 1 = corrugator supercilii; 2 = orbicularis oculi (orbital and palpebral parts); 3 = orbicularis oculi (lacrimal part); 4 = medial palpebral ligament; 5 = procerus; 6 = levator labii superioris alaeque nasi; 7 = levator labii superioris; 8 = nasalis (transverse part); 9 = nasalis (alar part); 10 = depressor septi; 11 = levator anguli oris; 12 = buccinator; 13 = mentalis; 14 = depressor labii inferioris; 15 = depressor anguli oris; 16 = platysma; 17 = masseter; 18 = temporalis; 19 = zygomaticus major; 20 = zygomaticus minor; 21 = sternocleidomastoid; 22 = occipital belly of occipitofrontalis. **(B)** Frontal view: 1 = corrugator supercilii; 2 = orbicularis oculi; 3 = medial palpebral ligament; 4 = procerus; 5 = levator labii superioris alaeque nasi; 6 = levator labii superioris; 7 = zygomaticus minor; 8 = zygomaticus major; 9 = levator anguli oris; 10 = nasalis (transverse part); 11 = nasalis (alar part); 12 = depressor septi; 13 = buccinator; 14 = depressor labii inferioris; 15 = depressor anguli oris; 16 = platysma; 17 = mentalis; 18 = masseter; 19 = temporalis. (From McMinn RMH, Hutchings RT, Logan BM: *Color Atlas of Head and Neck Anatomy.* Chicago, Year Book Medical Publishers, Inc, 1985, pp 12, 16. Used by permission.)

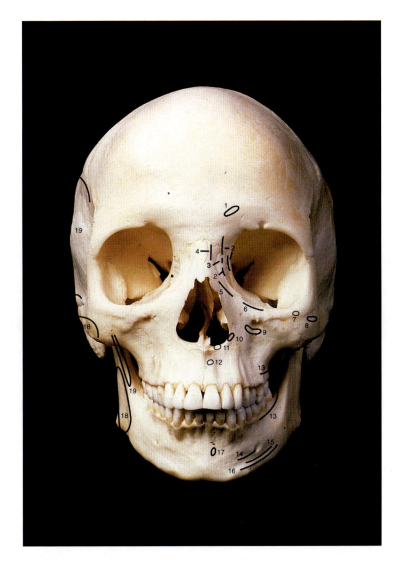

(B)

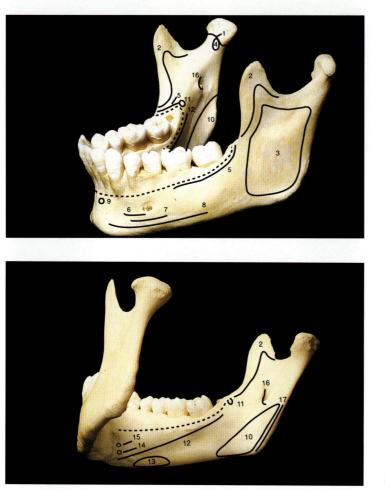

(A)

(B)

RELATED MUSCULAR ANATOMY

Although not considered an actual anatomical part of the joint itself, muscles are intimately related to joints in that all skeletal-type muscles (except for a few exceptions in the dermis and the muscles of facial expressions) pull across a joint in one form or another and cause that joint to work in the fashion it does. Taking a bit of poetic license, early anatomists envisioned the bellies of certain muscles as looking like the bodies of mice, with the narrowing and the gathering into a tendon at the end resembling a tail. Hence the diminutive term *muscle* comes from the original Latin root *mus,* or mouse. Of the three types, skeletal, cardiac, and visceral or smooth muscles, only the skeletal muscles are under the direct control of consciousness, which is why they are sometimes referred to as voluntary muscles. If enough poetic license is once again granted, the muscles of mastication may be thought of as pulling across the TMJ, originating on the upper of the two main bones of the head, the "craniomaxillary bone," and inserting on the lower of the two main bones, the mandible. They exist bilaterally, three pair to close, one pair to open. Muscles of mastication are of great interest to the clinician concerned with diagnosing and treating functionally induced TMJ arthrosis. They can be the first to detect the beginning stages of abuse of the malocclusion variety. Their telltale tenderness to palpation can be of great diagnostic value as to the severity and chronicity of the condition. Their imbalances of function and myostatic tension may be detected by the mute testimony of their chronic effects, i.e., by the shape of the dental arch form, or even by the full-scale anteroposterior facial dysplasias they may produce. And their painful eruptions of acute spasticity may act as a last-ditch warning of the advanced state of degeneration or levels of abuse to which the patient has been subjugated since this represents Nature's form of total biological rebellion to the functionally abusive state of affairs at hand. They are programmable, adaptable, palpable, controllable, autorepairable, and best of all for us treating clinicians, even functionally alterable! They are respon-

Figure 2–12 Muscle attachment sites of the mandible. **(A)** left superior oblique view; **(B)** left inferior oblique view. 1 = capsule of TMJ; 2 = temporalis; 3 = masseter; 4 = lateral pterygoid; 5 = buccinator; 6 = depressor labii inferioris; 7 = depressor anguli oris; 8 = platysma; 9 = mentalis; 10 = medial pterygoid; 11 = pterygomandibular raphe and superior constrictor of pharynx; 12 = mylohyoid; 13 = anterior belly of digastric; 14 = geniohyoid; 15 = genioglossus; 16 = sphenomandibular ligament; 17 = stylomandibular ligament. (From McMinn RMH, Hutchings RT, Logan BM: *Color Atlas of Head and Neck Anatomy.* Chicago, Year Book Medical Publishers, Inc, 1985, p 36. Used by permission.)

sible for the physical work and movement of mankind. When the most important ones of the body quit working altogether, we die.

The muscles of mastication have always been of concern for those involved in treating TMJ problems, for they almost invariably exhibit some level of acute or chronic myalgia due to imbalances in the occlusion and joint.[17-21] In most recent times they have generated new interest by virtue of their ability to refer pain to other nearby structures because of the presence of "trigger points." Travell defines a myofascial trigger point as "a focus of hyperirritability that, when compressed, is locally tender and, if sufficiently hypersensitive, gives rise to referred pain and tenderness, and sometimes to referred autonomic phenomena and distortion of proprioception."[22] Simplistically, they may be thought of as little "knots" in the muscle fiber that can be active or latent and may be locally sensitive or may refer pain to other areas. The pattern of referred pain is characteristic for each muscle, but even in spite of this, the confusion this lends to the diagnostic picture may be easily appreciated. Fortunately, these trigger points in the muscles of mastication tend to become latent or disappear altogether once the abuse that initially spawned them in the form of the imbalances of the malocclusion causing the TMJ problem has been corrected.

The Temporalis

The first of the three major closing muscles to consider is the temporalis. Although one muscle, it is commonly thought of in three parts. The entire muscle is a fan-shaped affair that originates along a curve above the temporoparietal and temporofrontal sutures of the temporal bone and inserts on the coronoid process of the mandible.[23] The anterior third of the muscle has fibers that run primarily vertically, and as a result, when they contract, they pull the mandible vertically.[24] The functionally distinct middle portion elevates and retracts the mandible, its fibers running at about a 45-degree angle to the Frankfort plane. The posterior third of the muscle has fibers that run almost horizontally, and as a result their contracture retracts the mandible with almost no elevation component and consequently acts as a direct antagonist to the inferior head of the lateral pterygoid (which attaches to the anterior condylar neck).[25-27] Although all three divisions of the temporalis muscle may work singly, they generally work in union, not for the sake of power in closing the mandible, but more so as a directing or guiding influence as the mandible closes. Obviously, overretraction of the mandible, as in occlusions that result in full skeletal Class II deep-bite situations, involves overworking of the horizontal fibers of the posterior third of the muscle, which must fight the pull of the inferior head of the lateral pterygoid, the horizontal fibers of the temporomandibular ligament, and the collateral ligaments, to force the condyle superiorly and posteriorly far enough to bring the posterior

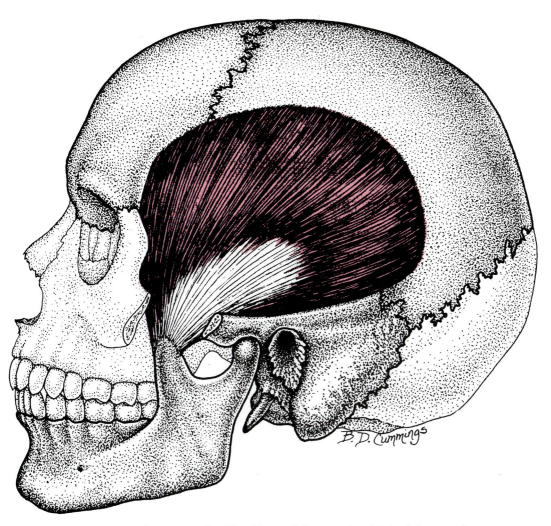

Figure 2–13   The temporalis. The fibers of the anterior third of the muscle are nearly vertical, the middle-third fibers are oblique, and the fibers of the posterior third are nearly horizontal. (From Travell JG, Simons DG: *"Myofascial Pain and Dysfunction, The Trigger Point Manual.* Baltimore, William & Wilkins, 1983, p 238. Used by permission.)

quadrants of the dental occlusion home. Closing on the anterior teeth obviously involves only the anterior third of the muscle. Interestingly, in edentulous patients or patients wearing dentures made in the usual fashion, i.e., thumb-on-chin construction bites, all of the temporalis muscle contracts on closure, whereas patients with well-balanced natural dentitions only require activation of the anterior third to comfortably and gently close the mandible! Although this muscle is often tender to palpation in TMJ patients, it is not generally as frequently or severely involved as some of the other muscles of mastication.

The Masseter

One of the two main muscles responsible for power strokes in closure of the mandible is the masseter. Some prefer to think of it as having a deep as well as a superficial origin. The main portion, or superficial origin, inserts at the anterior two thirds of the inferior border of the zygomatic arch, with the deep portion defined as inserting at the posterior one third of the zygomatic arch. The entire body of this rectangular muscle runs somewhat distally: it inserts at the inferior border of the mandible, with the superficial portion also attaching to the interior half of the outer border of the ramus and the deep portion attaching almost exclusively to the superior half of the outer border of the ramus.[28, 29] It is confluent via fascial connections to the medial pterygoid at the area of the gonion. Its main purpose is the powerful closure of the mandible vertically, although the slight offset of the direction of the fibers in an anterior direction from bottom to top allows for a modicum of anterior movement during closure also, although this component is not great. The deep portions of this muscle are aligned such that they are capable of slight retrusion of the mandible if they act without the benefit of any other fibers of the muscle. But again, action in this direction is not great. The main function of this muscle is still direct power closure of the mandible vertically with a slight anterior component associated with it. Nothing in this muscle is biomechanically designed to move the mandible up and back.

Figure 2–14 **(A)** Masseter muscle (superficial layer). **(B)** Deep layer of the masseter (superficial layer removed). Note the direction of pull of the main body of the muscle. (From Travell JG, Simons DG: *Myofascial Pain and Dysfunction, The Trigger Point Manual*. Baltimore, William & Wilkins, 1983, p 222. Used by permission.)

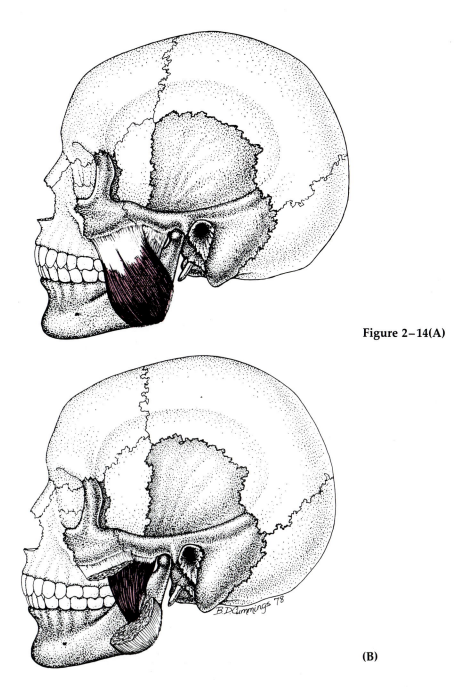

Figure 2–14(A)

(B)

The Medial Pterygoid

The other chief player in the mandibular power-stroke team is the medial pterygoid muscle, often referred to also as the internal pterygoid. It is the direct synergist of its "companion in closure," the masseter. It originates primarily at the medial or inner surface of the lateral pterygoid plate and even has a few fibers that originate on the palatine bone itself. Its insertion is at the internal surface of the angle of the mandible. Its fibers are oriented in the main belly of the muscle similarly to the masseter such that it can close the mandible, protrude the mandible, or when acting unilaterally, deviate the mandible to the opposite side.

An interesting observation is made by Travell and Levandoski[30, 31] concerning the relationship of this muscle to the complaint of ear "stuffiness" in some TMJ patients. It has been observed that the tensor veli palatini muscle is responsible for dialating the eustachian tube, and in order to do so it must push the medial pterygoid muscle to the side. In the normal resting state when the tensor veli palatini is inactive, the medial pterygoid rests against the eustachian tube, and keeps it closed. Stiffness of the medial pterygoid due to the action of active trigger points or other noxious stimuli common to a TMJ problem resulting from occlusal misguidance of the NRDM/SPDC variety can make the muscle so resistant to displacement by the diminutive tensor veli palatini that the strength of the smaller muscle cannot overcome the rigidity of the larger and blockage of the eustachian tube results. This can lead the patient to complain of stuffiness of the ears, referred to by a term ironically lyrical to the ear, *barohypoacusis*. A much more commonly observed event associated with this muscle in patients with TMJ problems is tenderness to palpation, for this muscle is almost invariably hypersensitive to digital pressure when the mandible is being forced too far back at full occlusion by the dentition.

The Lateral Pterygoid

Understanding the anatomy and function of the lateral pterygoid muscle is important to all those who treat common functionally induced

---

Figure 2–15 **(A)** The medial pterygoid muscle *(dark gray)* in relation to the lateral pterygoid muscle *(light gray)* in the lateral view. Part of the ramus and coronoid process of the mandible has been removed. **(B)** Coronal view of the skull from just behind the TMJs. (From Travell JG, Simons DG: *Myofascial Pain and Dysfunction, The Trigger Point Manual.* Baltimore, William & Wilkins, 1983, p 251. Used by permission.)

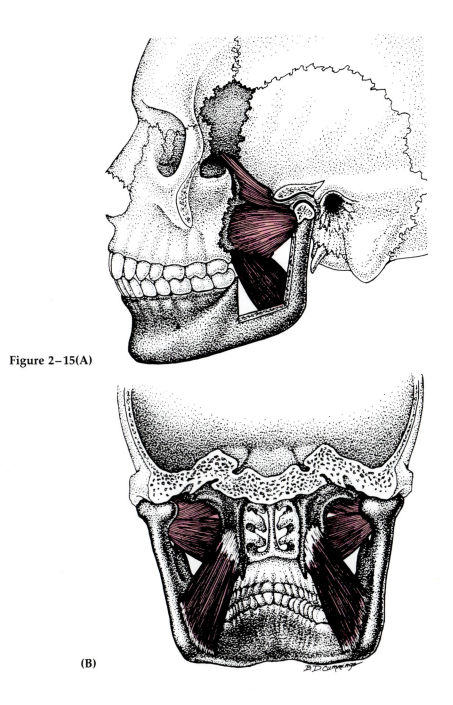

Figure 2–15(A)

(B)

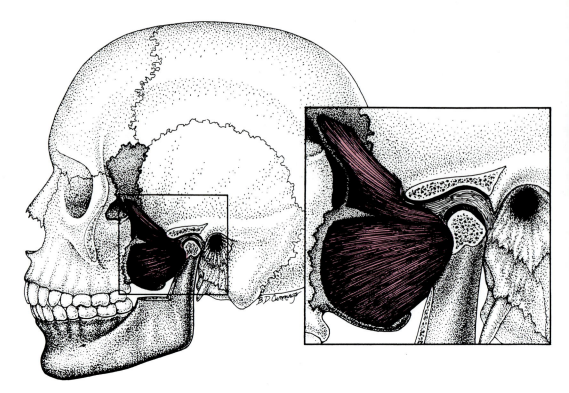

Figure 2–16   The lateral pterygoid. The coronoid process, zygomatic arch, and superficial portion of the TMJ have been removed. The superior head actually attaches to the anterior portion of the capsule and the pterygoid fovea. The inferior portion attaches to the neck of the condyle. (From Travell JG, Simons DG: *Myofascial Pain and Dysfunction, The Trigger Point Manual.* Baltimore, William & Wilkins, 1983, p 262. Used by permission.)

TMJ arthrosis. Sometimes referred to as the external pterygoid, the lateral pterygoid muscle is intimately involved, more so than any other muscle, with the actual working of the condyle-disc assembly during opening and closing movements of the mandible. It has mistakenly been referred to throughout the history of anatomical studies as one muscle when in fact in action and anatomy it actually represents at least two and often three. They act in a reciprocal manner on different portions of the joint to effect different ends.[32-36] There is a superior head that is the smaller of the two portions and an inferior head that is quite a bit larger. In the early days of the study of human anatomy, failure to understand the different functions of the two portions of this muscle initially led to confusion as to what it actually did.[37] That confusion has still not been completely resolved. The superior portion of the muscle originates from the infratemporal crest and the lateral surface of the greater wing of the sphenoid. The inferior portion of the muscle originates from the lateral surface of the lateral pterygoid plate.[38] This same inferior belly in turn inserts at the little fossa on the condylar neck just below the condylar head as well as at a short portion of the anterior surface of the shaft condylar neck. The superior head, however, is surrounded with controversy and misunderstanding as to just what it attaches itself to and what these attachments mean. There has long been a generally accepted opinion that the superior head of the lateral pterygoid inserts at the anterior edge of the intra-articular disc as well as a portion of the capsular ligament, with some additional fibers that also attach to the anterior surface of the neck of the condyle. However, there were those who rejected the notion that this portion of the muscle could have fibers attached to the condylar neck, the domain of the inferior belly of the muscle. They contended and supported with evidence from dissections that the superior head attaches *only* to the disc and capsular ligament. Another long-held opinion supports this viewpoint but does acknowledge that occasionally fibers may attach to the condyle below the capsular ligament. However, if and when this happens, they are of no functional significance.

The theory of the superior head of the lateral pterygoid muscle inserting into the anterior edge of the disc with the possibility of secondary fibers inserting into the little depression, or fovea, at the anterior base of the condylar head where the condylar neck starts is a time-honored definition that is well entrenched ubiquitously in the dental as well as anatomical literature. This, however, in light of more recent findings has become suspect because current evidence appears to indicate that such is not quite exactly the case. The controversial discoveries that have cast a new light on how this muscle is attached to the disc-condyle complex and just what it does to that complex once it is activated have come from half a world away, from "the land down under," and appeared in a landmark monograph written by Dr. T.M. Wilkinson[39] of the University of Adelaide, South Australia! After arduous and careful dissection of 26 human cadaver TMJs, Wilkinson made a series of rather startling and unexpected discoveries concerning the superior head of the lateral pterygoid and its relationship to the disc-condyle assembly. First of all, in all joints the insertion of the entire lateral pterygoid muscle is limited to the medial half of the condyle at the pterygoid fovea. Although other studies have been done on the gross anatomy of the ligamentous joint capsule, Wilkinson was the first to coordinate macroscopic dissection with microscopic examination of the anterior portions of the joint capsule. He describes a band of fibrous tissue that runs from the anterior edge of the articular facet of the capitulum continuously to the roof of the fossa. This uninterrupted band (due to the sagittally oriented plane of the cut) forms the floor of the superior joint space anteriorly and the floor of the inferior joint space posteriorly. As such, this band of fibrous tissue forms the anteromedial portion of the capsular ligament. The anterior portion, or toe of the disc, is confluent with this portion of the capsular ligament at its uppermost border. Wilkinson also discovered that about one third of the time the superior head of the lateral pterygoid exhibited a single insertion to the pterygoid fovea. It did so by one of two methods: either it attached directly to the bone via its own muscle attachment, or it attached secondarily by blending with the muscle attachment fibers of the inferior head. No fibers were seen to attach directly to the disc regardless of which of the two methods mentioned above the muscle used to attach itself to the pterygoid fovea. The capsular ligament below the toe of the disc attached itself to the superior aspect of the muscle, or what is referred to as the *roof of the superior head of the lateral pterygoid.* Thus in one third of the sample of joints studied the disc was attached to the joint capsule at its anterior edges, and the fibers of the anterior part of the capsule under the toe of the disc were united to the superior aspect, or roof, of the superior head. In the remaining two thirds of the joints studied, it was observed that the major insertion of the superior head was still at the pterygoid fovea but

---

Figure 2–17   (A) Sagittal section through the condyle. Note the arrangement and distribution of the fibers of the superior head of the lateral pterygoid muscle. The major portion of the fibers favor the bony attachment site at the pterygoid fovea of the condylar neck. (*MA* = maxillary artery; *DT* = deep temporal nerve; *RR* = regressive remodeling of the posterior slope of the articular eminence or tuberculum). **(B)** Sagittal section near the medial pole of the condyle. In this example the condyle is displaced posteriorly and the disc is displaced anteriorly. Note the clear distinctions and distributions between the upper head of the lateral pterygoid (*ULP*) and the lower head of the lateral pterygoid muscle (*LLP*). Again the balance of the distribution of the fibers of the upper head of the lateral pterygoid muscle favors the bony attachment site. (From Marguelles-Bonnet R, Yung J, et al: *Craniomandib Pract* 1989; 7:97–106. Used by permission.)

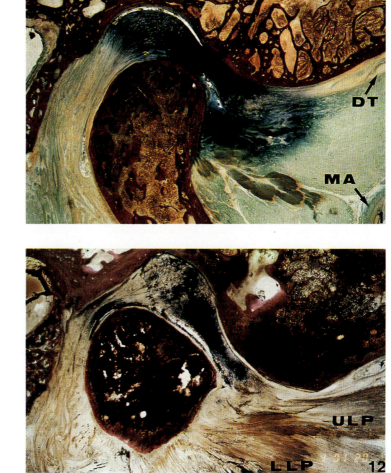

Figure 2–17(A)

(B)

the top 20% of the superior head's muscle fibers inserted into the capsular ligamentous tissue *below* the point at which the anterior edge of the disc attaches to the capsule. These fibers of the muscle then fused with the capsular fibers and passed on posteriorly in unison with the capsule to insert at the anterior edge of the condyle, but *not* the disc! The secondary insertion of muscle fibers in no way attached directly to the disc. They would have to penetrate the continuous surface of the cocoonlike capsular ligament in order to do this, but this was not observed. It was also observed that pulling on the fibers of the superior head of the lateral pterygoid muscle anteriorly caused both the disc *and* condyle to be pulled in an anterior direction. It was not possible to pull the disc anteriorly independently of the condyle regardless of the fact that tension in that direction was applied only to the fibers of the secondary insertion of the roof of the superior head. The disc could not be pulled down and forward over the head of the condyle directly by muscular force simply because no muscle fibers were attached to its anterior edge. The toe only blended with the adjacent capsular ligament anteriorly. Thus according to Wilkinson's findings, constriction of the superior head at the final moment of power-stroke closure is not an attempt by Nature to rotate the disc forward over the head of the condyle. Its purpose is to put a forward and upward force on the disc-condyle assembly, counting on the supportive ligamentous tissues to stabilize the disc on the condylar head, so that the whole disc-condyle apparatus is braced against the articular facet of the temporal bone (the slope of the eminence) with the condylar head cradled against the inferior central concavity of the disc, which in turn is positioned against the articular facet of the eminence so that the force vectors of occlusion pass squarely from the condylar head through the center of the disc onto the fortified cancellous bone of the temporal articular facet. But all this can only happen if the elevator muscles don't have to pull the mandible and condyle too far up and back to reach that occlusion. When this must occur because of malocclusion, something far different transpires both to the fibrocartilagenous and ligamentous structures inside the joint capsule as well as to the muscular and bony tissue adjacent to it.

Looking at how these two portions of muscle work tends to support this third opinion, for there is no dispute as to what the actions of the two heads are or that they work totally independently from each other at different times and to different ends. The function of the inferior belly of the lateral pterygoid is to pull the condylar neck, hence the whole mandible, forward and open. When contracture is bilateral, the jaw may be opened and/or protruded. When contracture is unilateral, the mandible will deviate to the opposite side. During all this activity the superior head remains totally passive! The superior portion does not have to contract to bring the disc down and forward with the condylar head. The supporting capsular ligament, the tension of the condyle against the disc, and the support of the collateral ligaments do that. It has also been proposed that the inferior belly even remains active during closure, progressively relaxing as the mandible retrudes in a fashion Wilkinson describes as the physiological equivalent of slowly "letting out the rope." Where the superior belly of the lateral pterygoid comes into play in turn is during the final moment of mandibular closure. It then constricts to keep a steady, opposing, coordinated tension on the disc-condyle assembly to keep it properly positioned and braced against the articular facet of the eminence at the final full-occlusion position in the fossa.

Any problem of distortion foreshortening the superior head of the lateral pterygoid due to abuse assists in displacing the disc forward. If in addition to this the condylar head must be forced too far superiorly and posteriorly by the occlusion to attain posterior occlusal stops, the phenomenon of the condyle being displaced off the heel of the disc and seating itself in the bilaminar zone ensues. This displacement of the condyle up and back subsequently opens up the anterior joint space, further making it all the easier and more necessary for the disc to be correspondingly displaced forward. Thus working reciprocally, one exclusively on the condylar neck, the other on the neck and only indirectly the intra-articular disc, at opposite times during the opening-closing cycle, the lateral pterygoid muscle cannot help but be thought of at least as two muscles and maybe even three instead of one.

One thing, clinically observable, that those dealing with patients with TMJ problems are readily aware of is that among the various muscles of mastication, the lateral pterygoid will generally show the greatest sensitivity to palpation.[40-43] There is some debate as to whether or not this muscle can be palpated directly or not by the examining clinician. The most current opinion feels that it can only be palpated indirectly due to overlaying and constricting anatomical interferences. To palpate the approximate area of the inferior belly of the lateral pterygoid, the patient must open the mouth slightly and deviate the mandible as much as possible to the side of the muscle to be examined to bring the ipsilateral coronoid process as far as possible away from the maxillary tuberosity of that side to make the buccal sulcus in that area as large as possible. The examiner then slides his finger along the roof of the buccal sulcus and upon reaching the end of the maxillary tuberosity area then presses the finger inward and upward toward the lateral pterygoid plate.[44-46] In patients suffering from functionally induced TMJ arthrosis due to occlusal misguidance, this procedure will invariably elicit an extremely painful response from the patient. Simple logic offers an explanation. The inferior belly of the pterygoid muscle pulls the condyle forward in the opening process. To overclose the mandible, which is what is required to drive the condyle up and back past the heel of the disc, the superior and inferior heads of the lateral pterygoids, which are attached to the condylar neck, are overstretched. Portions of them may even be tensed across the infe-

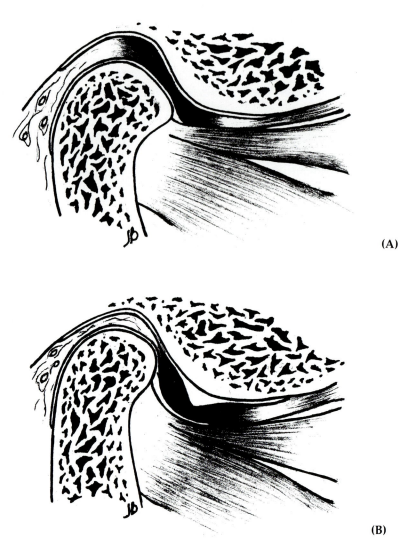

(A)

(B)

Figure 2–18 **(A)** Normal condyle-disc-fossa relationship. Note how the anterior band (toe) of the disc is attached to the roof of the superior head of the lateral pterygoid only indirectly via the anterior capsular ligament wall. **(B)** When the disc is anteriorly displaced, the posterior band (heel) of the disc is level with the anterior rim of the condyle, and the disc folds up through its narrow central zone. (Modified from Wilkinson TM: *J Prosthet Dent* 1988; 60:715–724.)

Figure 2–19 The Digastric **(A)** Lateral view; **(B)** frontal view. (From Travell JG, Simons DG: *Myofascial Pain and Dysfunction, The Trigger Point Manual.* Baltimore, William & Wilkins, 1983, p 275. Used by permission.)

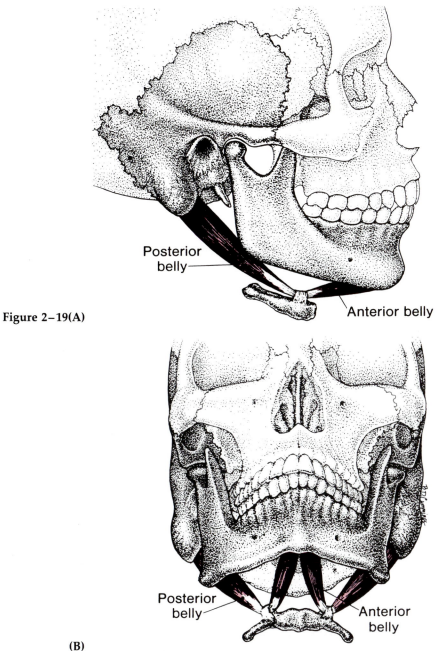

Figure 2–19(A)

Posterior belly

Anterior belly

Posterior belly

Anterior belly

(B)

rior border of the articular eminence, and the entire volume of anatomy associated with the pterygoid plexus is also tensed. It is common knowledge that excessive chronic traction situations of an abusive nature are the quickest way to hypersensitize muscular as well as related neural and vascular tissues to palpation. At either extreme, overcontraction or forced overstretching, muscles and their related supporting structures become sore. Such is the case of both the superior and inferior portions of the lateral pterygoid. They are chronically overstretched in severe condylar retrusion cases, while at the same time the superior head, which may have fibers indirectly attached to the disc, has its roof chronically foreshortened and as a result suffers cramping and hypersensitivity due to the opposite problem. To make things worse, there is the added effect of the large anterior joint space (due to posterior, superior condyler displacement) making it easy for a slippery disc well lubricated by synovial fluid to "squirt" down and forward in a state of anterior displacement (which helps keep portions of the superior head of the lateral pterygoid foreshortened). The anterior joint recess of the capsule must of course become distorted and distended to permit this forced anteromedial discal displacement. And then there's the added insult of the hard condylar head crushing into the soft retrodiscal bilaminar tissues, which by the way are tensed somewhat over the back of the condylar head due to the forward displacement of the anteriorly dislodged disc so that these sensitive, highly innervated tissues can get a good pounding. It is no wonder the origins of the name "TMJ pain-dysfunction" are so appropriate.

The Digastric

Another member of the "two-for-one club" is the digastric. Compared with the rythmic flow of the muscular anatomy of the head and neck and its beautiful relationship to function, the digastric appears on the surface to have been an anatomical leftover from the spare parts bin thrown in by Nature for good measure. Its odd arrangement makes it appear as if Nature were playing a figurative form of musical chairs with respect to attachment sites and the digastric lost. Actually, it serves a dual purpose, which is befitting a muscle with two separate bellies, and understanding its function and, most importantly, its symptomatology sheds a great light on the problem of understanding why TMJ pain-dysfunction patients suffer the way they do. The posterior belly of the digastric attaches to the mastoid process beneath the attachments of three other muscles of the cervical girdle, i.e., the sternocleidomastoid, the splenius capitis, and the longissimus capitis. From this site it travels forward and unites with the anterior belly at a common tendon that forms a short round connective tissue isthmus between the two. This tendon is attached to the hyoid bone through a fibrous connective tissue loop.[47] The anterior belly then tracks forward to attach to the lingual surface of the symphysis of the mandible in the area just below the genial tubercles.

The function of the digastric is indeed varied and is related biomechanically to whichever of its two hard tissue insertions remains stationary. When the mandible is fixed, i.e., braced against the interdigitation of the occlusion, the action of the digastric muscle elevates the hyoid bone, which is necessary for deglutition. Conversely, when the hyoid bone is braced by its own attending musculature and thus rendered stationary, the action of the digastric assists in depression of the mandible during mouth opening. However, this activity is secondary to the action of the inferior belly of the lateral pterygoid, which is generally the first muscle to come into action in mouth opening. Yet when maximum opening of the jaw is required (or forced opening against some form of resistance), the digastric is needed. What makes this muscle important to the clinician treating TMJ problems is that this muscle is always active when closure involves mandibular retrusion. Thus due to repeated acts of closing to an overly retruded position of posterior superior condylar displacement in retrusive deep-bite cases, against the tension and design intent of nearly all the other supporting musculature and ligamentous connective tissue of the joint to the tune of 2,000 incidents per day (the number of times many patients swallow in a 24-hour period), a tremendous physiological strain is placed on this slender muscle. As might be expected, it is generally quite sensitive to palpation in patients with these kinds of problems.

NEUROVASCULAR ANATOMY

The neurovascular anatomy of the TMJ exhibits some seeming paradoxes in its distribution. The TMJs are capable of generating formidable levels of both primary pain at the principle site and secondary pain in referred sites. Yet the disc has no primary nervous innervation. When peripheral joint circulation is restricted, as in cases of chronic intracapsular edema or severe superior posterior condylar displacement, condylar and eminential articular surface breakdown ensues (osteochondritis dissecans). If the restriction of circulation is great enough over a long enough period of time, actual osteoclastic remodeling of the cortical and medullary bone takes place (avascular necrosis). Yet the disc and articular surfaces of the condylar head and articular eminence have no direct vascular supply.

For purposes of simplification, the neurovascular anatomy of the

Figure 2–20   (A) Lateral view of the auriculotemporal nerve. (B) Weeping lubrication.

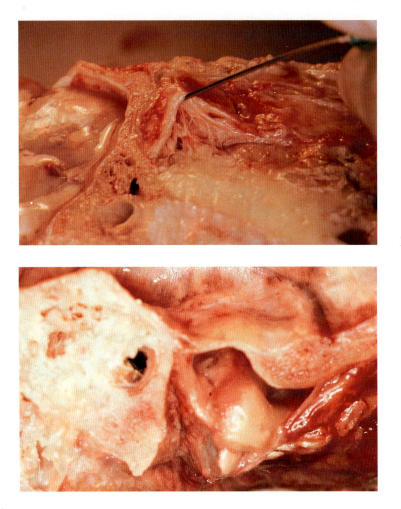

Figure 2–20(A)

(B)

TMJ may be divided into four parts, two of which are macroscopic and two of which may be thought of as microscopic. With respect to the latter, although the disc and articular surfaces have no nervous innervation, the ligaments and the capsule itself are highly innervated with nociceptors, as are the soft retrodiscal tissues of the all-important bilaminar zone. These are branches of the macroscopic component of the nervous innervation of the area, the auriculotemporal nerve, a branch of the mandibular division of the trigeminal. And the pathway of the auriculotemporal nerve courses directly through the posterior joint space!

As far as vascular supply on a microscopic level is concerned, the avascular disc and articular surfaces depend on "weeping lubrication" from the synovial fluid excreted from the inner surfaces of the synovial membranes.[48] This in turn is predicated on proper capillary supply to the peripheral capsular tissues. These arterioles and capillaries are branches of the macroscopic component of the vascular supply to the area, the superficial temporal artery, a branch of the external carotid. Again, the bilaminar zone is highly vascularized with capillaries and arterioles, and once again the pathway of the superficial temporal artery courses directly through the posterior joint space! Conceptually, the bilaminar zone, the posterior joint space through which courses the auriculotemporal nerve and superficial temporal artery, the retrocondylar area that is highly vascularized and highly innervated, is the most important anatomical area of the TMJ, at least from a clinical standpoint. It needs a certain amount of physical three-dimensional space for successful operation of its comparatively prodigious supply of nerves and arteries. When condyles impinge on this area at full occlusion, problems arise. Until treatments for functionally induced TMJ problems result in the complete decompression of this area at full occlusion, the case can never be considered fully resolved, for it will never be fully symptom free.

It must be remembered that the anatomy of the TMJ in particular and the maxillofacial complex in general may be thought of as being subdivided into basic categories of teeth, bone, and muscle with all of their related supporting connective, vascular, and neural tissues. These are artificial delineations conceived in the mind of man for the sake of description. They are not delineations of Nature. These components work together in a coordinated living biological functioning unit. They all contribute in varying degrees to varying biological demands of function. When things go well, they all function well. Likewise, when things go wrong each attempts to respond in some fashion according to its nature.

SUMMARY

The human TMJ in more ways than one is a pivotal anatomical entity in the maxillofacial complex. It stands figuratively as a structural Gibraltar strategically located between the two great anatomical conti-

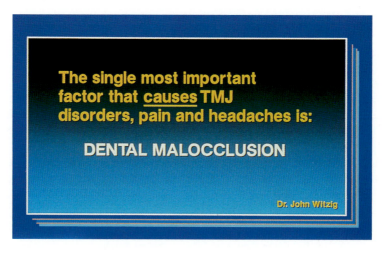

Figure 2–21   Evolution of an etiology.

nents above and below it. Its smooth and painfree operation is predicated first and foremost upon proper anatomical relationships not only within the joint itself but also between the joint and the occlusion. Systemic problems originating outside this relationship may on rare occasion attack the area to disrupt form and function. When this happens, as in cases of infection, neoplastic invasion, or physiological disorders such as rheumatoid arthritic breakdown, etc., treatments of a systemic nature are necessarily indicated. However, in a vast majority of cases, it will be found that an improper biomechanical and anatomical relationship is the primary cause of the pain and dysfunction of the joint and its surrounding structures. The critical concept that must be grasped by the treating clinicians is the relationship between the imbalances and malalignments of the occlusion and the resultant imbalances and malalignments that such an occlusion forces onto the disc-condyle-fossa assembly. Pain is Nature's way of alerting us to the presence of a disruption in the compatibility of this functional anatomical relationship. Our job as clinicians is to determine the nature of that anatomical malrelationship and, by means of properly coordinated treatments designed to address the teeth, bone, and muscle components of that particular relationship, restore the patient to a state of proper anatomy, hence proper function. The TMJs are the very foundations upon which the workings of the masticatory mechanisms of the body are built. With these foundational pillars of the stomatognathic system properly aligned once again, they may then provide the proper support for which they were originally intended. Then the pains will cease.

References

1. Coben SE: Growth concepts. *Angle Orthod* 1961; 31:194–201.
2. Coben SE: The integration of facial skeletal variants. *Am J Orthod* 1955; 41:407–434.
3. Coben SE: Growth in class II treatment. *Am J Orthod* 1966; 52:5–26.
4. Scott JH: The cranial base. *Am J Phys Anthropol* 1958; 16:319–348.
5. Kopp S: Topographical distribution of sulphated glycosaminoglycans in the surface layers of the human temporomandibular joint. *J Oral Pathol* 1978; 7:283–294.
6. Mongihi F: Abnormalities in condylar and occlusal positions, in Solberg WK, Clark GT (eds): *Abnormal Jaw Mechanics.* Chicago, Quintessence Publishing Co, 1984, pp 23–50.
7. Blackwood HJJ: Pathology of the temporomandibular joint. *J Am Dent Assoc* 1969; 79:118–124.
8. Sicher H: *Oral Anatomy.* St Louis, CV Mosby Co, 1949.
9. Enlow DH: *Handbook of Facial Growth,* ed 2. Philadelphia, WB Saunders Co, 1982.
10. Furstman L: Embryology, in Sarnat BG, Laskin DM (eds): *The Temporomandibular Joint,* ed 3. Springfield, Ill, Charles C Thomas Publishers, 1979, pp 52–69.
11. Rees LA: The structure and function of the mandibular joint. *Br Dent J* 1954; 96:125–133.
12. Toller PA: Temporomandibular arthropathy. *Proc R Soc Lond* 1975; 67:153–159.
13. DuBrul EL: *Sicher's Oral Anatomy,* ed 7. St Louis, CV Mosby Co, 1980.
14. Grant JCB, Basmajian JV: *Grant's Method of Anatomy,* ed 7. Baltimore, Williams & Wilkins, 1965, p 725.
15. Griffin CJ, Sharpe CJ: The structure of the adult human temporomandibular meniscus. *Aust Dent J* 1960; 5:190–195.
16. Thilander B: Innervation of the temporomandibular joint capsule in man. *Trans R School Dent* 1961; 7:1.

17. Bell WE: Recent concepts in the management of temporomandibular joint dysfunctions. *J Oral Surg* 1970; 28:596–599.
18. Bell WF: *Orofacial Pains,* ed 2. Chicago, Year Book Medical Publishers, Inc, 1979.
19. Gelb H: Patient Evaluation, in Gelb H (ed): *Clinical Management of Head, Neck and TMJ Pain and Dysfunction.* Philadelphia, WB Saunders Co, 1977, p 75.
20. Schwartz LL: Conclusions of the Temporomandibular Joint Clinic at Columbia. *J Periodontol* 1958; 29:210–212.
21. Travell J: Temporomandibular joint pain referred from muscles of the head and neck. *J Prosthet Dent* 1960; 10:745–763.
22. Travell J, Simons DG: *Myofascial Pain and Dysfunctions.* Baltimore, Williams & Wilkins, 1983, p 4.
23. Grant JCB: *An Atlas of Human Anatomy,* ed 7. Baltimore, Williams & Wilkins, 1978.
24. Munro RR: Electromyography of the muscles of mastication, in Griffin CJ, Harris R (eds): *The Temporomandibular Joint Syndrome,* vol 4. Monographs in Oral Science. New York, S Karger AJ 1975, pp 97–116.
25. Basmajian JV: *Muscles Alive,* ed 4. Baltimore, Williams & Wilkins, 1978, pp 101, 185–186, 380–384.
26. Mayers RE: An electromyographic analysis of certain muscles involved in temporomandibular movement. *AJO* 1950; 36:481–515.
27. Woelfel JB, Hickey JC, Stacey RW, et al: Electromyographic analysis of jaw movements. *J Prosthet Dent* 1960; 10:688–697.
28. Gray H: In Goss CM (ed): *Anatomy of the Human Body,* ed 29. Philadelphia, Lea & Febiger, 1973, p 389.
29. Shore NA: *Temporomandibular Joint Dysfunction and Occlusal Equilibration.* Philadelphia, JB Lippincott, 1976, p 61–62.
30. Travell J, Simons DG: *Myofascial Pain and Dysfunctions.* Baltimore, Williams & Wilkins, 1976, p 249.
31. Levandoski R: Personal communication, Feb 1988.
32. McNamara JA Jr: The independent functions of the two heads of the lateral pterygoid muscle. *Am J Anat* 1973; 138:197–205.
33. Lipke DP, et al: An electromyographic study of the human lateral pterygoid muscle (abstract 713). *J Dent Res* 1977; 56:230.
34. Mahan PE, Wilkinson TM, Gibbs CH, et al: Superior and inferior bellies of the lateral pterygoid muscle EMG activity of basic jaw positions. *J Prosthet Dent* 1983; 50:710–718.
35. Gibbs CH, Mahan PE, Wilkinson TM, et al: EMG activity of the superior belly of the lateral pterygoid muscle in relation to other jaw muscles, *J Prosthet Dent* 1984; 51:691–702.
36. Christensen FG: Some anatosurical concepts associated with the temporomandibular joint. *Am Aust Coll Dent Surg* 1969; 2:39–60.
37. Grant PG: Lateral pterygoid: Two muscles? *Am J Anat* 1973; 138:1–10.
38. Sobotta J, Figge FHJ: *Atlas of Human Anatomy,* ed 9, vol 3. New York, MacMillan Publishing Co, Inc, 1974, pp 212–213.
39. Wilkinson TM: The relationship between the disk and the lateral pterygoid muscle in the human temporomandibular joint, *J Prosthet Dent* 1988; 60:715–724.

40. Meyerowitz WJ: Myofascial pain in the edentulous patient. *J Dent Assoc S Afr* 1975; 30:75–77.

41. Franks AST: Masticatory muscle hyperactivity and temporomandibular joint dysfunction. *J Prosthet Dent* 1975; 15:1122–1131.

42. Greene CS, Lerman MD, Sutcher HD, et al: The TMJ pain-dysfunction syndrome: Heterogeneity of patient population. *J Am Dent Assoc* 1969; 79:1168–1172.

43. Kaye LB, Moran JH, Fritz ME: Statistical analysis of an urban population of 236 patients with head and neck pain. Part II. Patient symptomatology. *J Periodontol* 1979; 50:59–65.

44. Burch JG: Occlusion related to craniofacial pain, in Alling CC, Maham PE (eds): *Facial Pain,* ed 2. Philadelphia, Lea & Febiger, 1977, pp 170–174.

45. Johnstone DR, Templeton MC: The feasibility of palpating the lateral pterygoid muscle. *J Prosthet Dent* 1980; 44:318–323.

46. Shore NA: Temporomandibular joint dysfunction: Medical-dental cooperation. *Int Coll Dent Sci Educ J* 1974; 7:15–16.

47. Bardeen CR: The musculature, in Jackson CM (ed): *Morris's Human Anatomy,* ed 6. Philadelphia, Blakiston's Sons & Co, 1921, pp 378–379.

48. DuBrul EL: The biomechanics of the oral apparatus: Structural analysis, in DeBrul EL, Menekratis A (eds): *The Physiology of Oral Reconstruction.* Chicago, Quintessence Publishing Co, 1981, pp 21–38.

CHAPTER 3

The NRDM/SPDC Phenomenon: Physiology Gone Wrong

PATHOLOGY

To make the process of addressing patients with temporomandibular joint (TMJ) pain-dysfunction problems practical on a daily clinical basis, it is important for the practitioner to have a clear understanding of the range of possibilities that exist with respect to normal joint anatomy and function. One must understand what is considered generally acceptable before one can make rational judgments on what is unacceptable. Just as with other conditions, TMJ function and pathofunction displays a wide variance in the signs, symptoms, anatomical relationships, and pathological processes presented to the diagnosing clinician. However, the variation involved is not as endless as it may first appear to the novice. Yes, unusual cases do occur with unusual symptomatic pictures, etiologies, or treatment responses. Yet considerable clinical experience reveals that a certain pattern may be seen to underlie the entire spectrum of patients with functionally induced TMJ problems. There is considerable variation to many of the other dental problems we treat on a daily basis. Yet recurrent patterns of symptoms, signs, and treatment responses occur with respect to them also. No two endodontic procedures are exactly alike, yet they may be seen to follow a general pattern that allows the practitioner to easily determine what constitutes a normal course of events during treatment and what does not. No two full- or partial-denture cases are exactly alike. Yet in many ways most are the same. Physicians are used to the same thing. The common cold affects many people many ways with a rather wide range of signs, symptoms, etiologies, and durations. Treatments for the same also involve a fairly routine employment of common pharmacological agents. Variance is present, as in a "slight" cold or a "bad" cold, yet the boundaries of the disease and its treatments still fall within a reasonably limited set of parameters. The more patients a physician sees over the years, the more his clinical judgment will "sharpen" as to how to adjust for the variance exhibited. Strict diagnostic nomenclature, detailed and all-inclusive classification systems, and profuse scientific documentation of such maladies may constitute a pristine and erudite approach, yet such redundancy cannot remove the situation from its level of commonness. So too with TMJ problems that result from functional irregularities of the stomatognathic system. Yes, there is a wide range of causes and effects. But in spite of the variance represented from patient to patient, in spite of the different levels of severity seen from the mildest to the most severe, in spite of the complexities that can and do exist at times, patients with TMJ pain-dysfunction problems of a functional nature exhibit a consistency and general pattern of pathology, symptomatology, and treatment response such that recognition of the nature of these patients' problems and management of their conditions to a high level of success become a process entirely accessible to the common practitioner.

As stated previously, one must first understand the range and parameters of what is considered normal before one attempts to make judgments on what is abnormal. There are several important and commonly known facts concerning what in fact constitutes normal TMJ function. First of all, neither the TMJ nor its associated musculature should hurt nor make noise during function. All joints were made for movement, some were made to both move and bear a load. None of them should have to make noise or hurt the host in order to do so. They all should work smoothly, quietly, and painlessly within their normal range of motion. TMJs are no exception. Also, all joints should exhibit a characteristic radiographic picture of internal osseous anatomical shape and, most importantly for TMJs, spacial relationships between the opposing articular surfaces. Third, the condyle of the TMJ should both function and rest on the intra-articular disc at all times and nowhere else. Rotation and translation are important disc-mediated functions of the disc-condyle assembly, but the critical issue for the patient with TMJ problems is the status of the disc-condyle assembly during the full force loading of maximum, fully interdigitated, posterior-quadrant occlusion. If the condyle distributes these force vectors directly on the disc, the joint will in all likelihood do well. However, if these forces are chronically directed anywhere else in the joint, in all likelihood the joint will sooner or later do poorly, and a whole raft of attending signs and symptoms will ensue. The only thing capable of forcing the condyle to transmit the loading forces of full occlusion to areas other than the disc is some combination of dental arch/apical

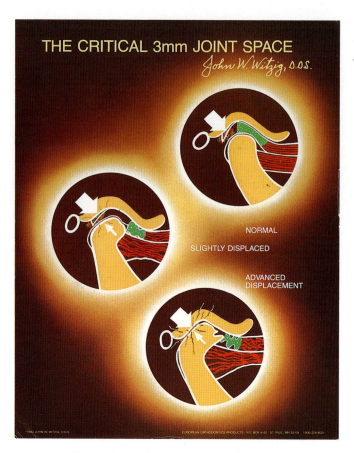

Figure 3–1 Critical 3-mm joint space.

base location and/or occlusal incisal interdigitation that guides the mandible back too far upon full closure. The status of the disc-condyle-fossa relationship is determined by the muscles during rotation-translation–type jaw motion. This relationship is alterable in the fashion that the muscles and their actions are alterable. This relationship during opening or closing (up until the teeth touch) does include the mitigating factors of learned or habitual activity; proprioceptive input from the periodontal ligaments of the individual teeth, muscles, and the joint structures themselves; reflex-type motor control; and even volition. Yet it is still the muscles that are the ultimate agents of control. However, this all changes at the moment when arch-to-arch dental contact is made. Once this happens at final closure, the proprioceptive (and in some cases even nociceptive) signals of the periodontal ligaments of the teeth begin to dominate, and the neuromuscular reflexive activity may have to be changed. As the inclined planes of the upper and lower teeth guide the mandible as a whole to the state of final fully interdigitated dental occlusion, the inclined planes of the teeth themselves and their overall relative anteroposterior and vertical spatial location become the determining factors of the disc-condyle-fossa relationship at final occlusion via new signals sent to the muscles. The muscles, as blind slaves to motor impulses modified by occlusal proprioceptive information, merely provide the power, the force that results in the physical vectors of mechanical loading that must be absorbed somewhere in some fashion by something within the joint. The intercuspation of the teeth determines the direction these force vectors will take and what will absorb them. Thus a relationship is generated that lies at the very heart of all functionally induced TMJ pain-dysfunction problems. The relationship of the condyle to the disc and fossa at full occlusion is determined by the relationship of the fit of the opposing occluding teeth. Joint form and position are a direct result of tooth form and position. The teeth ultimately determine how the disc-condyle assembly will relate; the disc-condyle assembly does not determine how the teeth will relate, at least not initially. It must also be remembered that this relationship of condylar position being determined by tooth position exists only during the "worst of times," i.e., during the intense pressures of full arch-to-arch interdental occlusion. This then allows for one of only two main types of circumstances to exist. Either the occlusion will force the muscles to lock up the disc-condyle assembly into a proper and acceptable relationship to the fossa and articular eminence at full occlusion, or the occlusion will force the muscles to lock up the disc-condyle assembly in a strained and improper relationship to the articular eminence and fossa. This may range from a mild discrepancy to one that is most exaggerated. Since the occlusion generates the governing proprioceptive stimuli that end up, via central nervous system (CNS) efferent/afferent circuitry, eventually being the source of control for what the muscles do, the "occlusion/condyle connection" may be conceptually thought of as a direct one-to-one relationship. The muscles are merely the mechanism that mediates this relationship and allows it to exist. How the teeth fit together is ultimately what determines how the joints fit together. If the occlusion can lock the mandible such that the condyle is properly positioned in the joint, things will generally be fine. If the occlusion locks the mandible such that the condyle is improperly positioned too far up and back in the joint (the only way the condyle can be improperly positioned by virtue of the anatomical design of the joint), there will be trouble. The inclined plane guidance of the teeth at final full-force occlusion cannot cause the mandible to be deflected too far posteriorly from the initial mandibular arc of closure that is first determined by the muscles without causing some sort of problem in the disc-condyle relationship. If the inclined-plane action of the teeth (occlusal-proprioceptive-afferent/motor-control-efferent CNS circuit) keeps the muscles "on course" and hence the condyle on the disc, the joint is functionally balanced and works fine. The teeth are happy, the muscles are happy, the disc-condyle-fossa assembly is happy, the retrodiscal bilaminar zone and all its arteries and nerves are happy, the ligaments and connective tissues of the joint are happy, and the patient is happy. But if the inclined-plane action of the teeth during heavy loading causes the mandible to seriously deflect posteriorly from what would have been a much more forward muscular/ligament/joint determined mandibular arc of closure, a whole "sea of troubles" wells up, and a functionally induced TMJ arthrosis to some level of severity or another results. If one will forgive the crude play on words and grant a little poetic license, imagine the muscles as "workhorses" of the stomatognathic system and the mandible symbolizing a cutter (no pun intended), "the horses know the way to carry the sleigh," if only at the end the teeth will let them have their way. When they don't, the muscles suffer (even though they try to adapt by shortening their lengths, etc.), the ligaments suffer, the disc-condyle assembly suffers, the helpless unprotected bilaminar zone suffers, and because of the complex relationship of stress and structure, the patient suffers. We can change all that.

DIFFERENTIAL PATHOLOGY

To begin a study of diagnostic procedures and treatment methodologies for TMJ problems, one must first begin by not only clearly understanding the ranges of normal joint anatomy and operation and defining what exactly the functionally related type of TMJ condition is, but also what it is not. We must understand the "what" (pathology) of what we are treating before we should endeavor to consider the "how" (treatment planning) of corrective measures. Under the broad field of craniomandibular disorders, there are many different diseases, malfunctions, and unnatural circumstances that can lead to pain and dysfunction in the head, neck, and TMJ area. Not only the joint itself but all other related supporting anatomical structures may reflect, in a given case, interrelated signs and symptoms. The main types of joint disturbance with which dentists concern themselves are primarily those of a functional origin. When a joint problem exists as a result of a maxillofacial structural or occlusal imbalance, it is that type of joint problem the dentist is most qualified to rectify. It is also by far the type that is most commonly seen.

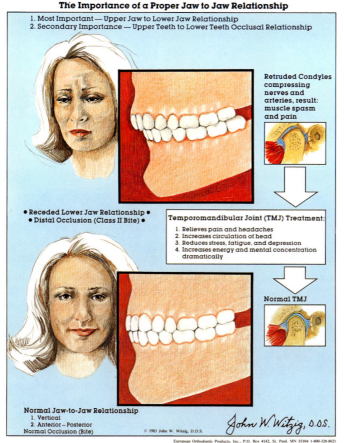

Figure 3–2 Importance of proper jaw-to-jaw relationship.

This is reflected in the very nature of the TMJ pain-dysfunction situation itself. It must first be accurately defined for just what type of pathology it is since that type of joint arthritis the functional joint orthopedics (FJO) methodology is most concerned with is not a disease, not a syndrome, but actually a condition. Although they are relatively infrequent in occurrence, true diseases and syndromes of the joint area do exist, but they are separate and distinct from the more common, functionally caused jaw arthritis seen to occur posteriorly in the TMJ area, which in turn results from structural and/or occlusal imbalance anteriorly in the occlusion. It is not for the mere sake of scientific definitions that these diagnostic categories are being delineated but rather out of a twofold desire to, first, help the practitioner better understand the complex nature of the problems he is facing in joint and myofascial pain-dysfunction treatment and, second, to help him also clarify the seemingly overlapping, confusing, and possibly misleading terminology of the TMJ puzzle.

Scarlet fever, malaria, whooping cough, and influenza are *diseases*. Mongolism, cleidocranial dysostosis, and gastrointestinal polyposis are thought of as *syndromes*. Diabetes, essential hypertension, and rheumatoid arthritis are often thought of as *disorders*. Obesity, baldness, allergies, and simple common fatigue are considered *conditions*. The *functionally* related TMJ pain-dysfunction phenomenon is a condition. It is just that it happens to be a traumatic condition. The word *condition* best describes it, even though this term is seldom used because the word has an inference of a naturally occurring process that implies a direct cause-and-effect relationship to improper nonpathogenic stimuli. Although the condition may in fact be compounded by coexisting or overlaying diseases, syndromes, or other disorders, TMJ arthrosis of itself it is merely the breakdown of a normally occurring natural process due to that process's inability to adapt to or compensate for a series of excessive and/or noxious stimuli. It is also true that the words "disease," "syndrome," and "disorder" are brandished about quite freely by the general populace of the medical-dental community with a certain time-honored acceptance. This condition is commonly referred to as TMJ syndrome, TMJ disease, myofascial pain-dysfunction syndrome, TMJ arthrosis, TMJ arthritis, TMJ functional arthritis, degenerative arthritis, functionally oriented TMJ osteoarthritis, and TMJ pain-dysfunction syndrome. These terms are in such common acceptance that it might seem trivial to banter semantics. It is only for the sake of a clear understanding in the mind of the practitioner dealing with this condition that the distinction is made. Once that understanding has been effected, as far as treatment planning to gain a desired therapeutic end is concerned, it makes little difference as to how the condition is named (unless one is trying to satisfy the demands of the seemingly endless quiddities of insurance forms). Once all the component parts of the problem—such as the pain, tissue change, dysfunction, secondary complications, or overriding disease states—are clearly relegated to their proper place in the diagnostic picture, the clinician is in the best position to deal with each of them regardless of which terms may happen to be used at that time or in that area to describe the condition. Patients are only interested in getting well.

FUNCTIONAL TRAUMATIC TMJ ARTHRITIS

As previously stated, the main arthritic condition that the FJO system of therapeutics is designated to address is the type of TMJ pain-dysfunction arthritis that is a result of improper function of that joint due to a sufficient occlusal or structural imbalance in the relationship of the upper and lower jaws to one another. This is the functionally induced condition that will serve as our main source of interest as dentists. It is ubiquitous throughout the main populace of general dental patients and may appear more often than we realize due to its insidious nature. There might be an orthodontic imbalance in the presence of reasonable structural balance, or there may be an orthopedic imbalance sometimes oddly in the presence of what at first may appear to be a reasonable orthodontic balance. Or both orthodontic and orthopedic imbalances may be present, all of which may bring about the improper functioning of the joint with its resultant muscular pain, joint pain, dysfunction, and derangement of actual internal joint structures due to a posteriorly deflected mandibular arc of closure and resultant displacement posteriorly of the condyle off the disc into the retrodiscal bilaminar zone, i.e., the phenomenon of neuromuscular reflexive displacement of the mandible causing superior posterior displacement of the condyle (NRDM/SPDC).

Accuracy in diagnosis has always been the key to successful therapeutics, and this is especially true of TMJ disorders. That accuracy is predicated on a thorough knowledge of the nature of the pathology that can affect the joint. The FJO system of treatment is an excellent method of treatment for TMJ problems, but only where indicated. A thorough understanding of the *signs* and *symptoms* the patient presents acts as our guide to what form of pathology may be present and therefore in turn is critical to the proper selection and therapeutic employment of FJO techniques. Incorrectly using FJO principles at the wrong time and place in treating such problems is a prime example of making the patient fit the technique. One of the clinician's old standby questions appears again to act as a guide, "What are the patient's, or in this case, the joint's needs?"

The chief area of concern of this particular text will be the proper function of the joint and what biomechanical processes in the occlusion result in the joint's dysfunction. This type of problem comprises the vast majority of TMJ conditions that present to the general dental office on a daily basis. It occupies such a dominant position in the field of etiological possibilities of TMJ problems that it should automatically be suspected first of all until definitive differential diagnostic evidence proves otherwise. The diagnostic methods now available make understanding the true pathology behind the TMJ problem a relatively easy matter of observing the clinical and radiographic findings and relating them to known relationships of TMJ anatomical, biomechanical, and physiological function and, even more importantly, dysfunction. It is the dysfunction of the sto-matognathic system, the dysfunction of the various subsystems associ-ated with it, the sensory, orthopedic, muscular, and neurovascular sys-tems, that forces clinicians to take the needed steps to erase the source of the problem and hopefully make a system of functional balance out of one that is in a state of dysfunctional imbalance. Studying the pathology of the TMJ from its most commonly occurring aspect is actually a study of the dysfunction of its various supportive anatomical and physiological systems. When this is done, one etiological agent emerges as the basis for understanding the effects observed on the patient, i.e., the NRDM/SPDC phenomenon. The occlusion and how it affects the joint and the muscles that work it—this is the heart and soul of the functionally oriented TMJ problem.

Sensual Dysfunction: Pain

The fact that TMJ dysfunction results in pain for the patient is prob-ably the single most important factor necessitating treatment. If a certain bodily part doesn't work right, it might be tolerated if no other serious ramifications ensue, but if it doesn't work right and hurts, something must be done! The pain associated with this problem is the most impor-tant symptom as far as the patient's outlook is concerned. It may be dull, intermittent, of variable yet persistent frequency,[1, 2] or sharp and stab-bing.[3] It most often expresses itself in the form of chronic recurrent head-aches or myofascial pain in the auriculotemporal area. It can radiate to the side of the head and neck. It might radiate to the gonial region, the sub-occipital region, the submandibular region, or the zygomatic arch. It can radiate to the parietal region, the frontal region, or often the supraorbital areas. It can be so insidious so as to hardly cause a change in a person's routine daily schedule,[4] or it can be so intense as to alter entire lives. In rare and tragic instances it has even ended lives. With no relief of chronic intense myofascial pain believed possible, a few unfortunate individuals have resorted to the ultimate step.

If a singular joint is involved due to imbalances causing posterior displacement and/or noxious stimuli to be transmitted to only one joint, the pain is almost universally unilateral to that side. If both joints are in-volved, the pain is usually bilateral. If both joints are involved, but one more than the the other, the pain is usually greater on the side of the more serious involvement. Nature can be reasoned out quite simply at times.

The pain generated also seems to follow a general pattern of being related to host resistance. A younger, healthy patient with mild joint in-volvement may only notice occasional flare-ups of headache-type pain in the head and neck area. An older patient with a more severely involved joint may experience moderate to severe headaches or joint pain 2 to 5 times per week or even daily. Some cases may be so severe that when the headaches reach their maximum level of intensity, they result in prostration of the patient. Host resistance wanes as the age of the individual increases. A common observation is that women complain of TMJ headache-type pain in a ratio of about 4 to 1 over men, especially menopausal women. This is why such concern is expressed over teenage patients or young children who notice TMJ headache-type pain. For if they are suffering when they are at their biological best, how much more so will they suffer as they progress to adulthood!

Pain may also be detected in the form of tenderness to palpation in the muscles of mastication and the joint area itself.[5, 6] Pressing in with the fingers over the joint area just anterior to the external auditory meatus may elicit a painful response in some patients. Palpation of the origin, belly, and insertion of the three main closing muscles like the masseter, medial pterygoid, and temporalis (anterior, middle, and posterior segments) will often reflect a certain degree of tenderness or sometimes outright pain. The medial pterygoids seem especially susceptible to this phenomenon. The lateral pterygoid also seems to be almost always very sensitive to approximated indirect palpation. (This may be observed by having the patient open slightly while at the same time deviating the lower jaw to the side of the lateral pterygoid muscle to be palpated. With the patient's mouth partially expanded in this manner, the examiner slides his little finger along the maxillary buccal alveolar sulcus such that the fleshy part of the finger travels up around the back side of the maxillary tuberosity in a direction up and in. Only gentle pressure is needed to elicit a response of considerable discomfort in most patients with TMJ problems.)

Other muscles that may also show tenderness to palpation are the anterior and posterior bellies of the digastric and the muscles of the neck and shoulder area, specifically the sternocleidomastoid and most notably the trapezius.[7, 8] This at first may seem surprising, but after careful consideration of the biomechanics of the head and neck, a simple explanation emerges. The body will often rally to the aid of an injured area through compensation actions by the surrounding components. Limping to avoid painful irritation of a sprained ankle is an ideal example. So it is with the head and neck. An improper structural or dental relationship of the jaws causes the muscles of mastication and joint to function abnormally. Since the muscles must "work around" these imbalances in the occlusion, they must often work in an uncoordinated and inefficient manner. Other complications that cause the muscles and joints to become compromised arise such as airway impingement due to mandibular retrusion (discussed later). To compensate for this, especially if that compromised state involves pain in its members, the head will be held on the spine in a slightly irregular fashion in an effort to assist in some small way with the confrontation of these noxious stimuli, as if the other muscles were attempting to come to the support of the overworked and painful parties. Since the head represents about a 10- to 12-lb weight, holding it perpetually at even an only slightly incorrect posture on the spine places an undue strain on the muscles that support the head, neck, and spine.[9] In these circumstances, what counts is not the intensity but rather the duration of the stress and strain placed on the supporting muscles. Hence, muscle fatigue and soreness in the neck and upper spine area might easily be a secondary characteristic of chronic TMJ problems. This is reflected in the head and neck posture of the patient. The head and shoulders of the patient with TMJ problems will often be seen to slump forward slightly. It is also reflected in the amount of spacing between the base of the skull and the dorsal spinous processes of the first two cervical vertebrae as observable on lateral cephalograms. In the mature adult the distance between the base of the skull at the basioccipital area and the superior surface of the dorsal spinous process of C1 should be about 9 to 12 mm. Likewise, the distance between the inferior surface of the dorsal spinous process of C1 and the superior surface of the dorsal spinous process of C2 should also be around 9 to 12 mm. Compromised, TMJ-induced, improper posture of the head, being that it is perpetually held forward, reduces these spaces, and it is felt by some that this can result in neural entrapment and/or muscle spasms, which are responsible for pain in the neck area. In a "domino" effect the entire spinal posture may be affected. The neural entrapment may also be responsible for the clinically observed phenomenon of referred pain to the back, shoulders, or even legs. Such symptoms have been observed to disappear once correct treatment for TMJ problems has been completed and proper function and correct muscular and structural balance have once again been restored to the maxillofacial complex![10]

In a more detailed study of pain, especially the pain of the patient with a TMJ disorder, a number of considerations emerge that the practitioner should bear in mind. Of all the goals of treatment for the patient with TMJ problems, deliverance from the various types of pain associated with the condition (or at least a serious reduction in its frequency and intensity) is the primary end of all treatments and the ultimate single standard by which the success of treatment is judged. True, preservation of structure, competency of function, and even restoration of damaged structures or lost relationships, either by natural or artificial measures, are important treatment goals of the highest magnitude also. But alleviation of pain cannot be challenged in its position of supremacy in the order of ends toward which the main body of treating clinicians strive. The pains may vary in location and will definitely vary in intensity, frequency, and duration, but they all are associated with the head and neck in general and the stomatognathic system in particular because they originate from the improper function of that system, an improper function that resolves itself to a matter of the accumulated effects of biomechanical and physiological abuse. Pain can originate from abused muscles, abused ligaments, abused nerves, abused blood vessels, and abused hard tissues. Since there are plenty of all of these in the head and neck, there are many sources for pain, and some pains don't even originate where they are supposed to! One of the most astounding phenomena associated with pain in the maxillofacial complex is that patients not infrequently perceive the pain at a site that is not the actual source. The process of "referred pain" takes place when one area in a muscle or ligament sends a signal to the brain that somehow crosses "biological wires" at a ganglion or some other location on the pathway to the brain; as a result the pain is actually perceived by the patient as originating in a completely different area, an area fortunately consistently associated with its own individual source.[11-19] This process reaches its zenith in the development of highly localized areas that are capable of generating referred pain. These little loci of hyperirritability are known as *trigger points*. When stimulated, trigger points may be painful at their own loci, they may refer pain elsewhere, or they may do both at once.[20-34] This phenomenon of pain referral, once perplexing and mysterious, is not so extraordinary in the light of modern-day knowledge of the principles of pain transmission.

The old concepts of pain being a simple matter of certain noxious types of stimuli activating sensory nerves that send biological electronic impulses to receptive sites in the brain have been elaborated to what is now known as the pain modulation process.[35, 36] This notion takes the basic principles of the older theory of direct impulse transmission and modifies them with the concept that pain impulses may be mitigated somewhat prior to perception in the CNS. It has long been known by the ancients of the Orient, and in various other fashions it has more recently been rediscovered by the West, that a number of different types of mild stimulation of sensory cutaneous nerves can have an inhibiting effect that diminishes deeper sources of pain.[37-42] There are a number of techniques that utilize this principle, i.e., massage, vapocoolants, analgesic balms, etc. There are also highly specific areas that when stimulated in certain precise fashions can have a total pain-inhibitory effect rivaling that of pharmacologically produced local or general anesthesia. This of course forms the basis for the ancient discipline of acupuncture. It is theorized that these phenomena work on a principle similar to the gate-control theories of the 1960s. It is as if the "switchboard" of receptor sites for pain in the CNS may be made to be so overloaded or jammed with the signals of minor stimuli that the impulses of the serious pain sources can't get through. Just how these techniques work is still uncertain, but there is no doubt as to their validity.

The existence of naturally produced morphinelike opioids called endorphins is also common knowledge.[43-45] These chemicals can be produced by the brain and pituitary gland under certain circumstances, and they have an inhibitory effect on pain. However, their action is limited, and the levels of concentration decrease in chronic pain situations.

Other factors also affect a patient's perception of pain. Attitudes or conditioning and emotional states can affect reactions to pain. Chronicity of pain or its repetitiveness and duration can also have an effect on the patient's perception of pain. Chronic recurrence can at times be more of a problem for the patient's total psychological reaction to the pain than its intensity. In a philosophical metaphor, "It's not the mountains in your life, but the grain of sand in your shoe that wears you down." Another mechanism that is ill understood is the process of idiopathic increased sensitivity to stimulation, known as the phenomenon of secondary hyperalgesia. Primary hyperalgesia is increased sensitivity to stimulation that results from a lowered pain threshold in the painful area.[46] However, in secondary hyperalgesia, no local cause is responsible for the hypersensitivity in the area. It is also a referred-type phenomenon, i.e., the pain or hypersensitivity occurs at a site somewhat distant from the primary pain source. The pain threshold is normal. It may be deep in the tissues but often is expressed as incidents of superficial hypersensitivity to touch. Confusingly, if located deeper in affected tissues, it manifests itself as tenderness to palpation. This is difficult if not impossible to distinguish from trigger point hyperirritability, common muscle soreness due to fatigue, muscle splinting, spasm, or inflammation without resorting to analgesic blocking. This will totally eliminate pain in the area if it is originating there as a primary source but will oddly only partially diminish the pain at the site of secondary hyperalgesia and will do nothing for the pain if it is referred or projected pain as from trigger points that have their primary source elsewhere. Trigger points, myospasm in its several forms, referred pain, and secondary hyperalgesia are all processes that involve the CNS and collectively are often referred to as "central excitatory effects." One thing these all have in common is chronic deep somatic pain sources in the maxillofacial complex. The more chronic the pain, the more prone the patient is to having these central excitatory processes occur. Referred pain and secondary hyperalgesia are a matter of biological electrical signals getting crossed either along nerve trunks, in the spinal cord, or in the brain centers.[47–52] They may even linger after the original source of deep pain is ameliorated. The various manifestations of myospasm ranging from mild to severe are a matter of Nature trying to protect these areas from further injury by means of immobilization. These mechanisms too may persist once the original noxious stimuli are removed before they eventually subside and things return to normal. Regardless of how confusing a picture of the occurrence, location, duration, intensity, and nature of the pain the patient describes or exhibits, correcting that primary source, i.e., the TMJ/occlusal functional imbalance, alleviates not only the pain of the primary sites but also eventually even the lingering ghosts of referred pain and secondary hyperalgesia in the secondary sites.[53–59] Pain is a cardinal diagnostic finding, a formidable pathological entity, and a commonly experienced yet still mysterious phenomenon. It is important to the clinician in TMJ therapeutics because it is the final barrier between the practitioner, his patient, and his success.

Basically, the pain resulting from imbalanced TMJ function results from overworked muscles (or muscles working in an uncoordinated and inefficient manner for which they were not designed), neural impingement, bilaminar zone compression, vascular interruption or interference, and excessive functional trauma to the muscles and actual joint structures themselves. This is why symptomatology of the TMJ pain-dysfunction problem may at first seem so complex. Basically it is nothing more than a variety of expression of one overall type of problem. Again, the NRDM/SPDC phenomenon is the chief etiological agent.

Orthopedic Dysfunction

The TMJs, like all joints in the body, should not only work pain free, but they should also work smoothly and quietly. Joint sounds or deviations of mandibular motion during opening or closing, either in the anteroposterior or sagittal plane, or alterations of mandibular movement in the more insidious forms of limited range of motion, are all signs and symptoms associated with joint pathology and dysfunction.[60-65] They are also directly or indirectly associated with the dysfunction of the orthopedic aspects of the joint. That is why before studying how the disc-condyle-fossa assembly might dysfunction in an imbalanced manner, it is

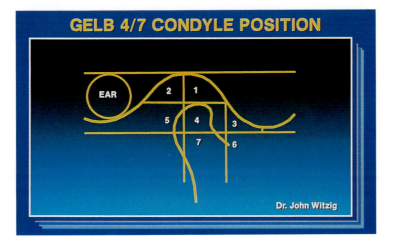

Figure 3–3   Gelb 4/7 position.

important to clearly understand how it should function in a normal fashion.

The first thing the modern clinician who treats TMJ problems should keep in mind is just where the condyle belongs within the confines of the glenoid fossa. It used to be thought that a concentric location of the condyle within the joint with equal anterior, superior and posterior joint spaces was the ideal and naturally occurring position at full occlusion, the starting point of the opening/closing cycle.[66] It is the considered opinion of not only your authors but also a great body of experienced clinicians that the concept of concentricity of condylar position within the glenoid fossa at full occlusion is for the most part apocryphal. It appears that the true ideal position of the condyle is in a slightly downward and forward position relative to the overall outline of the fossa. It is this location that the nationally known TMJ authority Dr. Harold Gelb describes as the 4/7 position.[67] This term is derived from the manner in which Gelb schematically slices up the TMJ into eight rectangular areas with a series of parallel lines. The bottom horizontal line of the diagram is drawn tangent to the inferior borders of the external auditory meatus and the most inferior position of the outline of the articular eminence. The uppermost horizontal line is drawn parallel to this bottom line, and it runs tangent to the most superior point of the outline of the dome of the fossa. A third horizontal parallel line bisects the distance between these two. A vertical line is then drawn perpendicular to these three horizontal lines from the aforementioned most superior point on the outline of the dome of the fossa. A second vertical line is drawn halfway between this point and the most inferior point of the outline of the articular eminence. The series of eight rectangles thus created is numbered right to left in descending order such that areas 1 and 2 represent the most superior positions of the glenoid fossa, areas 5 and 8 represent the most posterior portions, and areas 3, 4, and 6 represent the anterior portions. Ideally the head of the condyle should occupy basically the area of rectangle 4, with the neck of the condyle aligning predominately in area 7 at full occlusion. When this is the case, the forces of occlusion that load the joint are directed up and forward by the condylar head at about a 45-degree angle to Frankfort horizontal, which places these force vectors directly on the center of the intra-articular disc, which itself in turn is fortified by the heavy bony support of the articular eminence of the temporal bone. In such a circumstance, the anterior joint space is smallest and is filled completely by the central portion of the disc. The condyle is cradled very snugly in the center of the underside of the disc. The superior joint space is larger and is filled with a portion of the heel of the disc and the posterior attachments. The posterior joint space is filled with the posterior attachment and the nerves and blood vessels of the bilaminar zone. Basically the condyle is somewhat off center in a direction down and forward in the glenoid fossa. Nature can figuratively put up with this scenario all day since it is

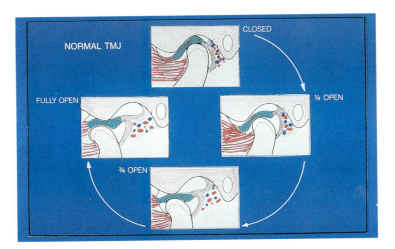

Figure 3–4 Normal condyle/disc relationship.

the common functional circumstance for which the joint was originally designed.

The Gelb 4/7 position is both the ideal rest position and the ideal fully interdigitated occlusion position. The rest position usually will be observed in the general populace of healthy patients to be even further down and forward than the functional occlusal position is, although the difference is not great and more due to translation than to rotation. The rest position is intimately related to the amount of "freeway space" present in the occlusion. This is defined as the interocclusal distance between the back teeth when the patient is in a relaxed state. The ideal locations for both function and rest positions are not loci of pinpoint dimensions but rather are ranges, not large, but ranges nonetheless in which the condyle may fall. One thing is certain, neither of these ranges is up and back in the fossa. It should also be remembered that the full occlusion position should *not* be a border position that is ligament determined, but rather it is a full-force position that is occlusion determined. The occlusion should be benign relative to the amount of superior and posterior displacement it forces on the condyle from rest to full occlusion. The less the difference, the better. The amount of freeway or interocclusal space between the upper and lower back teeth at rest varies from 1 to 3 mm interocclusal distance, although it may be more.

As the mouth is opened and the pressure is released from the full-force, occlusally determined, disc-condyle-fossa starting position, the condyle is securely positioned against the disc. Actually, it's the other way around; the collateral ligaments on the medial and lateral poles of the condylar head hold the disc firmly against the articular surface (capitulum) of the condylar head while at the same time muscular forces keep the entire disc-condylar assembly forcibly poised against the articular surface of the eminence (tuberculum). As the mouth opens, the condyle rotates against the bottom surface of the disc, and the disc-condyle assembly almost immediately begins to translate down the eminence, the upper surface of the disc sliding against the tuberculum's articular surface. The inferior head of the lateral pterygoid initiates the opening movement. The digastric comes into play only in much wider mouth-opening movements. Both condyles smoothly and effortlessly slide down the eminential pathway with no appreciable deviation or defection of the orthopedic midlines of the mandible to the maxilla. The elevator muscles, i.e., the masseter, medial pterygoid, and temporalis, are in a state of relaxation, as is the superior head of the lateral pterygoid, which is attached to the anterior edge of the joint capsule and pterygoid fovea of the condyle. As the simultaneous rotatory translatory action proceeds farther and farther down the eminential pathway, the tension of the elastic superior lamina (or ligament) progressively increases similarly to the steadily increased tension of a stretched rubber band. There might be a slight "bump" in the mandibular motion as the disc-condyle assembly slides over the apex of the eminential articular surface at maximum opening, a point at which the articular eminential surface rises slightly on the front side of the eminential crest. At this maximum range of opening, a border movement, the posterior attachment to the disc is stretched to its limit, and the assistance of the digastric is enlisted as the inferior belly of the lateral pterygoid is contracted to its maximum. The superior head is still at rest. The tension of the condyle against collateral ligaments is responsible for holding the disc-condyle assembly together.

In the reciprocal movement of closing an entirely different set of circumstance takes place. The elevator muscles, i.e., the masseter, medial pterygoid, and temporalis, activate and start to reverse the process. They bring the mandible closed and the disc-condyle assembly back up the eminential articular pathway once again. In so doing the tension of the posterior ligament is not counteracted by the activation of the superior head of the lateral pterygoid as formerly thought. This muscle remains passive until the final moment of closure. The disc remains in perfect position between the moving condylar head and stationary articular eminential pathway due to the tension of the posterior attachment and the collateral ligaments. Pressure of the condylar head against the inferior surface of the disc also helps in this process. Now something very important happens. The teeth come into contact. It may be in the posterior areas first. It may be in the anterior areas first. Nevertheless, when the teeth first touch, a governing mechanism is set off that is a product of the proprioceptive and tactile sensual information fed to the control centers of the brain from periodontal ligaments of the teeth. From that instant on until the point at which the teeth are in maximum interdigitation of full-force occlusion, the guidance of the mandibular arc of closure is *not* dictated by the proprioceptive information of the disc-condyle assembly of the joint and its surrounding ligaments and musculature, but rather is dictated strictly by the moderating influences sent to the muscles that originated in the inclined-plane guidance (or unfortunately, sometimes *mis*guidance) of the occlusion. In a balanced occlusion, this guidance brings the mandible home so that not only do all the teeth properly mesh upper to lower but they do so with the condyle still on the disc and with the entire disc-condyle assembly somewhere in the vicinity of the Gelb 4/7 position. There is no strain placed on any of the ligaments: the posterior attachment, the temporomandibular ligament, or the collaterals. The inferior head of the lateral pterygoid has finally completely relaxed. The digastrics are relaxed also. The masseter and medial pterygoids are in full constriction, with the temporalis constricting too, but also providing a guiding action. The force vectors of occlusion travel up and forward at about a 45-degree angle to the Frankfort horizontal right through the center of the disc and the well-fortified bone of the articular eminence. This is as it should be. The entire procedure, start to finish, happens smoothly, quietly, painlessly, and easily and may even be done with great reciprocating rapidity to which anyone having observed a nervous, gum-chewing football coach on the sidelines during a big game will readily attest!

To describe what happens in the "pathological" form of the opening-closing cycle in the patient with a TMJ condition, we must begin at the midpoint of the closing motion. All TMJ dysfunctional problems that are related to the occlusion follow this same basic pattern or abbreviated variations of it in the more advanced forms of the condition. It is simply a matter of degree. In the structurally imbalanced joint during the closing motion, the condyle is theoretically still on the underside of the disc as it is traveling up the eminential articular slope (although in advanced cases it may not actually be) to the home position of the start of the cycle. But as it nears this position, something improper happens. Actually, it's more of a matter of something that *is* proper *failing* to happen. As the condyle passes through the range of the Gelb 4/7 position and the transverse fibers of the temporomandibular ligament and the superior head of the lateral pterygoid become tensed to their normal limits, the posterior teeth fail to make contact. They are close to occluding with one another, but due to insufficient posterior vertical dimension of the occlusion, a small space still exists between opposing surfaces of the posterior teeth. This information is constantly being fed to and monitored by control centers within the brain. Sensing that the final occlusion has not yet been made and ignoring the plaintive signals from the muscles and ligaments of the whole apparatus that are beginning to strain, the motor control centers of the brain force the elevator muscles to "overconstrict" against the predesigned limiting tension of the now-strained horizontal fibers of the temporomandibular ligament, the overstretched albeit tensed superior head of the lateral pterygoid, and the supportive restraint to the disc of the medial and lateral collateral ligaments. This process forces the whole mandible to continue in its arc of closure in a superior posterior direction as it continues to seek the final stops of the insufficient posterior vertical dimension of occlusion. The posterior component of this overretraction process is grossly intensified by one of the true villains to the TMJ, anterior incisal interference, i.e., inclined-plane action in the anterior teeth that guides the mandible even more posteriorly as it overcloses and seeks the posterior occlusion. This forces the condyle to continue its labored path, against the built-in restraints of the local anatomy of the area, in a superior posterior direction. As it does so, two very important things happen. First, by default, the anterior joint space becomes increasingly large as pressure between the articular surface of the condylar head and the central concavity of the disc lessens and is gradually shifted to the much more biomechanically unstable thicker posterior band or heel of the disc. This occurs in spite of the resistance to such initially offered by the collateral ligaments, etc., that tend to resist such disjunction of the disc-condyle assembly. The second thing that occurs is that the superior head of the little lateral pterygoid muscle, which is attached to the anterior portion of the capsular ligament and condylar neck, responds to the initial attempts at excessive superior posterior travel of the disc-condyle assembly by either reflexively shortening up as a matter of self-preservation to avoid being overstretched or torn, or merely provides passive tension indirectly on the disc via the capsule by virtue of its own natural resistance to elongation. Just which of these two or whether some combination is responsible for the restraint the muscle places on the superior posterior movement of the disc is unclear. But there can be no mistake as to what happens next, and what happens lies at the very heart of the TMJ pain-dysfunction etiological picture. The posterior teeth have still not made arch-to-arch occlusal contact, hence the musculature continues to overclose, enlisting the extra services of the posterior and middle positions of the temporalis and even the digastrics to assist in the extra posterior component of closure needed to bring the mandible home occlusion-wise. With the enlarged anterior joint space (and distended anterior capsular recess) now providing the place, the increasing tension of the superior head of the lateral pterygoid providing the means, and the abused and elongated ligaments of the area surrendering all forms of resistance, the continued muscle-induced and occlusion-misguided forcible movement of the condylar head in a superior posterior direction pushes the capitulum of the condylar head "over the hump" of the mechanically unstable thickened heel of the disc, and with the condylar pressure on its back side, the muscle-induced tension on its front side, and a nice big anterior joint space to drop into provided by the forcibly vacated condyle and distended anterior capsular recess, the slippery intra-articular disc squirts down anteriorly over the front side of the condylar head, and the back side of the condylar head seats squarely on the posterior attachment and highly sensitive bilaminar zone as the posterior teeth finally make contact. To complicate things even further, the mandible has been so overly retruded that all the attached viscera it carries with it cause an increased pressure in the throat area, with a sensation of airway impingement being noted by the brain. To compensate for this, the brain tells the girdle of the muscles of the neck and the shoulder muscles to posture the head forward on the spine slightly by about 10 degrees to compensate for the visceral impingement on the airway, another biomechanically unstable and strained relationship.

The ligaments of the joint are abused and strained. The superior head of the lateral pterygoid has been abused and strained. The normal elevator musculature has been overcontracted past ideal working lengths and has been strained. Supportive musculature that isn't even supposed to be associated with normal mandibular closure has been enlisted, overworked, and strained to help retrude the mandible to its overclosed position against the initial restraint of the design intent of the anatomy of the area. And on top of all this, the force vectors of such a forced overconstriction and disarticulation of the area, which can be of the most intense variety, are not absorbed by a nerve-free fibrocartilaginous shock-absorbing intra-articular disc in the normal superior *anterior* direction but are redirected mercilessly to the hapless retrodiscal bilaminar tissues in an improper superior *posterior* direction. This happens during chewing, swallowing, and the most brutal of all phenomena with respect to punishment administered to the joint, bruxism! The proprioceptive and sensual information fed to the brain by the protesting muscles, ligaments, and joint structures "fall on deaf ears" as far as the control centers of the brain are concerned. Chewing, i.e., getting the back teeth together to extract nutrients from coarse foodstuffs, is a function deeply associated with survival of the species and has been for millions of years. As such, it is a function that receives top priority in the operation of the body. The brain is more than willing to compromise the well-being of the joint for the sake of making up for the inadequacies of the posterior occlusion. Anterior incisal interference merely forces the entire complex to make an even greater compromise. The muscles, ligaments, and internal joint structures are forced to take the abuse in spite of the nociceptive signals they plaintively send to the brain. They are forced to continue to do the bidding of the brain as dictated by the mechanics of the occlusion until the participants are forced to resort to a desperate form of rebellion in the form of complete myospasm, which is effected by Nature in acute situations in hopes of preventing the ultimate response to all this abuse, i.e., the actual physical breakdown of the component parts. But the need to chew ever returns and is demanding, and in the end rebellion is useless, and the stomatognathic system is sometimes forced to pay that ultimate price of physical degeneration after a long and painful battle. The occlusion-directed NRDM/SPDC phenomenon—it's a mighty misery.

Once the condyle has seated itself off the back edge of the disc in the bilaminar zone (Gelb 2/3 position) at full occlusion, the scene is set for one of the most pathognomonic findings associated with improper stomatognathic function, joint sounds.

Joint Sounds

The second most important characteristic of the patient with TMJ problems is the occurrence of joint sounds during function.[68–75] Even the lack of sounds can be a very significant finding if accompanied by the first and most important symptom—pain. Joint sounds without the concomitant presence or history of pain may lull both the patient and practitioner into an attitude of lack of concern, and maybe in some cases justly so. But whenever joint sounds occur during opening and closing of the jaw, it is a sign of some degree of internal derangement and an incorrectly operating joint structure.

There are two main types of joint noise, crepitus and "clicking." Both are intimately related to the status of the functional anatomy of the joint itself.

Clicking   Until the present, clicking of the TMJ upon opening and closing of the jaw has been one of the most widely observed, poorly understood,[76] often surprisingly ignored, and yet clinically significant findings of the routine dental examination. It is nearly always present in one form or another in patients with TMJ problems who have a structural imbalance of the skeletal Class II deep-overbite type. The phenomenon of joint clicking or "popping" has a proclivity for occurring in the late teen

---

Figure 3–5 **(A)** Face and TMJ manifestations of jaw-to-jaw relationship. **(B)** Normal mandible position. **(C)** Abnormal mandible position. **(D)** Sagittal section of a normal healthy TMJ. With the teeth in the full intercuspal position, note the position of the condyle in relation to the glenoid fossae and articular eminence. Also note the famous 3:1:2 ratio of discal thickness from posterior to anterior. LC = posterior limit of lower compartment; LLP = lower head of lateral pterygoid muscle; ULP = upper head of lateral pterygoid muscle; AR = anterior recess of lower compartment of anterior band or "toe" of disc. **(E)** Sagittal section of a TMJ with a posteriorly displaced condyle. Note the small posterior joint space with tissue compression. BZ = bilaminar zone; AR = anterior recess; LLP = lower head of lateral pterygoid muscle. (Parts D and E from Marguelles-Bonnet R, Yung J, et al: *J Craniomandib Pract* 1989; 7:102. Used by permission.)

**How the Face and TMJ are Affected by the
Jaw to Jaw Relationship**

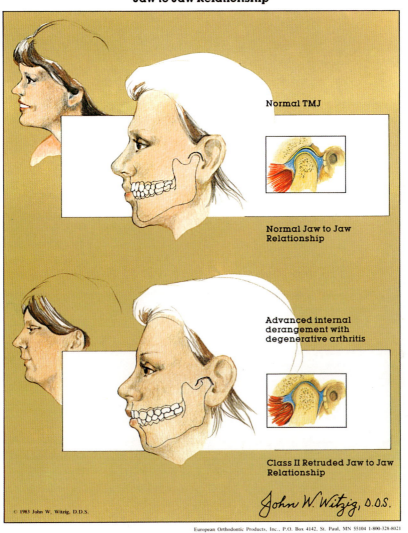

Normal TMJ

Normal Jaw to Jaw
Relationship

Advanced internal
derangement with
degenerative arthritis

Class II Retruded Jaw to Jaw
Relationship

© 1983 John W. Witzig, D.D.S.

European Orthodontic Products, Inc., P.O. Box 4142, St. Paul, MN 55104 1-800-328-8021

Figure 3–5(A)

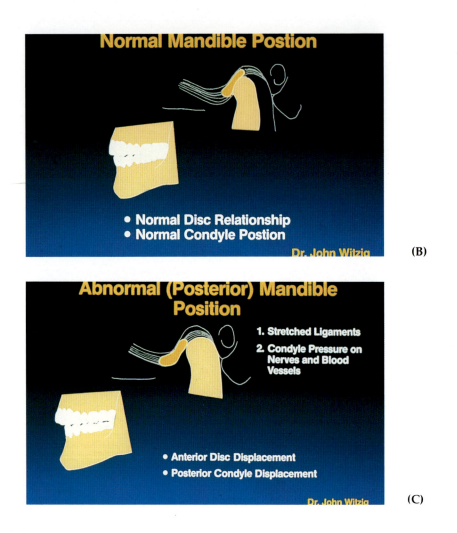

(B)

(C)

(D)

(E)

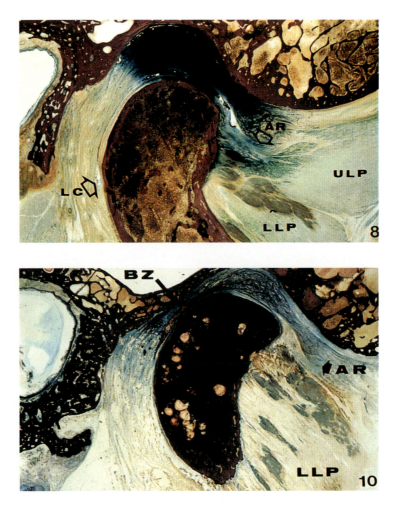

and adult patient but seems to be less present in younger children, although it can occur in any age group. One report even cites a newborn with a slightly audible click (probably an aberration). Audibly, the click is nearly always reciprocal, i.e., the joint "pops" or clicks at a given point in the arc of opening and conversely clicks again at about the same point in the arc of closure, albeit usually less audibly. Sometimes the closing click is so soft as to be only detectable with a stethoscope as a soft "thump." It may even be totally inaudible, but functionally it is there. By virtue of what causes opening and closing clicks, it is a structural necessity that if an opening click is present, a closing counterpart in some form or another, whether audible or not, must also be present. The presence of a reciprocal click is a sign that the full opening range of movements is still present and that the patient is not as "bad off" as he might yet become if situations are allowed to worsen. But remember, properly functioning TMJs simply shouldn't make noise when they work!

The cause of the click is a product of the anatomical shape of the disc and its stereoscopic relationship to the head of the condyle at the beginning of the opening movement. A midsagittal cross section through the fibrocartilaginous intra-articular disc front to back would reveal that it is biconcave on the surfaces that articulate with the head of the condyle and the articular eminence. At the posterior end, or "heel," of the disc it widens out to its thickest dimension. At the anterior, or "toe," end of the disc, it may or may not widen out slightly. Dual posterior ligaments (superior and inferior) are attached to the bulbous posterior heel of the disc. The superior ligament or lamina is elastic and attaches to the posterior dome of the fossa. The inferior ligament curls down and attaches to the posterior neck of the condyle. It is not elastic. Portions of the superior head of the lateral pterygoid may be attached to the anterior toe portion of the disc only indirectly via the anterior capsular tissue plane of the capsular ligament. The general, all-around shape of the fibrocartilaginous disc is not unlike that of a cross section of a common red blood cell.

Figure 3–6 Cryosection of a TMJ. This section reveals the beginning stages of joint degeneration due to posterior condylar displacement at full intercuspal occlusion. Note the demarcation of the disc (arrows) and the more posterior position of the condyle (C) in relation to the fossa (F) and articular surface of the temporal bone (T). Also note how the condyle is beginning to bend over. (Courtesy of Dr. James Colt, Denver.)

Figure 3–7 Advanced joint degeneration. Note the more severe posterior displacement of the condyle, its bent-over contour, the thinned posterior band or "heel" of the disc (arrow) with the loss of the more conventional 3:1:2 ratio of discal thickness, and most importantly, the severe compression of the retrodiscal tissues of the bilaminar zone. (Courtesy of Dr. James Colt, Denver.)

Figure 3–8 TMJ clicking.

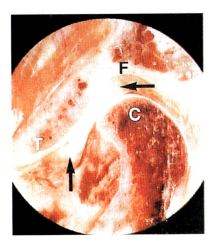

Figure 3–6

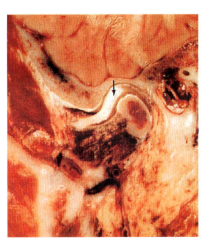

Figure 3–7

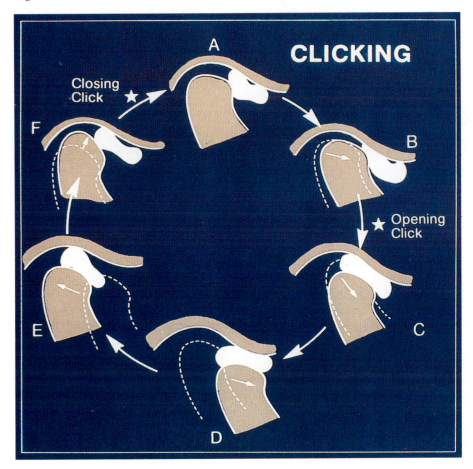

Figure 3–8

Under normal circumstances in an uncompromised joint, the mesio-superior portion of the head of the condyle, or capitulum, rests snugly and securely "smack dab" in the center of the concavity of the inferior surface of the intra-articular disc. The disc, in turn, is securely positioned, at about a 45-degree angle with respect to the horizontal, against the slope of the eminence, or tuberculum. At no time during rest or full occlusion does the disc sit horizontally across the dome of the fossa. Only the posterior band or heel of the disc ever occupies this area, and only in the anterior half of it. The concave superior surface of the disc stabilizes the whole apparatus of disc and capitulum against the convex tuberculum. The thickened heel portion is, among other things, an effort of Nature to stabilize the condyle in the center of the disc and prevent migration of the head of the condyle superiorly and posteriorly, which would result in impingement on the highly vascular and sensitive bilaminar zone. This is not the circumstance that exists, however, in the case of a joint with functional clicking. The above ideal anatomical relationship does not, in fact, exist in the routine patient with TMJ problems but is structurally compromised. For a variety of reasons previously alluded to, when the teeth are in maximum interdigitation, a position that represents the starting point for the arc of opening in the patient with a functional click, the head of the condyle starts out in a relatively more superior posterior position than is normal in the TMJ. This position is such that the condyle does not rest in the center of the concavity of the underside of the disc but is resting up past the thickened heel of the disc superiorly and posteriorly. When the capitulum rests in such a manner, it is said to be riding off the disc. The mandibular arc of opening involves essentially the coordination of the two basic types of movement: pure rotation of the condyles within the joint, as in very minor opening movements, and full-scale translation of the condyle and disc assembly down the slope of the eminence, as in major opening movements. In a patient where the condyle is riding off the disc, as the condyles begin to rotate at the beginning of an opening movement, no joint sounds are heard. The condyles at this point are merely rotating on the posterior ligaments and against the back edge of the heel of the disc. Then, as the translation component of the opening arc begins to take place, the head of the condyle moves forward while the disc remains relatively stationary due to increased tension from the surrounding supportive ligaments and the posterior attachment. As the condylar head advances, it slides over the thickened bulbous heel of the disc, and once past it, the normal tension and "tightness" of the supporting ligaments of the capsule and surrounding musculature cause the condyle to quickly "snap" into the concave depression in the center of the disc, thus producing the distinctly audible click. From then on the condylar head translates normally down the slope of the eminence of the glenoid fossa to its maximum opening. Upon closing, the reverse takes place. The condyle and the intra-articular disc, in which is cradled the articular facet area of the capitulum, travel up the slope of the

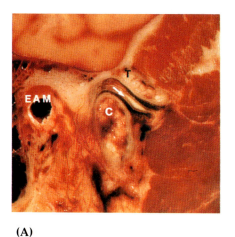

(A)

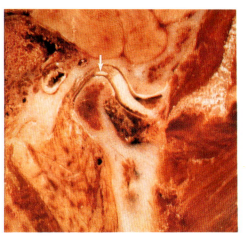

(B)

Figure 3–9   "Disc ironing." **(A)** Cryosection of a right lateral view of the TMJ with a chronically posteriorly displaced condyle (C). Note the thinning of the posterior band or heel of the disc (arrow) and enlarged anterior joint space due to the relative distal location of the condyle (C) from the articular eminence of the temporal bone (T). EAM = external auditory meatus. **(B)** Another TMJ with posterior displacement of the condyle, disc "ironing" at the heel, and keratinization of some of the tissues of the bilaminar zone (arrow). (Courtesy of Dr. James Colt, Denver.)

eminence to approximately the same point in the path where the opening click occurred, at which time the disc stops its ascent, but the condyle keeps going superiorly and posteriorly. As the condylar head passes over the heel of the disc, it makes another, usually less audible click and rests in its final position "riding off the disc." The difference between an early click on the opening motion and a late click is a product of the level of abusive elongation of the surrounding ligaments, especially the elastic posterior superior lamina. The more elongation and distortion that has occurred, the later the click since the click occurs when the tension of the posterior attachment and other supportive connective tissues of the capsule becomes great enough that they stop the advancing condyle from pushing the disc ahead of it in its descent down the articular slope of the eminence. When the tension becomes great enough, the disc stops, and the condyle hops back on once again and in so doing produces the sound.

An observation of a single opening click with no apparent closing click is a modified form of reciprocal clicking that is conceptually the same. This single opening click phenomenon usually occurs due to the somewhat thinner or distorted shape of the heel of some discs. At the beginning of the opening movement in the single click situation, the condyle is off the back edge of the disc, which itself is displaced down and forward in the fossa due to the elongation of supporting ligaments, distortion of the anterior recesses of the capsule, deformation of the superior head of the lateral pterygoid, and the availability by default of extra anterior joint space because of the posterior displacement of the condyle. As the opening motion begins, the condyle may push the disc ahead of it a short way until tension on the disc due to the progressively tensed posterior ligament, etc., becomes great enough to halt it temporarily while the condyle slides over the relatively diminutive posterior band or heel to produce a small click. As the condyle continues down the eminential pathway, the disc-condyle assembly remains in a normal relationship, and conventional forces maintain this proper disc-condyle relationship throughout the remainder of the translatory sequence. At near completion of the reciprocal closing cycle, the posterior lamina loses its ability to exert tension on the disc due to its elongation. Hence, due to the increased availability of anterior joint space, tension of the superior head of the lateral pterygoid on the connective tissue "toe" of the anterior capsular area that is uncompensated for by the now-lax posterior lamina, and the relatively thinned posterior band, the disc not only loses contact with the condyle as the condyle keeps going farther superiorly and posteriorly, but the action takes place without enough friction of the condyle over the flattened heel of the disc to cause an audible sound as it "falls off" the disc on into the bilaminar zone.

At both ends of the "clicking spectrum" there are considerations that must be made. The first is in the area of a totally quiet joint. Some patients have classic TMJ signs and symptoms except that there is a noticeable absence of joint sounds of any type during function. This may result from two types of circumstances. The first is that associated with what may be termed "disc ironing." Under certain conditions the disc may have suffered functional abuse from the condylar head for so long that its posterior band has been worn flat or otherwise distorted such that there is not enough of a bump at the back edge to generate a sound as the condylar head passes back and forth over it during the opening-closing cycle. Some discs may never have had that thick of a posterior band from the beginning. The disc is displaced anteriorly in a fashion consistent with the previously described scenario of condylar displacement up and back with concomitant discal displacement down and forward. During function the condyle will recapture the disc for a portion of the opening-closing cycle, but it falls off at the end of the closing motion at full occlusion. There is simply not enough change in contour between the back edge of the disc and its center to cause an audible click as the translating condyle correspondingly regains and loses it. But one important finding always accompanies such circumstances as those representing this form of quiet joint that is a result of disc ironing: there is a full range of opening. This is not the case in the other form of quiet-joint TMJ arthrosis of a functional nature.

In some joints the posterior ligament of the disc as well as other associated ligaments are so elongated from the abuse of excessive elongation and distortion that the condyle, which starts out off the back edge of
the disc at full occlusion, merely pushes the disc ahead of it during the
entire course of the opening movement and never regains it. The disc
constantly moves down and forward ahead of the condyle and "jams up"
in an obstructive mass of discal and connective tissue at the base of the
eminential articular slope in the anterior recess of the capsule of the joint.
Not only does this prevent the condyle from regaining the disc, but it also
prevents the condyle from traveling any farther along the articular pathway, hence the whole opening motion of the mandible or at least the
translatory phase of that opening is stopped cold. The anterior recess of
the capsule also becomes distorted and enlarged to accommodate the con-
glomeration of discal and associated ligamentous tissues referred to in
colloquial terms as "a balled-up disc." It represents a disc that is perpetually jammed ahead of the translating condyle, thus limiting that range of
translation itself. A modicum of rotation is possible, but even that becomes limited due to common visceral congestion below the mandibular
border at the base of the throat and neck. The posterior attachment has
no influence in this process at all because of either being elongated to an
exceptional degree or having been shredded, mangled, or otherwise severed from the disc altogether. The disc is perpetually displaced forward in
such a condition, and the amount of opening possible for the mandible is
grossly reduced due to the limited ability of the condyle to engage in the
translatory portion of the cycle. The interincisal opening in such instances
is seen to hover only around the 23- to 27-mm range, and what opening
of the mandible that does exist is restricted almost exclusively to the rotational phase. This condition is referred to as a "clinical closed-lock" type
of situation, a term that is a bit of a misnomer. There is nothing locked
about it. It is true that there is a jamming of the disc-condyle assembly
due to the fact that the disc is perpetually pushed ahead of a condylar
head that cannot count on surrounding ligamentous structures to stabilize the disc enough so that the condyle can hop back into it again.
But there is still some limited degree of translation and a fair amount of
rotational-type opening possible. The terms *lock* and *closed* are inappropriate and misleading (like so many types of TMJ terminology). Closed-lock
actually represents a state of limited opening with a nonreducible disc in
which only rotational movement of the mandible may be expressed. It
should not be confused with frank myospasm, which will lock the jaws
shut or limit their movement to only several millimeters of opening between incisal edges of the upper and lower anteriors.

The term *anteriorly displaced disc* is also a bit misleading. Generally a
disc that is displaced anteriorly and inferiorly in conjunction with a
condyle that is of course displaced superiorly and posteriorly is also most
often displaced somewhat medially. Displaced discs quite often are mor-
phologically altered, or will be if they remain displaced long enough. All

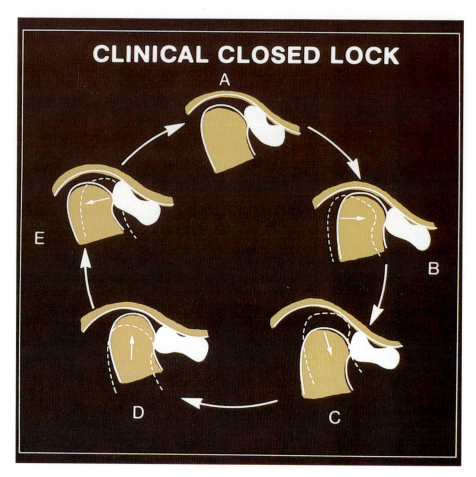

Figure 3–10   TMJ clinical closed lock.

Figure 3–11   Cryosections of TMJs with advanced stages of internal derangement. **(A)** Left TMJ, lateral view, beginning stages of "balling up" of the disc (arrow). **(B)** Left TMJ, lateral view, more advanced example of "balled-up" disc (arrow) due to chronic posterior condylar displacement (C = condyle; F = fossa; T = articular surface of temporal bone). **(C)** Anteroposterior view (coronal view) of the beginning stages of medial disc slippage (C = condyle; T = roof of fossa and articular surface of temporal bone). Note the proximity of the lateral pole of the condyle to the temporal bone due to medial displacement of what should be intervening articular disc material. **(D)** Advanced stages of a totally medially displaced disc (horizontal arrowhead) Note the lack of protective disc material between the top of the condyle (capitulum) and the temporal bone (vertical arrowhead). (Courtesy of Dr. James Colt, Denver.)

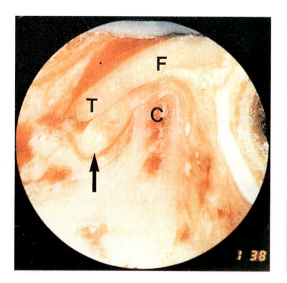

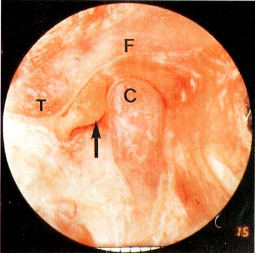

Figure 3–11(A)   (B)

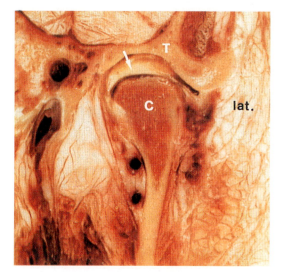

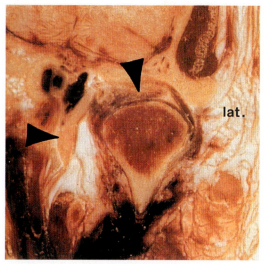

(C)   (D)

discal derangements imply a disc that is somehow pushed too far forward over the head of the condyle at full occlusion. There are two basic forms of derangement. In the first or milder form, the disc is anteromedially displaced in conjunction with superior posterior condylar displacement. (You cannot have one without the other.) However, the disc is recapturable by the condylar head at some point on the opening translatory path. The earlier that this recapturing of the disc by the condylar head takes place during the opening movement, the milder the case is, and the greater the chances for a complete return to normal once the occlusion is corrected. The later the click, or recapturing, the more difficult it is to return the joint to normal operation, at least from a biomechanical standpoint, but not from a pain-relief standpoint. Getting the condyle out of the bilaminar zone and preventing condylar intrusions onto sensitive retrodiscal tissues are the primary actions responsible for relieving the patient's pain symptoms and as such represent the clinician's primary goal. Recapturing the disc with the condylar head and keeping the two together at all times during both function and rest is a noble but nevertheless secondary goal. Not all discs are recapturable at the end of successful treatment, successful that is in that the patient's primary complaint of chronic pain in its various manifestations in the maxillofacial complex have been greatly reduced or eliminated altogether. Clicking may not be eliminated in every patient. In some it will remain. But it must also be noted that *not all clicking is pathological.* Sometimes there may be slight irregularities on the condylar head, on the eminential articular facet, or even within the disc itself that cause a slight click or "bump" during normal function. If no other signs or symptoms are present or if a slight click remains after successful treatment, heroic efforts at eliminating such minor sounds are unjustified. Patients don't care that much about unresolved minor clicking, but they do care about unresolved major pain.

The more advanced form of derangement causing balled-up discs and limited opening is not so much of a displacement as it is an outright dislocation. This balling-up type of derangement is the primary factor responsible for the clinical closed-lock– or limited-rotation-only–type opening situation just described. In this more severe situation, the disc cannot be regained by the condyle and actually prevents the condyle from translating to any appreciable extent by acting as a blocking or damming mechanism preventing forward condylar translation by virtue of the congestion of "balled-up" discal and ligamentous material at the base of the articular eminence. In spite of the severity of this situation, routine FJO methods of treatment often resolve these circumstances with an astoundingly high level of success. Although the posttreatment condyle cannot be made to ride on the disc again, it nevertheless ends up riding on substitute tissues. The important thing is that it can be kept out of the bilaminar zone, and that means pain-free joint function once again for the patient, the primary goal of all TMJ treatment plans.

Crepitus Crepitus or crepitation is the tragic and natural conclusion of joint abuse taken to an extreme.[77, 78] It is the sound of denuded bone on bone. Years of traumatic occlusion or superior posterior displacement of the condyle can destroy either the disc itself in the form of perforations or the disc's posterior ligamentous attachments if the condyle chronically rides far enough off the disc. The noise of crepitus results from contact of the head of the condyle with either the dome or slope of the tuberculum or articular eminence without the benefit of any intervening shock-absorbing and lubricating articular disc cartilage. A torn or severed posterior ligament allowing the disc to be displaced forward, "out of the way," permitting the contact of capitulum to tuberculum, is often associated with the rotation phase only or limited jaw opening. Without the protection of an intervening cartilagenous disc, the hyaline cartilage of the head of the condyle and the articular cartilage lining the dome and slope of the tuberculum or articular eminence may become scored, roughened, and cytologically irregular due to the stress of chronic abuse. It must be remembered that the TMJ structure, when functionally intact, is a natural shock absorber, and as such it is designed to accept the pressures generated during normal functional occlusion. But it must also be remembered that the stomatognathic system is capable of generating enormous forces for very brief periods of time and turns the condyle-fossa relationship into almost a hammer-and-anvil situation during heavy, prolonged occlusal function. If these forces are intensified and multiplied by bruxism (as they almost always are) and the physiology of the intracapsular structures is compromised by poor "weeping lubrication" of synovial fluid or the circulatory strangulation effects of chronic inflammation with its attending high-pressure intrasynovial edema, over a period of years or a lifetime it is no wonder that cartilagenous discs, posterior attachment tendons, and condylar heads break down under such chronic biomechanical and physiological maltreatment. As the ligaments continue to be improperly stretched, the posterior ligament can be eroded, perforated, or even partially torn loose from the heel of the disc. This may lead to not only the crepitus of bone-on-bone articulation in the joint during function but also concomitant osteoarthritic bone remodeling of the head of the condyle. This in turn can result in condylar flattening and/or lipping. Ironically, this could cause a temporary period where the patient appears to function better. The limited opening due to disc jamming or the clicking will in either case both disappear as the condyle is free to rotate and seemingly translate to adequate, albeit reduced degrees of opening. But the condyle is riding on the bone of the eminence. The disc is never "recaptured" but rather remains perpetually squeezed forward out in front of the head of the condyle as a crumpled, distorted cartilaginous remnant. Distortion of the uppermost portions of the superior head of the lateral pterygoid is commonly present in severe TMJ arthrosis. It is the distortion of the roof of this little muscle along with forced distension of the anterior recess areas that will cause the remnants of the now posteriorly unattached disc to be displaced forward and slightly medially. The external lateral collateral ligament is also usually overstretched enough or, in extreme cases, even sufficiently torn so as to permit the movement of the disc in this direction. This allows the head of the condyle to be forced in an unrestricted fashion to the most superior posterior position in the glenoid fossa at full occlusion, for there is in such circumstances a complete absence of the stabilizing or braking action of the disc, its bulbous heel, and attending superior head lateral pterygoid action. The remaining bilaminar tissues are then left to absorb the shock of the forces of occlusion that will be transmitted to them through the head of the condyle. Chronic mechanical irritation of this area leads to chronic inflammation. This not only disturbs the function of the superficial temporal artery and auriculotemporal nerve complex or neurovascular bundle that pass through this area, but the physiological action of chronic localized inflammation also has the potential, if severe enough, to initiate the process of bony degeneration of the head of the condyle and/or dome and slope of the eminence around the glenoid fossa. This process is cytologically similar to the bony breakdown of osseous tissue around any other area of chronic soft-tissue irritation and inflammation. As the bones go through the osteoarthritic breakdown and remodeling process, their surfaces roughen and may produce osteophytic changes in their surfaces or other osteoarthritic irregularities, and the rubbing of these opposing surfaces during function produce the "woeful groans" of bone on bone. Crepitus is always a sign of long-standing and severe superior posterior displacement of the condyles and an advanced level of intra-articular degeneration.

Imitation sounds   At this point in our discussion of joint sounds detectable by the examiner in the patient's TMJ, it would be appropriate to discuss a sound that is not a true sound at all in that it is not a sound generated by air waves as the result of motion of an object; rather it is a perceived sound, detected only by the patient, and it doesn't come from the TMJ but is auricular in origin. It is the phenomenon of tinnitus. It is defined as a subjective perception by the patient of noise in the ears such

Figure 3–12   Crepitus as a result of perforations in the posterior attachment. **(A)** A lateral view of the left TMJ shows perforation in the posterior attachment of the disc. **(B)** Axial view of the posterior attachment covering the condylar head. Note the perforation in the center. **(C)** Condyle with a notch of necrotic bone due to abuse of bone-on-bone articulation of the condyle with the eminence in the area of the perforation. The hemostat is lifting the disc up off the condylar head. (Courtesy of Dr. James Colt, Denver.)

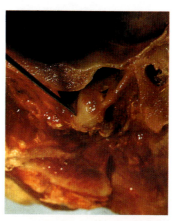

Figure 3–12(A)

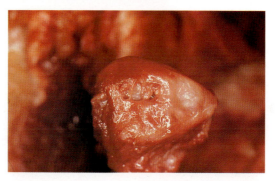

(B)

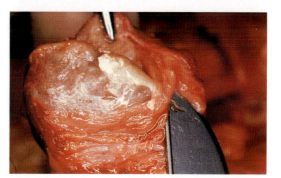

(C)

as ringing, buzzing, or hissing. It is a commonly registered complaint of many patients with TMJ problems.

In the early days of clinical TMJ investigation, J.B. Costen's original definitions of the TMJ syndrome included symptoms that were both auricular and temporomandibular in nature. And in spite of the fact that the treatments he employed only addressed the bite, they often not only relieved the joint problems but also the auricular components as well! Yet in the days prior to World War II, the health care profession seemed just as "turf conscious" as it is today, so the authorities of the time insisted that the treatment of TMJ problems should be under the jurisdiction of the dentists whereas the auricular symptoms should be the domain of the otolaryngologists. Although this may have at first seemed theoretically reasonable, history (as well as precise anatomical investigations made a generation after Costen described his findings) has proved that such divisions may not always turn out to be totally compatible with reality.

Barring such rare things as acoustic neuromas or viral infections of the cochlea itself, tinnitus has been looked upon as a relative enigma by the medical professions. Like Mark Twain's weather, everybody talks about it, but nobody does much about it. Very little has been done by the medical profession with respect to proposing sound (no pun intended) methods of accounting for or treating the problem. The dental discipline, however, has learned to look at this particular symptom from a different perspective.

It has long been known that the mandibular joint has been intimately connected to middle-ear structures throughout the evolution of the mammalian species. In the lower vertebrates, the jaw articulation has direct connections to the incus and malleus bones. In modern man the eustachain tube, which connects the inner ear to the posterior portions of the nasopharynx, is under the control of the tensor palatini muscle. The tensor tympani muscle flexes the eardrum as a form of protection against the trauma of high-decibel sound waves. These two muscles are innervated by nerves that arise from the mandibular branch (V_3) of the trigeminal nerve. More interestingly, the deep auricular artery branches off the

---

Figure 3–13   (A) Meniscomalleolar ligament. A sagittal section through the medial pole of the right TMJ shows the malleus (M), meniscomalleolar ligament, (MM), foldings of the upper fibers of the bilaminar zone (F) and the auriculotemporal nerve (AT). Insert: AE = magnification of anterior extension of disc. (From Marguelles-Bonnet R, Yung J, et al: *J Craniomandib Pract* 1989; 7:102. Used by permission.) **(B)** The pterygotympanic fissure (also known as the petrosquamous fissure or the squamotympanic fissure) is demarcated by the black arrow. It allows for confluence of the posterior fossa area with the region of the middle ear. (Courtesy of Dr. T.J. Spahl, St. Paul, Minn.)

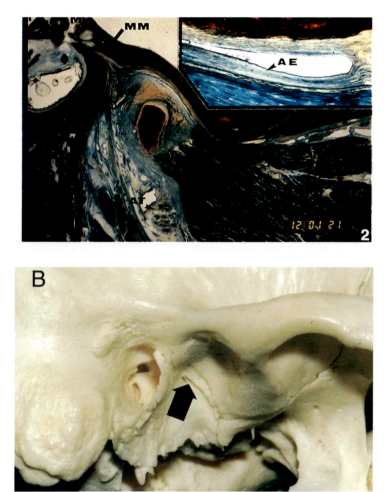

Figure 3–13(A)

(B)

maxillary artery near the union of the maxillary artery with the external carotid and follows the course of the auriculotemporal nerve through the posterior joint space area and between the cartilage and bone of the acoustic meatus to supply the outer surface of the eardrum. Even more interesting, the anterior tympanic artery, which also branches off the maxillary artery close to the deep auricular, ascends behind the capsule of the joint to travel through the petrotympanic fissure to the eardrum. Yet what may be the most noteworthy relationship of all was discovered in the early 1960s by O.F. Pinto, who first showed how the connective tissue of the joint capsule is connected to the malleus. He described the mandibular malleolar ligament (sometimes referred to as the miniscomalleolar ligament or simply Pinto's ligament) as a ligamentous connective tissue connection beginning at the posterior discal laminar tissues and extending up through the tympanic fissure to the tympanic cavity where it attaches directly to the malleus. It is the malleus that in turn is directly connected to the tympanic membrane.

The exact mechanism by which posterior condylar displacement initiates tinnitus and the role the meniscomalleolar ligament plays in the process in some patients is unclear. It may be a matter of impaired circulation and/or direct physical pressure of a mechanical and/or hydraulic nature. But the anatomical relationships described above certainly add to the indictment of the superiorly posteriorly displaced condyle as one of the leading etiological agents, especially when coupled with the fact that this particular problem has been consistently observed to disappear once the condyle has been adequately and permanently decompressed.

Altered Mandibular Movements

Muscular restriction of movement   The main factors responsible for the restriction or deviation of movement of the lower jaw are the condition of the muscles and the status of the condyle-disc-fossa relationship. One of the signs of an extremely acute TMJ arthritis is the very limited opening associated with muscle trismus. As a protective reflex, the muscles rally to the aid of the acutely traumatized joint and/or its supportive components by going into various degrees of spasm to immobilize the joint in an effort to facilitate the body's attempts at healing. This is one of the more advanced levels of myogenic response to injury. The muscles are often quite sore, as is the joint. Attempts at forcing the jaw open past a given point of restriction will elicit a painful response, and the muscles and joint are usually quite sensitive to palpation. This sequence of events is similar to the pain and restricted movement associated with a sprained ankle. This type of *acute* TMJ arthritis is a common sequela of acute trauma such as a blow to the chin or the difficult or prolonged surgery required to remove impacted mandibular third molars. The muscle trismus may also be unilateral, and it may be so severe as to prevent the occlusion of the posterior teeth on the affected side, another example of the protective mechanism where the muscles attempt to come to the aid of the joint the only way they can. This type of limited opening is muscular in origin, usually of reasonably short duration and also usually responsive to conventional palliative measures.

Joint-initiated restriction of movement Jaw movements may also be restricted as a result of the status of the condyle-disc-fossa relationship. The anterior displacement of the disc will result in the condyle being able to operate normally in its initial rotation and translation phases of opening. The head of the condyle can just as easily mechanically rotate on the posterior attachment while riding off an anterior displaced disc as it can if it were positioned properly in the center of the inferior concavity of a normally positioned disc. But if the disc is displaced so far forward in the fossa as to prevent the condyle from jumping back up onto it again during the translation phase of opening, the condyle will jam the disc ahead of it as it tries to translate in its path down the slope of the eminence. Thus no true condyle-on-disc translation is possible, only condyle-on-posterior-attachment–mediated movement with a disc ahead of it can occur. This can appear in the complete absence of any joint sound or can be accompanied in more advanced stages of degeneration by crepitus and is diagnosed by measuring the amount of opening between the incisal edges of the upper and lower anteriors. Jaw opening in such cases is limited and will measure from 24 to 27 mm at maximum. This amount of opening is definitive for a clinically-closed-lock situation. For a normally functioning joint permitting proper rotation *and* translation, the maximum opening should be nearly twice that of the closed-lock situation, i.e., at least 40 to 45 mm and most often more.

Joint-initiated deviation in mandibular movement Muscle trismus limiting jaw movement is a sign of acute problems or a sudden dramatic intensification of chronic problems. Limited jaw opening due to a perpetually anteriorly displaced and functionally nonrecapturable disc, indicated by a 24- to 27-mm maximum opening suggestive of the clinically closed-lock situation, is a sign of chronic bilateral problems. Yet, there are other types of irregular and/or midline shifting jaw movements that involve combinations of the above phenomenon that at first might seem to present a confusing picture clinically until the signs and symptoms are broken down into their simpler components.

The first type is jaw movement associated with reasonably noticeable clicking. The patient may open the lower jaw to its full 40- to 45-mm or greater maximum degree of opening, but the path to that maximum opening position is irregular or "jerky," as opposed to the fluid arc of opening of normally functioning joints. This is a result of the sudden snapping of the head of the condyle past the thicker heel of the disc and down into the center of the disc's central concavity. The higher the crest of the heel, i.e., the thicker the heel, and the lower the central concavity, the greater will be the drop or snap of the condylar head as it slides over that heel and recaptures the center of the disc. Correspondingly, the louder also will be the audible click. But this also will effect a more noticeably irregular "jerk" in the arc of opening and closing of the mandible at the points where the condylar head passes to and fro over the heel of the disc. This is especially noticeable when the process takes place at different points bilaterally in the opening and closing arc of movement from one joint to the other. This can result from one condyle being retruded enough in its glenoid fossa as to be riding off the disc while the other remains in its normal relationship. This is referred to as torquing of the mandible. It could also occur if the clicking is severe in one joint and mild in the other. From a frontal viewpoint during opening this will cause the mandible to deviate laterally a very slight amount as first the one condyle hops on to the disc, then the other. Patients will sometimes deviate their mandibles very slightly upon opening so as to favor the more affected side and help soften the snap that occurs at that point. Yet since the patient can obtain maximum opening, at which point both condyles have come to full translation and are in full contact with both discs, the deviations of the mandible away from its theoretically straight line arc of opening and closure may be subtle and therefore difficult to observe clinically.

A joint-initiated deflection of mandibular movement that is impossible to miss clinically is when only one joint suffers unilaterally from a clinically closed-lock situation. In this type of case the mouth may open normally to about the 24- to 27-mm limit as the condyles go through their initial phase of opening. The one superiorly posteriorly dislocated condyle of the affected side rides on the posterior attachment ligaments up in the bilaminar zone of the unilaterally affected joint, while the other properly positioned condyle rotates normally in the unaffected joint. At about the 20- to 30-mm point in the arc of opening, if the patient tries to open his mouth further, there is a marked deflection of the mandible to the side affected by the closed-lock condition. The nonrecapturable, permanently anteriorly displaced disc blocks the further translation of the condyle on that side. The patient may force some slight translation-type movement, but this is only a result of jamming the disc ahead of the

---

Figure 3–14 (A) Condylar path measurements transposed to line drawings (after Farrar). A = early opening click; B = intermediate opening click; C = late opening click; D = tracing of patient with "clinical closed lock"–type of disc interference, which is similar to a normal tracing, albeit of shorter range. (From Solberg WK, Clark GT: *Temporomandibular Joint Problems, Biologic Diagnosis and Treatment.* Chicago, Quintessence Publishing Co, 1980, p 156. Used by permission). (B) The mandible will deviate to one side (the side of the anteriorly "jammed" disc) when the opposite joint is still capable of *fully* translating with or without clicking.

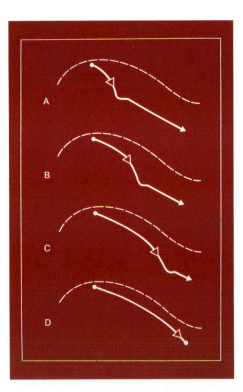

Figure 3–14(A)

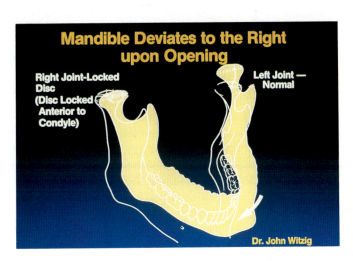

(B)

condyle slightly and usually results in discomfort to the patient. A combination of subclinical muscle trismus and anterior and inferior discal displacement prevents the condylar head from hopping back up into the center of the discal concavity. Since the normal side is free to translate properly and the affected side is locked or jammed at the rotational limit of opening, the mandible makes a drastic shift to the locked side during attempts at full opening. The normal linear distance a condyle may translate in a correctly functioning joint is in the range of 11 to 14 mm. The condyle of a joint in a clinically closed-lock condition may be restricted to translate only a few millimeters, if at all, due to the forward jamming at the disc, and even then it may be done only with considerable strain and discomfort to the patient.

A mandible with its condyles in the normal joint relationship opens, closes, and operates smoothly. Any deviation or aberration in the arc of movement when viewed either frontally or laterally is generally indicative of some form of joint disc-condyle malrelationship or derangement.

Muscular Dysfunction

In the previous section we alluded to muscular function and its relationship to orthopedic function and dysfunction. In that discussion we tried to concentrate on the orthopedic components of the TMJ complex. However, this is difficult to do because the biomechanical function of the joint cannot be succinctly separated into neat, compartmentalized categories. Rather, bones, muscles, ligaments, nerves, and blood vessels all work together as an entire functioning unit—what Dr. Melvin Moss refers to as a "functional matrix."[79-82] At least that's the way Nature seems to reveal it. Yet for the sake of better understanding, such categorization becomes handy, although it cannot exist without a certain amount of overlapping of subject matter.

As previously stated, healthy, normal TMJs working in conjunction with a well-balanced or at least benign occlusion should function smoothly, quietly, and painlessly. The same should be said for the associated musculature that works the whole apparatus. True, there may be isolated instances where a temporary dysfunction of a system may occur due to a direct cause-and-effect circumstance. Unusual stresses, strains, or functional demands may bring about such incidents, as may acute trauma. Under such conditions the pain and discomfort or even restricted function of the stomatognathic system are perfectly understandable and acceptable as normal responses of an otherwise healthy system. But when discomfort and dysfunction recur on a consistent basis, the condition is no longer considered a normal response and therefore becomes unacceptable.

The muscles of mastication are key elements in the TMJ pain-dysfunction problem, and the cardinal effects they display when they are truly involved in full-scale TMJ arthrosis situations are what give the condition its name. When muscles become involved in TMJ problems, they express their displeasure in primarily two ways: pain and dysfunction. For a muscle, pain may be expressed in the form of tenderness to palpation or movement, or it may exist in the form of outright discomfort in the complete absence of any palpation or movement. Dysfunction of muscles is observed when they display less-than-normal strength or reduced ranges of motion or they just plain quit working altogether (a physiological form of rebellion known as myospasm). Both forms of expression of their condition, pain and dysfunction, are graduated by degrees from mild to severe, and their level of expression is directly correlated to the level of severity of the condition in which they are involved. Looking at their form and function on a more detailed level readily explains why they react the way they do.

The muscles of mastication are of course skeletal muscles, the muscle type that comprises the major percentage of muscular tissues of the body, the other two major types being cardiac and smooth muscle. Of the skeletal muscles, there are two major types: type I muscles, which have fibers that contract slowly but are fairly resistant to fatigue, and type II muscles, which are capable of more rapid contraction but fatigue more quickly. Of type II muscles there are two subcategories. Type IIA fibers, also called fast-oxidative glycolytic fibers, differ histochemically from type IIB muscle fibers, which are referred to as fast-contracting glycolytic fibers.

The muscle tissue itself is composed of a collection of bundles of fibers called fasciculi. Each fasciculus contains a number of parallel cell fibers called sarcoplasm, which themselves are composed of bundles of myofibrils. It is at the level of the myofibril that the actual work of muscular action is accomplished, for these long threadlike cytoplasmic structures contain the myosin and the action proteins that together with adenosine triphosphate (ATP) are responsible for the actual contraction of the muscle element itself.[83] The smallest organizational unit of muscle fibers is the motor unit, which consists of a varied number of muscle fibers of one of the three types previously mentioned that are all innervated by a single motor neuron. The skeletal muscles of mastication contain motor units of all three types in each muscle: I, IIA, IIB. However, some muscles contain more of one type over another. Muscles associated with power strokes, like the masseter and medial pterygoid, have a high percentage of type II fibers. They generate an enormous contractile force but are subject to tiring quickly. Other muscles, like the lateral pterygoid, that are designed for holding action are dominated by type I fibers. These tire less easily but unfortunately are more prone to shortening due to myotatic problems or a lack of inverse stretch reflex activity (discussed subsequently). This as we shall see shortly has a definite role to play in the development of anteriorly displaced discs and reciprocal clicking.

When it comes to muscle contraction, several other facts should be kept in mind. First is that a muscle motor unit activation is an all-or-none response. This at first seems contradictory to commonly observed muscle action such as precise movements or long-term holding (isometric) actions. Yet these muscle actions are possible with a system built on all-or-none response units due to the ability of these units to shift the work demand of that particular muscle from one group of units to another. Activated groups of motor units may be stimulated in somewhat random fashion throughout the body of the muscle without activating adjacent motor units. The activation is capable of progressively being shifted from area to area and group to group in a sequential alteration of activation and relaxation. In this manner the burden of work the muscle must do as a whole is spread out among the various members in such a way that the various motor units go through alternating periods of activity and rest. Thereby the action desired may be carried out without fatigue of any particular group of contributing motor unit members. True fatigue sets in the muscle as a whole when the work load demanded of the muscle is greater than the ability of the various motor unit groups to exchange activity. When this happens, the muscle starts to take action to let the host know that within its sheaths things are not physiologically happy.

The pathway from the totally relaxed muscle, through simple muscle tonus, muscle discomfort and stiffness (splinting), to frank muscular spasm and immobility, like functionally oriented TMJ problems in general, is continuous. Its various manifestations are merely a reflection of the severity of the situation at hand.

Simple muscle tonus is the muscles' natural tension designed to resist unwanted elongation in a relatively passive state. Tonus keeps things from going totally limp. When the tension or tonus of a muscle is increased, it is said to be hypertonic; when decreased, hypotonic. This is all based on the myotatic reflex (discussed subsequently in the section on reflexes). Tonus is intimately associated with entities called muscle spindles, which when stretched beyond a certain point reflexively cause the muscle to tense or contract to a state of tonus. The sensitivity of these self-regulating muscle spindles can be increased by fusimotor activity, which shortens them. The tonus of a muscle in general can be affected by such things as sensual information from the dermis or muscosal tissues, and it can be intensified by CNS sources as well as somatic and even psychological factors. Emotional stress can make an individual not only psychologically "tense" but also muscularly tense because it definitely increases muscle tonus.[84]

Muscle tonus in the maxillofacial complex serves to keep the muscles in a state of active alert in preparation for contraction; it also serves to maintain a positive contact between the opposing articular parts of the joint despite the influences of gravity or other forms of negative pressure. It is also intimately related to resting muscle length, hence the vertical dimension of occlusion. Muscles are less efficient when they are forced to operate at a length different from their ideal resting length.[85] Therefore, changes in the vertical dimension of occlusion require a change in resting muscle length and tonus. This ability of the muscles to change their tonus to adapt to changes in vertical dimension help maintain an ideal resting length, hence maximum efficiency of operation is preserved.[86] This forms the basis for the generation of the concept of the Class II neuromuscular sling associated with malocclusions of the skeletal Class II deep-bite variety that suffer from a lack of posterior vertical dimension. Part of the treatment must consist of altering the resting muscle length and corresponding tonus to adapt to a new, more compatible increased vertical that is in turn an important aspect of all mandibular advancement cases. Even if the case appears to be Class I due to a long mandibular length, if the condyle is up and back too far in the fossa at full occlusion, not only must the correction consist of alteration of the dentition so that the occlusion locks the mandible in a more "bilaminar zone–favoring" forward position, but the treatments should also provide assistance in retraining of the "Class II–type," existing neuromuscular sling of masticatory musculature to a new tonus and resting length position compatible and efficient with the new posttreatment occlusally determined vertical and the new disc-condyle-fossa relationship. Functional appliances have been indisputably proved to change musculature in this fashion better than anything else.[87–102]

The next step beyond the normal muscle-tensing activity represented by muscle tonus and the nearly identical, albeit intensified condition of hypertonicity is an even more intensified level of tonicity known to the academic community as "protective muscle splinting."[103] Muscle splinting consists of an advanced state of tonicity that exhibits discomfort or pain on movement or contraction of the involved muscles and a feeling of stiffness and/or weakness. It is essentially a CNS-initiated protective mechanism that Nature very slyly uses to warn the host of impending injury or abuse and to remind the host of the unpleasant and recent history of the same. Muscles that are overworked, associated joint structures that they operate that are abused, and ligaments that restrict their actions and are traumatized collectively can elicit the response of protective muscle splinting. This is one of the body's ways of rallying to the defense of an injured member. Although no major structural damage of the muscle is apparent and no major dysfunction is exhibited when the muscle is used, the discomfort, pain, stiffness, or weakness acts as a deterrent to activity. It is as if Nature is trying to immobilize the area surrounding the injured or distressed component so that attempts at repair and healing may proceed in an undisturbed fashion.

Muscle splinting disappears once the source of mechanical abuse, fatigue, proprioceptive stimuli or sensations of change, or other physiological jeopardy is no longer present. Although the patients perceive the pain and stiffness in the involved muscles themselves when those muscles are in a state of protective splinting, it is a CNS-initiated response as evidenced by the complete and placid relaxation of these hypertonic muscles in the deeper levels of general anesthesia. Muscle splinting is a commonly observed phenomenon, a well-known example of which is a sprained ankle. The trauma of overstretching of the ligaments and connective tissue of the ankle causes localized pain, swelling, and a stiffness of the joint, all of which encourage the host to refrain from loading, moving, or otherwise mobilizing the joint. However, this is due to an acute trauma type of situation. Muscle splinting can also occur in the muscles of mastication when they or the joint structures they mobilize are subjected to chronic forms of noxious stimuli such as muscular overcontraction, ligament elongation, discal displacement, bilaminar zone trauma, prolonged improper excessive loading of the joint due to bruxism, and chronic inflammatory reactions due to the disruption of the disc-condyle complex common to most functionally oriented TMJ problems. It is a credit to the incredible resiliency of the human body that more muscle splinting does not occur than is observed in many patients with TMJ problems. Yet all too often the clinician will hear statements like "My jaws get tired and hurt when I eat coarse foods." Instead of a sprained ankle, in this case an occlusion that drives the condyle off the disc, strains the associated ligaments, and traumatizes the sensitive retrodiscal bilaminar tissues results in a "sprained joint," if you will. But one of Nature's responses to such a condition is still the same: the common phenomenon of the stiffness, weakness, and soreness of protective muscle splinting. Yet if this does not act as enough of a warning and should the noxious stimuli and localized abuse continue, Nature then resorts to even stronger measures with respect to the muscle's response.

The natural conclusion and end result of the path of steadily increasing tonicity that begins with muscle tonus, progresses to hypertonicity, intensifies to muscle splinting, finally results in frank muscle spasm. Myospasm is the involuntary and painful contraction of a muscle with associated rigidity. There are several types of myospasm, and all but one are indicative of the end stages of long-term abuse of a member. It is also a sign of the body's last-ditch muscular-oriented efforts to protect that member before final tissue breakdown begins. Short myospasms, such as a cramp in the arch of the foot or a muscle of the leg, are called clonic muscle spasms, are of quite short duration, and except for the momentary pain associated with them, are relatively innocuous. However, the myospasms that are of longer duration are more serious and are an obvious indication of trouble. There is the initial tonic spasm, which is a reaction to an injury or abuse, and the cycling myospasm, which is the result of long-standing tonic spasm that causes such distress within the subject muscle itself that it becomes its own source of noxious stimuli acting to self-perpetuate the spasm. Isotonic spasm, like isotonic muscle contraction, causes a shortening of the involved muscle, hence a distortion of the muscle activity, what there is of it. Isometric muscle spasm, like isometric contraction, tends to rigidly hold the muscle at the same length and resist stretch. This in turn also acts to restrict movement.

One other factor to remember with respect to the entire pathway of muscle tonus, protective muscle splinting, and myospasm is that all of these manifestations of muscle activity are involuntary in nature. This leads one to consider the closely associated mechanisms of muscle reflexes. The occurrence of reflex activity is closely associated with just how the *dysfunction* of functionally abused TMJs is manifested.

There are a number of reflex muscular activities that occur within the maxillofacial complex. A few are of special interest to the clinician attempting to understand the basic nature of TMJ pain-dysfunction conditions. The first is the stretch, or myotatic, reflex alluded to previously. The purpose of this involuntary reflexive activity is to tense or contract a muscle slightly as it is being stretched. The agents responsible for mediating this reflex are the muscle spindles, mechanoreceptors interspersed among the muscle fibers. They are activated by passive stretching of the surrounding muscle fibers and serve as monitoring agents responsible for keeping the muscle tonus proper at all times during both rest and function.[104] Of course, at periods of high tonicity, as in the form of isotonic contraction of a muscle during working movements, their services are totally unnecessary, their activity ceases altogether, and they remain quiet. The myotatic reflex is responsible for keeping the muscles in a state of proper tonus so that positive contact is maintained at all times between the resting joint structures in spite of the negative pressures effected on the area by gravity. Thus reflexive muscle tonus (contraction) counteracts the effect of gravity on the mandible to keep it positioned such that there is always positive contact of the condylar head against something in the glenoid fossa. Hopefully, it will be the intra-articular disc. Interestingly, there is a paucity of muscle spindles in the inferior head of the lateral pterygoid and anterior belly of the digastric.[105] Upon careful reflection, the wisdom of Nature in this regard becomes clear. These muscles must be capable of total flaccidity in the final phase of the power stroke to full occlusion because any tension on their part, reflexive or otherwise, would interfere with full occlusion of the teeth. This is especially true in the case where the mandible must be pulled up and back further than normal due to a lack of the posterior vertical dimension of occlusion and/or anterior incisal misguidance. In such circumstances the condylar head and neck are being forced in the direct opposite direction of the pull of both the inferior and superior portions of the lateral pterygoid muscle. Therefore total flaccidity on the part of the inferior portion is required because any form of contractile tension in that part of the muscle would be counter-productive to such an effort. However, there is a price to pay for such freedom. Posterior condylar displacement in these circumstances results in an overly stretched and traumatized lateral pterygoid muscle. But this is only for the inferior head of the lateral pterygoid. Something quite the opposite happens, ironically, to the superior head in NRDM/SPDC situations, and it involves another type of muscular reflex or, more correctly, the lack of it: the inverse stretch reflex.

It is necessary at times for a muscle to become completely relaxed and momentarily lose all tonus whatsoever, as in the case of being stretched its full resting length. If total flaccidity could not be obtained, the muscle itself instead of the surrounding ligaments would be the limiting agent of movement, and movement beyond that length in the form of forceful stretching could cause actual physical damage to the muscle tissue itself. Hence Nature cleverly came up with the inverse stretch reflex. It is a commonly observed phenomenon in not only humans but many other species as well. The agents of transmission of this reflex are the Golgi tendon organs, mechanoreceptors found in the tendons of muscles that are sensitive to the amount of distortion present and have an overall dampening effect on all forms of muscle contraction, especially the muscle tonus resulting from myotatic reflex activity. The reflexive total relaxation that occurs during hard stretching counteracts and overrides the tonus produced by the myotatic reflex action, and the muscle may then in turn be stretched to its full resting length with impunity. Thus the inverse stretch reflex is a protective mechanism designed to erase the tonus of the myotatic reflex. But it is more than that. In allowing for hard, full resting length stretching of a muscle, it also helps preserve that resting length. The resting length of a muscle is variable as per the dictates of its function. A muscle that is not occasionally stretched to its absolute limit tends to lose its current resting length and will shorten over a period of time, a phenomenon referred to as *myostatic* contracture.[106] Prevention of muscle shortening and changes in muscle resting length due to myostatic contraction is the theoretical basis for explaining the purpose of such phenomena as yawning and normal occasional clenching of the teeth. Yawning imparts an inverse stretch reflex to the elevator muscles of mastication, and normal periodic clenching of the teeth does the same to the superior head of the lateral pterygoid (in a manner discussed in more detail later). This is what is the basis for the theoretical concept of the shortened musculature of the Class II neuromuscular sling associated with classic mandibular retrusive deep-bite skeletal Class II malocclusions. Occasional inverse stretch reflex–mediated, full resting length, hard stretching of a muscle prevents myostatic contracture from occurring; thus the resting length of a muscle is preserved and, indirectly, its overall length. The iron pumpers are right, "Use it or lose it!"

With this in mind, it may now be readily understood why the

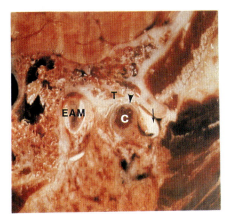

Figure 3–15   Anatomical cryosection of the right TMJ, lateral view. This illustration depicts rotational anterior disc displacement and superior posterior condylar displacement at full intercuspal occlusion, physiologically and biomechanically "the worst of times" for the joint. Note the anteriorly displaced and distorted disc (small arrow), the proximity of the condylar head (C) to the temporal bone (T), and the resulting intense impingement on the retrodiscal tissues of the bilaminar zone (larger arrowhead). EAM = external auditory meatus. (Courtesy of Dr. James Colt, Denver.)

condyle can be forced up off the back edge of the disc in NRDM/SPDC types of malocclusions. As the condyle is forced too far superiorly and posteriorly in the fossa by the muscles in an effort to gain the deficient posterior vertical dimension of occlusion, the chronic elongation of the supportive ligaments allows for the easy displacement of the disc down anteromedially into the enlarged anterior joint space. This results in distortion and elongation of the anterior recess of the capsule. This also could result in a repeated inability of the roof of the superior head of the lateral pterygoid, which may be indirectly attached via the anterior capsular wall to the front end of that disc, to reach its full resting length. This can result in myostatic contracture and a shortening of a portion of the muscle that no inverse stretch reflex is capable of counteracting. Remember, the posterior attachments have become somewhat elongated also and have lost some of their elastic properties. Thus the disc never has the chance to be retracted fully up onto the condylar head unless the condyle first compromises by moving down and forward in an attempt to regain it. But this can only occur in the translatory phase of opening, a time when having the condyle riding on the disc is not that important for the joint. When the disc-condyle assembly should be intact is in the full occlusion position. This is when simple clenching, with the condyle bracing the disc on the articular eminence, enables the roof of the lateral pterygoid to maintain its full working length. But the combination of the head of the condyle being inaccessible to the disc due to its proximity to the superior and posterior areas of the dome of the fossa, the distension of the anterior recess of the capsule, and the shortened resting length and myostatic contracture of the roof of the superior head of the lateral pterygoid, all acting to help keep the disc anteromedially displaced, makes the accomplishment of this goal of condyle on disc at full occlusion impossible to achieve. Thus it may be seen that common muscle reflex activities can contribute to the overall expression of the TMJ pain-dysfunction picture, but if that isn't enough, other naturally occurring actions of the muscles worsen the situation once superior posterior displacement of the condyle and attending anteriomedial displacement of the disc start to take place. And these normal muscle actions come into play at the worst conceivable time during the TMJ functional cycle, the point of full-force maximum interdigitated occlusion!

It is common knowledge that the superior head of the lateral pterygoid is passive, except for the exhibition of normal muscle tonus that is a product of the myotatic reflex; and this passivity remains as the condyle advances down the articular eminence in translatory motion due to contraction of the inferior belly of the lateral pterygoid. The superior head of the lateral pterygoid only activates to apply stabilizing traction to the disc-condyle assembly upon closing mandibular movements.[107–110] However, there is some confusion as to which type of closing activity stimulates the muscle to contract. And as luck would have it, the type of closing activity that does cause the superior head to contract results in a "worst-case scenario" as far as maintaining the integrity of the disc-condyle complex is concerned. In addition to remaining inactive throughout opening movements, the superior head of the lateral pterygoid also remains inactive during closing movements of the mandible when no resistance is encountered by the teeth! These are referred to as empty-mouth movements. During such activity, as long as no resistance is encountered and no type of power stroke is required, the rearward tension of the elastic posterior lamina on the back edge of the disc and the myotatic-generated forward tension of the muscle tonus of the roof of the superior head on the front edge of the capsular ligament-disc are enough of an equalizing source of control of the disc to keep it properly poised between the condylar head and articular facet of the temporal bone during the entire empty-mouth cycle of opening and closing translation. When the superior head of the lateral pterygoid is actually activated is when resistance, either in the form of tooth contact with a bolus of food during mastication or tooth contact with other teeth during bruxism, is encountered during a closing or clenching motion. This requires a power stroke, and all power strokes excite the superior head to contract at the final moment of closure to provide positive superior and anterior traction to the disc-condyle complex.[111] Resistance against a bolus of food in the far posterior regions of the dental arches will temporarily put an inferior traction on the condyle, thus creating a temporary enlargement of the anterior joint space. In the normal, balanced TMJ that is not victimized by misguidance of an interfering malocclusion, this resistance-generated widening of the anterior joint space as the mandible closes and as the condylar head travels up the eminential pathway is only of a momentary duration. While it is occurring, the tension imparted to the anterior capsule and ligamentous disc assembly pulls (or more correctly rotates) the disc down over the condylar head just enough so as to fill in this temporary joint space enlargement and keep positive contact between the condylar head and its inferior surface as well as between the articular facet of the eminential pathway of the temporal bone and its superior surface. This takes place advantageously for the joint at the handy thickened heal of the back edge of the disc. But here is where there exists parting of the ways in the action of the normal, healthy, functionally balanced joint and the abnormal, unhealthy, functionally imbalanced joint.

In normal function the moderating influence of the superior head of the lateral pterygoid on the disc-condyle assembly is passive enough to allow this unit to continue up the path of the eminence and resecure the capitular surface of the condyle once again, which in this case doesn't travel too far out of the range of the disc's ability to do so. A superior head fully relaxed at full resting length is required to allow this to happen. It is most important to note that the most recent research states that the activity of the superior head is latent throughout the entire sequence of the power stroke right up to the moment just before full-force occlusion of the posterior teeth is realized. It then reaches its maximum level of contraction just as the teeth make contact, a point in time during which in turn maximum forces are being generated within the joint. It *continues that contraction* as long as the elevator muscles are still at maximum contraction and applying maximum load to the articular structures. The entire superior head of the lateral pterygoid does *not* relax until all the other elevator muscles in the power stroke that are associated with that particular incident of mastication or *bruxism* have relaxed. This is so because such activity is necessary to stabilize the entire disc-condyle assembly through the entire power stroke and especially at its completion. For it is at this point, when the elevators are at full-force contraction, when the superior head of the lateral pterygoid is at full contraction, and as a direct result, when the condyle is securely braced in the middle of the disc, that all the convex and concave surfaces of the articular components are in maximum biomechanical stability and therefore are best prepared to absorb the powerful force vectors of full occlusion.

It now may be seen why such a normally well balanced activity can produce the most untoward results for the joint when the right combination or, more accurately, *wrong* series of events occurs to produce condyle-disc displacement. As the disc is being moved down over the front of the condylar head as the head ascends into the fossa during the

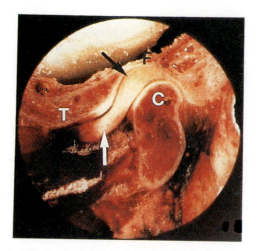

Figure 3–16   Anatomical cryosection of the left TMJ, lateral view: The trauma of bruxism. Note the loss of discal contours and the 3:1:2 ratio. Also note remodeling and distortion of the condylar head (C), enlarged anterior recess (white arrow), and thinning of what should be a bulbous heel of the disc (black arrow). Also note the denser bone of the articular eminence of temporal bone (T) and the severity of the superior posterior condylar displacement relative to the borders of the glenoid fossa (F). (Courtesy of Dr. James Colt, Denver.)

resistance-filled power stroke, thus creating for that disc a larger-than-normal anterior joint space, the condyle is perched somewhat precariously against the thickened posterior band or heel of the disc. Where things go wrong is at that point where the disc is unable to ascend the slope far enough with the condylar head because the condylar head is pulling away from it in a superior *posterior* direction until final occlusion is realized. This results in a perpetually enlarged anterior joint space. Additionally, the round surface of the condylar head ascending against and past the round and slippery surface of the heel of the disc represents an increasingly unstable biomechanical situation that, as the condyle is continually forced superiorly and posteriorly within the fossa, eventually reaches a point of no return and the disc can no longer negotiate its surface. The two opposing rounded surfaces of the condyle against the posterior band suddenly displace the disc; this is anteromedially assisted possibly from its front end by the distended anterior recess and the contracting roof of the superior head of the lateral pterygoid on the anterior wall of capsular tissue (because the action of the power stroke is still going on) and also assisted posteriorly by the condylar head that forces its way into the upper and backmost portions of the glenoid fossa. Thus with this area occupied, there is no more room for anything else, and this disc is forced down and forward. This displacement of the condyle up and back and the disc down and forward persists as long as the power stroke is in effect and all the elevator muscles and superior head of the lateral pterygoid are contracting. The inferior portion of the superior head attached to the condylar fovea must overstretch, as must the inferior belly, to permit the extra condylar regression. But alas, no help is in sight for the disc-condyle assembly even once relaxation takes place. It's too late. The posterior ligaments are elongated, and the roof of the superior head is shortened due to myostatic contraction resulting from an inability to take advantage of the maximum inverse stretch reflex to maintain its resting length and tonus. The clenching required to do this is predicated on full dental occlusion, which is what forces the condyle too far up in the fossa in the first place. The only way to get the condyle back on the disc is to initiate a translatory movement and allow the condyle to "go down after it." The sooner it catches up to it, the better. But in the full-occlusion (bruxism) position, the condyle is forced too far up and back out of range for the disc to negotiate it due to muscular, ligamentous, and stereoscopic joint space distortion. Some ligaments are elongated, as are some muscles. Some things are made larger: the anterior recess of the capsule, the anterior joint space, and the condylar portion of the articulation against posterior attachments. Some things are made smaller: the posterior joint space and the roof of the superior head of the lateral pterygoid muscle. The vicious cycle of reciprocal clicking eventually takes its toll. The more it occurs, the more it is induced to occur, and the easier it becomes for the joint to fall into it. Excessive superior posterior intrusion of the condyle into the fossa simply cannot be handled by the joint. It was never designed for such, nor will it long tolerate it once it occurs. It comes from malocclusion. Yet even this relationship is misunderstood, and once again muscles become the main focus of attention in clearing up the matter.

It is often erroneously thought that the teeth actually physically force the mandible posteriorly in occlusal, inclined-plane misguidance situations as the muscles of mastication are attempting to attain posterior occlusion. Such is not the case. If it were, the muscles would gradually overcome the interfering anterior teeth and force them out of the way while maintaining proper orthopedically dictated disc-condyle relationships during closure. Anterior teeth are easy to move, especially in an anteroposterior direction, as anyone the least bit experienced in clinical orthodontics has observed. If the muscles of mastication, which are capable of generating enormous forces during power strokes, were governed in their operation only by the dictates of the joint, they would soon bludgeon any interfering anterior teeth that might guide the whole mandible posteriorly upon closure in either a labial or lingual direction, or a combination of both, to eliminate the misguidance so the mandible might close to full posterior occlusion in a fashion anteroposteriorly compatible with proper disc-condyle-fossa relationships. But, as previously stated, this is not what actually transpires. In another example of protective reflexes, the instant the teeth touch, certain inhibitory reflex muscle activity occurs within the elevator muscles. The proprioceptive and tactile nervous innervation of the periodontal ligament is famous for its exquisite sensitivity. As the first contact of teeth upon closing occurs, the nerves of the periodontal ligament fire a signal that reflexively decreases the contractile power of the closing power stroke motion in the elevator muscles and makes them more subject to more precise forms of neuromuscular reflexive government in the final portion of the closure to full occlusion. This inhibitory reflex is a diminutive form of the more formidable nociceptive inhibition reflex that is associated with the sudden collision of teeth with hard objects in food and causes a painful sensation to the victimized unsuspecting teeth and a sudden reflexive opening of the jaws.[112-115] In the milder form of the reflex, tactile information from the periodontal ligaments initiates reflexive inhibitory action to the closing muscles while still permitting the motion to reach completion in full, albeit slightly tempered, maximum interdigitated occlusion. Such sensory information also permits the brain to make adjustments in the mandibular arc of closure. Fine motor control is provided by muscles like the temporalis so that the path to full occlusion is "dental-collision" free. Thus it protects the teeth. But it does so at times at the expense of the joint. The muscles, *not* the teeth, are what provide the true active physical guidance of the mandibular arc of closure. The teeth are responsible for initiation of the guidance through the neurological signals they provide to the brain. The actual work of directing that arc of closure to full occlusion is a product of the muscles. All the movements of the condyle are a direct result of neuromuscular mechanisms that are generated as a result of the tactile sensations of the teeth as they contact one another in the initial inclined-plane relationships of the act of closing together. This is why posterior displaced condyles are always associated with overworked musculature, for it is this musculature that is responsible for pulling the mandible that far back against the design intent of the disc, the associated ligaments, and even the muscles themselves. The teeth call the signals, and the muscles do the work.

Neurovascular Dysfunction

It is difficult to separate the function and dysfunction of the muscles and osseous components of the TMJ from each other for discussion purposes since the action of the one group is so intimately related to the action of the other. Yet there is a third area of concern that must be considered when attempting to understand the overall symptomatic picture that patients with TMJ problems routinely present, that of neurovascular dysfunction. Nervous innervation of both sensory and motor types as well as adequate vascular supply is critical to proper function of the TMJ. They each in their own way also suffer certain consequences when the joint is in a chronic state of malocclusion-initiated dysfunction of the superior posterior condylar displacement type. Even though the area where neurological and vascular dysfunctions might occur is limited, the effects of the symptomalology they are capable of producing under select circumstances is far-reaching. Another factor that will be noted concerning neurovascular dysfunctions of the TMJ is that observing the symptomatic effects of these dysfunctions often can be relatively easy but explaining the exact physiological causes is quite another matter. Yet that should not deter clinicians in their efforts to obtain proper functional balance to the maxillofacial complex and disc-condyle-fossa relationship, for once this is attained, the vast majority of neurological and vascular dysfunctions directly associated with improper joint function will sooner or later right themselves.

One of the first neurological symptoms to be noted is not a dysfunction but an actual normal function: that of pain. Pain is transmitted to the brain via sensory nerves. Ligaments are well innervated with nociceptors or pain fibers that are sensitive to stretching or improper elongation. Likewise, muscles that suffer acute or chronic abuse can emit pain sensations due to the protective reflexes of muscle splinting (common stiffness and soreness), which are readily recognizable, and due to the direct one-to-one cause-and-effect relationship of etiological agent-to-tissue response, which is easily understandable. However, there are a series of neurologically mediated symptoms that are not so easy to understand, at least not on a simple cause-and-effect basis, because their exact etiological agents and localized physiological mechanisms are cloaked in uncertainty. This general area of symptomatology has become known by the somewhat ambiguous term of *referred pain*. It is this phenomenon that has led the main body of the TMJ investigators into an illusory and labyrinthine archipelago of etiological impostors and diagnostic dead ends. The symptom-analyzing chaos of this meticulous quest was multiplied by the awareness that a relatively rare occurrence of a tumor, generalized degenerative arthritis such as rheumatoid, or other systemic condition might mimic the general cephalalgia, cervicalgia, and/or myofascial pains of the routine patient with TMJ problems. However, these other conditions almost invariably exhibited a direct, logical, and easily understandable one-to-one relationship with their respective prime etiological agents. Yet due to the disguising effects of referred pain and other factors, the vague and often nondescript headache and neck ache pains of the patient with TMJ pain did not! Even in our modern day of advanced knowledge of the functionally induced TMJ arthrosis, we must still occasionally resort to the theory to account for the manner in which the varied symptomatic picture of pain distribution appears in the patient with TMJ problems. This, however, does not deter those familiar with FJO methodology from implementing the technique on an unprecedented level of success to eliminate the patient's pains, whether they be either primary or secondary in nature. Although the secondary or referred pain of either muscular or neurological origins is puzzling and difficult to fully understand, fortunately for both the patient and the practitioner, such pains are quite often easy to fully resolve. When it comes to the question of what is the most common etiological agent by far that is responsible for the multisymptomatic and varied nature of the physical complaints of patients with TMJ problems, functional joint compression is the cause, and therapeutic joint decompression is the answer.

Referred pain can originate from both the muscles of mastication and the supportive musculature of the cervical girdle by means of the mechanism of trigger point formation. Referred pain can also come from simple, direct mechanical pressure from the condylar head on the auriculotemporal nerve bundle in the posterior fossa area. The auriculotemporal nerve is a branch of the mandibular division (V_3) of the famous trigeminal or fifth cranial nerve. It is also known to have anastomoses with branches of the facial nerve (VII). Thus the two great cranial nerves of the maxillofacial complex and all their associated neural centers and ganglia are capable of being interconnected with each other in a giant complex as far as perception of a stimulus originating in the auriculotemporal branch is concerned. It is theorized that referred pain can follow the distribution of the trigeminal nerve and possibly even the facial nerve due to noxious mechanical stimulation of the auriculotemporal and other mitigating neurological factors that will be discussed shortly.

It is also known that pain may originate in the muscles themselves due to the fatigue and cramping represented by common muscle splinting, but from this point onward, the actual physiological causes of some of the more well known types of pain patterns that patients with TMJ problems might exhibit start to become somewhat theoretical. Although the actual mechanisms of the origin of pain patterns in specific areas of the head and neck that such patients may be commonly observed to experience must sometimes be explained by considered opinion and etiological theory, there is nothing theoretical about the relief and improved function these patients experience on a long-term basis once that prime etiologic culprit, the superiorly posteriorly displaced condyle, is corrected back down and forward to its correct position in the fossa again by common FJO techniques. Other than the pains of muscle splinting and trigger point formation within the muscle itself and the pains of ligament elongation, which may be only temporary during acute traumatic situations, the principal cause of TMJ-type headache pain ultimately resolves itself down to a matter of pressure. The pressure can be on nerves and/or arteries. It can even originate from pressure on nerves within the arteries as in vascular distension situations. The pressure may be of two types: simple direct mechanical pressure as that represented by a hard object like the condyle applying physical force to a soft object like the bilaminar zone, or it may be manifest in what turns out to be a far more pernicious form, that of hydraulic pressure. Pressure of both mechanical and especially hydraulic types can cause pain in localized areas; in more distant anatomical areas, it can initiate the phenomenon of referred pain; it can disrupt normal anatomical function; it can restrict circulation; it can inhibit neurological function; and if allowed to persist long enough under the proper set of qualifying circumstances, it can destroy connective tissues, articular cartilage, and even bone. Recognizing its sources and effects and counteracting and eliminating its actions are the daily diagnostic and treatment-planning forte of the successful TMJ clinician.

Mechanical pressure on the neurovascular bundle of the bilaminar zone, of course, is a product of the interference of the malocclusion (or occlusal misguidance) on the mandibular arc of closure. That arc is strictly muscle and joint determined until the teeth first touch and the proprioceptive (and sometimes even nociceptive) neurological stimuli cause the muscles to alter their actions and, as a result, alter the mandibular arc of final closure such that a superior posterior displacement of the condyle at full occlusion is effected. This might be thought of as a relatively short, albeit intense form of trauma to the joint. Taking a bit of poetic license and stretching semantics a bit for the sake of a more easily comprehensible comparison, such circumstances as this might be thought of in terms of frequent periodic mechanical *microtrauma* to the TMJ. The duration of the moment of full functional occlusion is actually quite brief, although the frequency of occurrence can be prodigious to say the least. The real villain with respect to the biological damage that can be done due to direct mechanical pressure is no doubt the phenomenon of bruxism. The intense physical pressure it is capable of producing combined with the steady prolonged periods of its occurrence can quickly result in this paranormal functional activity becoming a source of *macrotrauma* to the disc, posterior attachment, supportive connective tissues of the joint, and the condylar head. As previously stated, not much is known about the long-term effects of direct mechanical pressure on the auriculotemporal nerve, hence the theory that referred pain may result at given locations throughout the distribution of the entire trigeminal nerve. It is known that mechanical pressure from the condylar head can reduce circulation through the superficial temporal artery in retrusive condylar situations by as much as 90% during full closure. In the short-term instance of mastication, such intermittent forms of direct mechanical pressure might not seem to be a problem, but in the long-term instance of the bruxism situation, we might be looking at an entirely different matter. Yet the worst-case scenario considers the nemesis of the combined effects of mechanical pressures to initiate the damage followed by the biological firestorm of the hydraulic pressure of chronic, trauma-induced, noninfectious intracapsular inflamation that prevents proper circulation-mediated attempts at cellular repair.

It is known that the articular surfaces and the disc of the TMJ are avascular in nature. They are of a microscopically pourous nature and depend on free-flowing, weeping lubrication of the synovial fluid for their cellular nutrition. It is also a commonly observed fact that opening the superior joint space during a surgical procedure on a TMJ that is suffering from such functionally induced noninfectious capsular inflammation will result in synovial fluid being ejected from the incision site under great pressure, the hydraulic intracapsular pressure of traumatic inflammation. This chronic state of inflammatory hydraulic pressure that is a result of built-up synovial and inflammatory fluids within the joint capsule cannot help but have a deleterious effect on not only the internal (intrasynovial) joint structures but also the nerves and arteries passing through the posterior joint space, i.e., the auriculotemporal nerve and superficial temporal artery. How much will such chronic forms of trauma-induced, bruxing-intensified, inflammatory pressure restrict normal arterial circulations and neurological function in the posterior joint space of such a joint? No one knows for sure, but the signs and symptoms observed in the patient when such conditions are present paint a fairly logical picture of cause and effect. One might want to think of the mechanical pressure produced by condylar displacement superiorly and posteriorly as a form of damage done by trauma on a macroscopic level. However, the more universal hydraulic pressures of built-up inflammatory fluids and increased synovial pressure should be thought of in terms of damage done as the result of restricted nutritions on a microscopic level. This represents the end stages of the joint degeneration process because once mechanically initiated and hydraulically sustained trauma and restricted circulation start taking their cellular toll, we begin to enter the morbid domain of osteochondritis dissecans and blatant avascular necrosis. Physiological principles are universal even for cartilaginous and osseous tissues. If you wound a cell and then fail to feed it, it dies.

"All nature is but art unknown to thee;
All chance, direction which thou canst not see;
All discord, harmony not understood;
All partial evil, universal good;
And, spite of pride, in erring reason's spite,
One truth is clear, Whatever is, is right."

Alexander Pope, 1688–1744
English poet

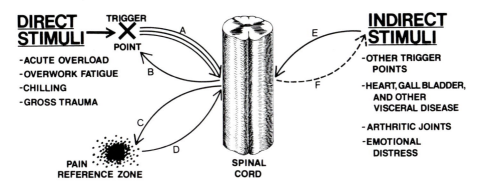

Figure 3–17   Trigger point phenomenon. This illustration depicts the theoretical basis behind the activity of trigger points in muscles and other tissues. The triple arrows (A) from the actual site of the trigger point in the muscle to the spinal cord represent the multiplicity of effects originating at the trigger point. Arrow B signifies the completion of a feedback-type neural circuit that is evidenced by the self-sustaining attribute of many trigger points. Arrow C represents the ability of trigger points to refer pain secondarily to a distant site. Arrow D represents the influence on the trigger point of therapeutic techniques such as stretch and spray with vapocoalants. Arrow E represents the activating effect of indirect stimuli on the trigger point; dashed arrow F denotes the effects of trigger points on visceral function (From Travell JG, Simons DG: *Myofascial Pain and Dysfunction, The Trigger Point Manual*. Baltimore, Williams & Wilkins 1983, p 15. Used by permission.)

REFERRED PAIN OF MYOGENIC ORIGIN

While considering the various forms of neurological and vascular dysfunctions of the maxillofacial complex that could contribute to the symptomatic picture of head, neck, and facial pains of patients with TMJ problems, one broad area that demands at least a modicum of discussion is the observation of referred pain of myogenic origins. Many factors contribute to the process by which the functionally induced TMJ arthrosis patient becomes symptomatic, but the agent that opens the door to let most of them in is malocclusion that forces vertical and posterior overclosure of the mandible. And all orthopedic considerations of condyles slamming into tender bilaminar zones aside, an untoward consequence of such overretrusion of the mandible is the stress that particular process places on the muscles of mastication. Overwork and overconstriction do not make them happy. They may easily become sore in their own right due to a distal driving malocclusion of a deep overbite variety. Yet, in addition to this, such abuse also allows for the formation of those mysterious little foci of hypersensitivity that not only are painful themselves but also are capable of referring pain to distant areas in a manner not totally understood. Such highly localized areas are referred to in modern times as "trigger points," and their existence definitely contributes to the varied and confusing symptomatic picture that the patient with TMJ problems often presents. Dr. Janet Travell, one of the world's foremost authorities on trigger points, defines them as "a focus of hyperirritability in a tissue that, when compressed, is locally tender, and if sufficiently hypersensitive, gives rise to referred pain and tenderness (and sometimes to referred autonomic phenomena) and distortion of proprioception." Figuratively, they might be thought of as little knots in the normally smooth and flowing thread work of the muscle fiber. They may be sore by themselves when activated by some form of noxious (abusive) stimuli, or they may be in a quiescent state only sore to palpation. Once they form, like any knot, they can sometimes be hard to get rid of. They can remain dormant. They are ubiquitous in the general populace, a price of being human. Just how they form or what constitutes their exact nature is unknown. But of their existence, there is no doubt, nor is there any doubt that when activated they have the uncanny ability to somehow refer pain to a specific distant area characteristic to themselves. Thus occurs the beguiling phenomenon of pains in a site of perception that may not be the true site of origin. Trigger points, once detected via adroit manual palpation, may be treated directly by means of certain injection techniques, etc., or they may be treated indirectly. Fortunately, once the muscle abuse adjacated to the muscles of mastication in the overly retrusive mandibular arc-of-closure–type TMJ patients is treated via mandibular advancement FJO-type techniques, the problems of trigger point hypersensitivity and referred pain are observed to generally subside.

The existence of myofascial trigger points and their significance has been widely observed and studied in many of the disciplines of the healing arts.[116–126] They most often arise in muscles where they may be only mildly troublesome painwise, or they may be so hyperirritable as to cause the most excruciating pain. They may also cause a painless and slight restriction of movement, or they may severely restrict a particular muscle's normal performance. They may also form in skin, connective tissue, and even periosteum. Along with referred pain, the most common characteristic associated with trigger points by far is that they may also on occasion result in stimulation of autonomic responses in the referred site. These "autonomic concomitants," as they are called, occur in the distant referred pain zone, and depending on the anatomical area affected by the trigger point, may result in localized vasoconstriction, lacrimation, salivation, secretion of nasal mucous, and pilomotor stimulation ("gooseflesh"). Even proprioceptive irregularities might occur due to trigger point activity, such as tinnitus, vertigo, and slight ataxia problems. Generally, however, active trigger points mostly express themselves in the form of musculoskeletal pain.

The concept of the trigger point did not spring forth upon the health care profession in a sudden burst of clarity and resolution but rather emerged gradually out of a fog of confusion and highly variable and ill-defined terminologies dating back to the 1840s. Early investigators theorized that small callouses formed in muscles and this accounted for highly localized areas of tenderness that elicited pain and felt like little cords to digital palpation. Early in the 20th century it was observed that small gelatinous hardening could be palpated in muscle tissues in deep anesthesia and even after death until the point where rigor mortis stiffened everything. In the early 1940s several investigators began to realize that pain in certain areas was not always generated at the site of perception but rather originated in a distant tender spot in the same muscle or even different muscles altogether. Trigger point locations (areas at one time referred to as myogelosis due to the high-viscosity gelatinous feel of the little trigger point nodule in the tissue) started being charted along with the specific sites of referred pain characteristically associated with them. This work reached its zenith in the landmark contributions of people like Dr. Janet Travell and Dr. David Simons.

Among some of the terms used in the past to describe the trigger point phenomenon as a whole, or portions of it, were "myalgic spots," "sonarticular rheumatism," "muscular rheumatism," "rheumatic myalgia," "fibrositis," "myositis chronica," "pressure point," "nerve point," "fibropathic syndrome," "muscle indurations," "myodysneuria," and "myofascitis," to name a few. In addition to a lack of agreement in terminology, considering that trigger points that form in abused tissue can refer pain to other areas and also considering that clinicians in the past (and present) have been invariably prone to concentrating their diagnostic and therapeutic efforts at the secondary site (the site of the perceived pain) instead of the primary site (actual trigger point location), it is no wonder confusion has dominated the area for so long. Does the patient have a true bursitis, tennis elbow, spinal osteoarthritis, tension headache, etc., or does the patient have trigger points that are activating and referring pain to these locations, thereby merely mimicking these conditions? Could both be occurring at once? The fog has been thick indeed.

Myofascial trigger points have certain basic characteristics that should be kept in mind. A brief review of these clinical characteristics and the related findings upon direct examination would be essential to gaining a broader understanding of why patients with TMJ problems present with the symptomatic pictures that they do and why they respond to treatment the way they do.

First of all, trigger points may be thought of as being of one of two major types, active or latent. Active trigger points can cause both pain and dysfunction of the muscle of origin. The dysfunction involved takes the form of (1) restriction of movement and/or (2) a weakness of the affected muscle. It will at once be noted that this is a very analogous scenario to the previously described phenomenon of muscle splinting. La-

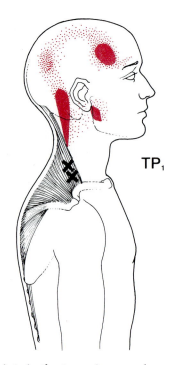

Figure 3–18   Trigger points in the trapezius muscle, a specific location site referred to as TP₁ (X's), when activated refer pain to specific sites in the head and neck. Solid red denotes essential referred pain zone; stippled areas denote the "spillover zone". (From Travell JG, Simons DG: *Myofascial Pain and Dysfunction, The Trigger Point Manual.* Baltimore, Williams & Wilkins, 1983, p 184. Used by permission.)

tent trigger points, on the other hand, do not cause pain, at least not generally, but are "clinically silent." They can cause a painless restriction of movement and weakness of the affected muscle, however. Latent trigger points can erupt periodically due to overwork, overstretching, chilling of the particular muscle concerned, or even emotional stress to cause pain once again for the patient. Another agent capable of reactivating latent trigger points is the presence of an arthritic joint! Latent trigger points may also remain silent in the main body of the muscle tissue for years after resolution of the initial problem only to reactivate upon stimulation (insult) as previously described to cause pain again. Much of the stiffness and reduced range of motion of old age is theorized to be due to the accumulation of latent trigger points. Although both active and latent trigger points develop at all ages and in both sexes, women are more prone to their development than men are. Those individuals also prone to trigger point formation are those in sedentary life-styles who only occasion-

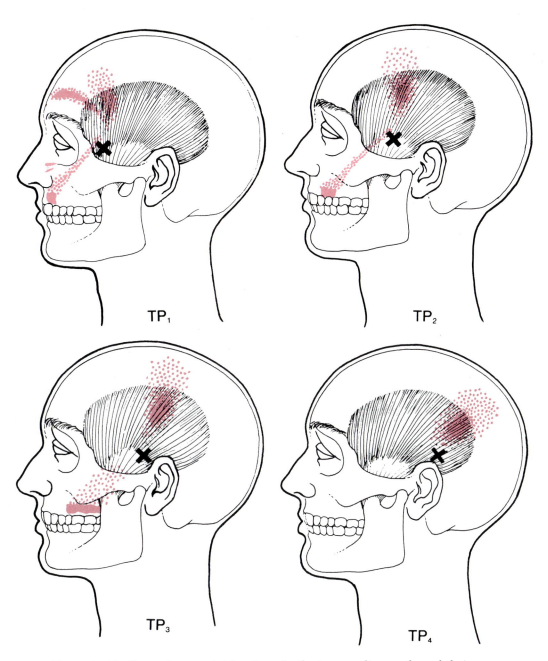

Figure 3–19   Four trigger point locations in the temporalis muscle and their essential-zone and spillover-zone referred pain patterns. (From Travell JG, Simons DG: *Myofascial Pain and Dysfunction, The Trigger Point Manual.* Baltimore, Williams & Wilkins, 1983, p 237. Used by permission.)

ally indulge (overindulge) in sustained physical exercises, i.e., weekend athletics.

As previously stated, trigger points have a characteristic pattern of occurrence and refer pain in patterns to other reference zone locations characteristic of each muscle. The pain is usually low grade and dull, although it can be so intense as to be incapacitating to the host. This referred pain (reference zone) site can be intensified by accurate digital pressure of proper magnitude at the site of origin (trigger point area). The more the trigger point is irritated, the greater the intensity of the referred pain. Secondary trigger points might even develop in adjacent musculature that is chronically enlisted to provide protective splinting or spasm in the aid of the primary muscle suffering the original injury.

Trigger points may be activated commonly by overstretching either quantitatively or qualitatively past customary ranges of motion. Overworking of muscles is also a common offender, as is any other form of muscular trauma. Chilling of the muscle activates trigger points to make the muscles that contain them stiff and sore. This accounts for the susceptibility of senior citizens to cold drafts. This author remembers a time early in his career when he slept beneath an open window when a cold front passed through overnight. The pain and "spasm" of the right trapezius and other adjacent cervical musculature upon waking the next morning was so intense that his head and shoulder could not be voluntarily put in a normal posture. Thus he painfully went to work his first day as a private practitioner in a distorted posture, resembling Quasimodo, Victor Hugo's "hunchback of Notre Dame." It took nearly 2 days to return the muscles to normal. Muscles are especially vulnerable to developing trigger points or reactivating latent ones due to chilling when muscles are in a state of exhaustion as a result of excessive exercise or are suffering from postexercise stiffness. This accounts for the heavy stockings dancers often wear during rehearsals.

It must also be remembered that although myofascial trigger point sensitivity can vary from day to day and even from hour to hour, the signs and symptoms of trigger point activity can also linger long after the resolution of the initial insulting circumstances. Trigger point formation may eventually resolve after completion of treatment to a state of clinical silence. But the potential that any remaining latent trigger point might be reactivated to bring back "the old pains once again" always remains.

The location of an individual trigger point is usually associated with a portion of a muscle referred to as a "taut band." These are stringy or cordlike areas within a muscle that exhibit increased resistance to digital palpation. They have also been described as a "ropiness" in the muscle. The taut band is not an area of localized muscle spasm because it exhibits no unusual electromyographic (EMG) activity. The bands, of course, run parallel to the direction of the fibers of the main body of the muscle and feel tense when palpated. Their feel to a technique of perpendicular snapping palpation has been likened to the imagined feel of plucking a guitar string that is covered by a layer of fleshy soft tissue. These taut bands associated with trigger point location oddly remain even after death, until rigor mortis sets in, but have been observed to disappear within minutes after direct and correctly localized trigger point therapy! The tautness of the band (which is usually 1 to 4 mm in diameter) is most easily detected when palpated repeatedly across its length at various locations along the length of the muscle. However, this method of palpation makes detection of the trigger point more difficult. Their location (and there may be more than one) would be the points at which the sensitivity to this form of taut band palpation was greatest. Trigger point areas of hyperirritability are on the order of approximately 1 cm^2 in area or less. A more definite way of palpating the trigger point along the length of a taut band in a muscle is via the "stripping" technique. In this method the operator runs the tips of his fingers along the length of the taut band in a slow, deep-stroking massage-type fashion. A lubricating medium on the skin greatly facilitates this process. As the fingertips approach the location of the trigger point in the taut band, a small gelatinous nodular sensation or tiny lump will be detected. This requires practice and an adroit digital technique. Interestingly, when the longitudinal palpation technique is used, if it is repeated a sufficient number of times, the nodular sensations along the taut band (or bands because a muscle may exhibit multiple taut bands) indicative of the location of trigger points may be observed to disappear. The concomitant trigger point sensitivity to palpation and its associated referred pain patterns may also be seen to subside. This phenomenon formed the basis for massage-type therapies and their abilities to relieve pain and restore limited function of muscles long before modern medicine discovered the trigger point phenomenon.

The reason longitudinal deep massage-type digital palpation along the length of the taut band in a muscle more readily reveals the nodular feel of the exact trigger point location better than does cross-fiber, "plucking-type" palpation along the band's length (where the trigger point locations are more often detected as the most hypersensitive loci) is due to the structural characteristics of the trigger point itself. Although latent trigger points have no detectable cytological characteristics microscopically other than a sporadic "fat dusting" or accumulation of microscopic lipid droplets in the surrounding tissue, more active trigger points have various microscopic interstitial morphological findings associated with them. In addition to the previously mentioned localized accumulation of fat droplets, biopsy specimens of highly active trigger point nodules have exhibited "contracture knots," a "clublike" distortion of contracted myofibrils adjacent to an empty sarcolemmic tubule. The nuclei of muscle cells were observed to seem to accumulate in chains or clusters, especially near areas of high vascular supply. There was a marked localized loss of muscle striation and a high degree of variability of the intensity of muscle fiber staining in microscopic slide sections. Fiber degeneration was present, and in the most severe cases (highly active trigger points) lipid accumulation and connective tissue replaced muscle fibers.[127, 128] Ultramicroscopic studies revealed a generalized breakdown of myofibrils, extralength sarcomeres, and intracellular lipid buildup in some fibers. In advanced cases ruptured sarcomere remnants were detected along with accumulations of collagen in areas of frank necrosis.[129] Something unpleasant is obviously going on within the muscle tissue when trigger points form.

After careful consideration of the above, it soon becomes clear as to why cross-fiber palpation reveals only the taut band whereas longitudinal, deep-stroking, massage-type palpation along the length of the taut band gives the impression of a small gelatinous nodule at the site of the trigger point. As the fingertips are moved on the skin slowly and adroitly along the length of the taut band in the muscle (which must be passively stretched for this procedure), a "milking effect" is produced that pushes the tissue fluids ahead of the fingertips. This also leaves a small discernible area of blanching of the skin immediately behind the fingertips. The very same process is no doubt occurring in the muscle's taut band beneath. Thus, in a manner similar to the venous constriction that raises small nodes at the sites of venous valves, the myogenous debris adjacent to the highly localized area of minute muscle tissue damage that is represented by the trigger point wells up in reaction to the milking action of longitudinal digital palpation. Of course, such a procedure, known as flat palpation, is only possible if the taut band is being pressed between the fingers and underlying bone.

A technique handy for examination of the muscles of mastication, most of which are palpable from two sides, involves pincer-type bidigital palpation. The belly of the muscle being examined (in a state of passive stretch, i.e., stretched enough to be only on the verge of causing pain) is grasped between the thumb and index finger, and with the fingers squeezed, the muscle is rolled back and forth between the fingers to detect the taut band. Once located, the band(s) may be palpated along the length of the entire muscle to locate trigger points by direct feel and/or patient response.

Two phenomena that may occur when a trigger point is palpated are the "local twitch response" and the so-called "jump sign." It must be remembered that a taut band is surrounded by normal relaxed muscle fibers (although a number of taut bands may exist so close together in severely involved muscles that they seem to blend into one). The localized twitch response occurs when a trigger point in that taut band is firmly palpated and the muscle fibers associated exclusively with that particular band constrict slightly or twitch. Occasionally the twitch may be vigorous enough to actually effect a jerk of the body part that the muscle operates. This should not be confused with the jump sign (and confusion does exist with respect to use of these terms), which is a sudden and acute painful response of the patient to the stimulation of a highly active trigger point.

Therefore, in light of the above, it may be seen that proper palpation of a trigger point may simultaneously elicit a local twitch response, a jump sign, and even a referred pain pattern (if the pressure applied is accurate enough, firm enough, and of sufficient duration). If the trigger points are active ("hot") enough to cause pain in a resting muscle, even without being palpated, digital palpation of these trigger points often produces (or *re*produces) the patient's referred pain pattern. Pain will initially be perceived at the site of the trigger point. The referred pain pattern does not occur immediately, however, because there is usually about a 10-sec delay involved.

Modern treatment of the direct and active type for trigger point problems depends heavily on what has been referred to as the "workhorse" of myofascial therapy, the stretch-and-spray technique utilizing vapocoolants. This method has been observed to inactivate "hot" trigger points more rapidly and with less patient discomfort than do local injection, dry-needling techniques, or ischemic compression methods. In simple, single muscle problems of fairly recent onset, full return to pain-free function is usually accomplished with several applications of vapocoolant to the skin over the particular muscle while the muscle is in a state of passive stretch. In more complicated anatomical areas containing multiple muscle groups, this techniques serves as a practical and efficient method of addressing a number of muscles all at once, which makes for significant progress in an overall treatment plan of pain relief. Another advantage of the stretch-and-spray technique is that exacting accuracy of application of the vapocoolant is not required. The stretch of the muscle (taut bands) is far more important than is the accuracy of vapocoolant application. It has also been observed that simple, gradual, and persistent gentle stretching of a muscle has a greater chance of quieting down or inactivating painful trigger points than does spraying without stretching. In spite of this, the usual pattern of treatment of this type is to first spray, then stretch out the muscle, and then spray the stretched muscle once again.

The passive stretch of the muscle required for the success of this technique at first poses a bit of a dilemma to the treating clinician. To thoroughly deactivate trigger points with the stretch-and-spray technique, the muscle must be stretched to its *full normal length*. Yet the reason the muscle is to receive such treatments in the first place is that it has suffered some sort of abuse or damage and the resultant trigger point formation has caused pain and restriction of movement. That means that full extension to its normal length is prohibited by the pain it would induce. Therefore, this natural limit must be approached sequentially by a series of spray-stretch-spray steps. Thus full extension is attained *gradually*. The involved muscle is passively stretched with slow steady pressure to the point at which the patient notices "tolerable discomfort." Overstretching at this point would induce painful protective myospasm problems. As the tension in the muscle is released due to the action of the vapocoolant, the operator (sometimes enlisting the aid of the patient) slowly and gradually continues to extend or stretch the muscle to keep the tension on it constant until its full range of extension is achieved, with sweeps of vapocoolant applied along the way as is needed. Once full pain-free extension is achieved, the return to normal resting length must also be smooth and gradual, with every effort made to avoid loading the muscle immediately.

Should a muscle become arrested during this process short of its full range of extension (the myogenic equivalent of getting stuck), continued vapocoolant spraying may not succeed. Several alternative treatments that may be utilized in this instance are, first, to spray the surrounding musculature to also deactivate latent or active trigger points in the adjacent muscles that may also be involved by virtue of exhibiting restriction of motion, a restriction that would prevent the specific muscle concerned from reaching its full extension. Second, the muscle may have to be treated with a hot pack for a few minutes to "recharge the system" so that subsequent vapocoolant spraying may once again become effective. One may also have the patient move the muscle(s) through several full range-of-motion cycles (as full as possible without pain, that is) before resumption of the stretch-and-spray technique. Gradually, full extension of the muscle is usually achieved (which is when spraying has its best effect) when such sequential methods are used in severe range-of-motion limitation situations.

The method found to be generally most successful in the stretch-and-spray technique involves spraying the target area in sweeps in the direction of the muscle fibers (taut bands) at about a 30-degree angle to the surface of the skin from a distance of approximately 18 in. The parallel sweeps with the spray should all be along this one direction only. They should begin at the attachment of the muscle containing the taut bands (and hence the trigger points also), sweep along the belly of the passively stretched muscle(s), and travel toward the area of referred pain. The referred pain area is then also sprayed. A slight overlap of the wet portion of the spray in successive sweeps is best. Two or three sweeps overlapping in such a manner usually is all that is required to cover a muscle adequately. Caution must be exercised, however, so as not to frost the skin, which can lead to chemical burn–type ulcerations. The mechanism by which the vapocoolant effects relief of pain and eliminates restriction of movement is through "tactile stimulus jamming" of the neurological circuitry concerned with pain transmission. But again, freezing surface layers of dermis is not required. The whiteness of the skin observed when the dichlorodifluoromethane (Fluori-Methane) vapocoolant spray evaporates is due to the sebum the coolant dissolves from the skin's pores. When frequent applications of vapocoolant are employed, the sebum can be easily replenished with common commercial hand creams.

Although the spraying with vapocoolant implies a certain casualness of application, it is surprising how much accuracy is actually required in

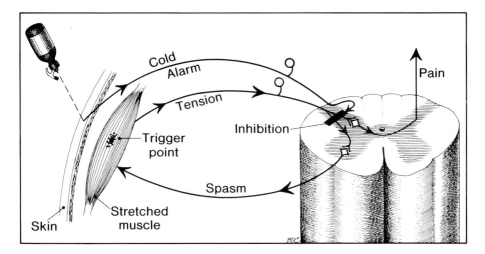

Figure 3–20 Schematic representation for the theoretical basis behind the observed effectiveness of the vapocoolant spray technique on deactivation of trigger points. The sudden stimuli of the vapocoolant spray on the skin over a primary trigger point site deeper in the underlying muscle inhibit the pain and reflex spasm that would otherwise prevent the passive stretching of that muscle. The black bar in the dorsal horn of the spinal cord symbolizes this inhibition (From Travell JG, Simons DG: *Myofascial Pain and Dysfunction, The Trigger Point Manual*. Baltimore, Williams & Wilkins, 1983, p 72. Used by permission.)

spraying the skin over a muscle at maximum extension. Being off target by as little as several centimeters may easily result in only a partial release of the tension that might be fully released in the muscle if the vapocoolant stream were more precisely directed. Sometimes the muscle tension is not released until the spray is extended all the way to cover the entire reference area of referred pain.

Once the stretch-and-spray technique deactivates the trigger points, they are no longer sensitive, and they no longer refer pain or restrict muscular extension. The tactile sensations of the vapocoolant facilitate the stretching of the affected muscle(s) by inhibiting pain and spinal stretch reflex mechanisms.

The advantage of the stretch-and-spray technique for the TMJ clinician is not only in pain relief of sore cervical musculature but also in the instances where trigger points seriously restrict mouth opening due to temporalis, medial pterygoid, and masseter muscular restrictions.

Yet as helpful as the stretch-and-spray techniques are in deactivating trigger points, reducing both primary-source pain and secondary referred pains in muscles, and restoring the full range of extension to those restricted muscles, there are times when the musculature does not fully respond to these methods as desired. In such instances, as the pain subsides, restriction of the full range of motion remains along with a certain amount of muscle stiffness, and the muscle seems less and less responsive to stretch-and-spray treatment. Thus the full painless maximum extension of muscle cannot be realized. Under such circumstances the clinician may choose to employ the second most popular form of treatment for trigger points: the "injection-and-stretch" technique.

Trigger point injection therapy is not as popular among clinicians as the easier methods of stretch-and-spray for several reasons. First of all, the exact site of the trigger point to be injected must be determined. This can be difficult for those inexperienced in taut band and trigger point palpation. Injection of trigger points may also result in an increase in soreness of the muscle for several days around the injection site. Ironically, this may intensify rather than eliminate referred pain patterns from trigger points that might remain in the injected muscle. This, of course, is a much less likely sequela of stretch-and-spray techniques. Nevertheless, the injection of trigger points has emerged as a modality in addressing myogenic pain.

The actual act of puncturing the trigger point with the tip of the needle seems to be an important component of the injection technique. Methods include dry-needling, injection of saline, or injection of local anesthetic. Dry-needling requires the greatest degree of accuracy of penetration. Due to the fact that no anesthetic is injected, however, breaking up trigger points with the needle tip in the dry-needling technique can prove most painful to the patient. Injected saline results in the same problem. Local anesthetics, of course, eliminate most of the pain of the trigger-point injection. However, although local anesthetics require the least amount of accuracy in placement, they may result in localized areas of muscle necrosis. Experienced clinicians who employ trigger point injection techniques prefer 22-gauge needles for the "feel" they provide of the structures being penetrated. For more sensitive patients or in cases where resultant ecchymosis may be an unsightly problem, 25-gauge needles may be substituted. But experts feel that the 27-gauge needle is too flexible for such procedures because it has a greater tendency to slide and deflect around the core of the trigger point in the taut band and provides fewer tactile sensations to the operator as to the consistency of tissue being penetrated.

Dr. Travell lists the following steps as a standard regimen for trigger point injection:

1. With the patient recumbent, always use a sterile technique to inject the trigger points with 0.5% procaine in isotonic saline until the area becomes nontender.
2. Immediately after the injection, passively stretch the muscle as parallel sweeps of the vapocoolant are directed over it.

3. Apply hot packs for a few minutes to reduce postinjection soreness.
4. Have the patient actively move the muscle through its complete range of motion.
5. If any local trigger point tenderness or restriction of movement remains, stretch and spray the entire myotatic unit, agonists, and antagonists.

(For a more detailed discussion of stretch-and-spray and injection-and-stretch techniques of trigger point therapy, the reader is referred to the classic text on the subject *Myofascial Pain and Dysfunction: The Trigger-Point Manual* by Drs. Travell and Simons.)

It should be noted that the stretching component is also an important part of the injection technique, as it is with that of the spray-and-stretch method. It should also be noted that when trigger points are injected with local anesthetic, it is best to use the lidocaine type without vasoconstrictor.

Although the mechanisms by which the injection technique deactivates the trigger point are ill understood, several theories have been proposed. First, the needle may actually mechanically disrupt the structure of the trigger point nodule itself. Once the neuromuscular loop that originates at the trigger point itself is interrupted, pain in the area, the referred pain, and the tension or ropiness of the taut band disappears. Another consideration is that the release of certain elements, such as potassium due to muscle cell damage, may cause a depolarization-type biochemical block of nerve fibers in the area of the trigger point. Another possibility theorized is that the fluids injected irrigate the trigger point area sufficiently so as to remove neural sensitizing toxins that may have accumulated to form the trigger point. But this does not explain the high success of dry-needling. It may well be a combination of these and other factors as yet unknown.

Other less widely used methods of directly addressing specific trigger point formation sites are massage, ischemic compression (sustained firm digital pressure over a trigger point of sufficient intensity and duration to deactivate it) stretching techniques without the benefit of the use of vapocoolant spray, moist heat, ultrasound, biofeedback, transcutaneous electrical stimulation, and pharmacological agents.

Thus it may be seen in light of the above that myofascial trigger points contribute to the musculoskeletal aches and pains of mankind. They are surprisingly overlooked as a source of referred pain patterns by members of the medical profession, and their presence in the maxillofacial complex has brought great consternation and diagnostic confusion to members of the dental profession. Scientific methods of treatment have been developed over the last 50 years that adequately address the trigger point problem in the muscles. Yet there still remains the problem of what *causes* them to form in the first place. This brings us back to the muscles of mastication, the muscular component of the teeth-bone-muscle triangle of the maxillofacial complex, and their relationship to the NRDM/SPDC phenomenon.

Trigger point treatments described above of the active and specific type, even though effective at relieving primary and secondary referred pains and restoring full ranges of extension and function of the affected muscles are, at their most basic level, essentially symptomatic in nature. The taut bands and their diminutive nodular-like trigger points are clearly defined entities to be sure. But they are merely "companions in crime" to other agents that bring about the classic headache, neck ache, and myofascial pains the patient with functionally induced TMJ arthrosis exhibits. Upon careful reflection, the relationship between the primary and secondary referred pains of the head and neck brought on by trigger point activity and the retrusive mandibular arc-of-closure problems of an NRDM/SPDC situation gradually becomes clear.

As Dr. Travell states, "Obvious inadequacies of body structure that perpetuate trigger points should be corrected before proceeding with intensive trigger point therapy." She further states, "Recovery of full function involves more than trigger point inactivation by stretch-and-spray. The muscle has learned dysfunction that restricts both its range and strength: It must relearn normal function."

A severe Class II retrusive mandibular situation is an inadequate occlusal relationship. A condyle forced up off the back edge of the articular disc into the bilaminar zone at full occlusion is an inadequate joint relationship. Overconstricted, overworked muscles that must effect this end against the entire design intent of the stomatognathic system and the initial limitations of joint anatomy create an inadequate muscular relationship. Teeth that interdigitate in such a way as to result in such a scenario, the NRDM/SPDC phenomenon, represent an inadequate occlusal relationship. Such "obvious inadequacies of body structure" do indeed require correction prior to intensive trigger point therapy, for it is just such an aggregate of inadequacies that sets the stage for the formation of multiple trigger points in the muscles of mastication in the first place. And it has been clinically observed that once the malocclusion has been corrected, once the joints have been adequately decompressed, once the muscles have been retrained, relengthened, and rehabilitated to a new occlusion that locks the mandible/condyle unit correctly down and forward, the pains that might result from trigger points throughout the maxillofacial complex are seen to drastically subside or cease altogether. With time this "passive" form of treatment of trigger points by means of the elimination of the muscle-abusing, retrusive-type malocclusion that spawned them results in their silence. But it must also be remembered that trigger points and their referred pain patterns are not the only agents responsible for headache and neck ache pains in the patient with TMJ problems. There are others.

"CAROTID PRESSURE REDISTRIBUTION" THEORY

The "carotid pressure redistribution" theory is one of the more interesting speculations on certain pain patterns that occur in the patient with TMJ pain. It has been observed that many patients complain of "sinus headaches," pain in the paranasal sinus area, and/or pain in the supraorbital region. This can occur in children, which often leads a well-meaning and concerned parent to seek an ophthalmic examination in the fear that glasses may be needed. This may or may not be the case. If so, the glasses will help the child see better but won't eliminate the headaches. When a patient's eyes cannot accommodate or focus well enough, the patient simply cannot see well. This has nothing to do with headaches. Occasionally the paranasal sinuses may suffer from acute sinusitis, but this is transient (7 to 10 days) and intensified by postural hypertension, i.e., bending over and touching the toes for 10 to 15 seconds and then quickly straightening up. Increased pain in the cheek, infraorbital, or nasal sinus area is all but pathognomonic for a maxillary sinus infection of some sort. A chronic paranasal sinus blockage can also cause similar headache pains because pathology in the nasal chambers seldom if ever causes pain at the original site but rather refers pain to the proximal parasinus area. However, such true sinusitis is easily discovered via routine otolaryngological diagnostic procedures.

Pains also are reported by patients with TMJ problems as arising in the temporal regions and the posterior auricular areas. These areas of headache are easily explained by simple muscle-splinting procedures that could result from the exertions of overretracting the mandibular arc of closure. The proximate source of pains of the frontal and supraorbital areas are a bit more difficult to decipher. The theory of carotid redistribution offers one possible explanation. As the mechanical and hydraulic pressures in the posterior joint space are increased due to condylar intrusion and chronic trauma-induced inflammation, the circulation through the superficial temporal artery can be progressively restricted. The histochemical needs of this muscle increase as its work is increased because of not only the usual demands of function but also the extra demands of abnormal function, i.e., bruxism. As a result the muscle calls for more circulation to bring additional nutrients and carry away surplus by-products of metabolism, which are building up within its tissues (lactic acidosis). However, this circulation is impaired due to the aforementioned pressure on the area of the superficial temporal artery that passes through the area of the posterior joint space. This allows the needs of the temporalis muscle to increase steadily without satisfaction. As a result it correspondingly calls for still more. Sensing this, the external carotid artery relaxes slightly to allow a greater volume of blood flow in an effort to answer these needs. Yet the restriction on the superficial temporal not only does not allow this increased blood flow to reach the far reaches of the temporalis muscle but causes a steadily increasing backpressure to spread out through the other branches of the external carotid, i.e., the posterior auricular and occipital, which run in a posterior direction, and the maxillary, which branches off in an anterior direction. One of the first branches of the maxillary artery is the middle meningeal artery, which not only serves the inferior aspect of the temporal lobe of the brain but also anastomoses with the lacrimal artery, which is part of a complex in the orbital cavity consisting of the dorsal nasal, anterior and posterior ethmoidal, supratrochlear, supraorbital, posterior ciliary, and anterior ciliary arteries. The arteries of this complex are all branches of the ophthalmic artery. Thus the areas of pain distribution described by many patients with TMJ problems as being in the supraorbital, frontal, or deep temporal area are all served by a series of arteries that are all but directly connected to the proximal end of the maxillary artery. It has long been common medical knowledge that so-called vascular headaches result from arterial distension and engorgement with blood. This is why the traditional treatment for such conditions has always involved the use of ergotamine or similar-acting arterial constrictors. Vascular distension of certain arteries is capable of generating formidable levels of pain in these arteries. Pharmacological agents that force constriction of these arteries relieves the pain of the increased blood pressure against the distended arterial wall. It seems some arteries as well as the bowel are very sensitive to excessive amounts of pressure within their lumina.

Returning to our backpressure theory, if this increased pressure of blood attempting to force its way through a restricted superficial temporal artery results in an increased arterial wall pressure being redistributed through the other branches of the external carotid, it could result in increased diastolic pressures in the middle meningeal artery and the arteries of the orbital cavity complex. These areas do not have the same need for blood as the temporalis does. They may try to resist the increased pressure by constricting for a while until they become exhausted, or the blood may simply force its way through the system and force distension as diastolic pressure increases. Either way, the final result is the same: painful distension due to hypertension against the arterial walls of the vessels that are distributed through these areas! The posterior auricular and occipital arteries may suffer the same fate. Since the pains described by patients follow predictable and fairly well defined anatomical areas that correspond to known arterial distributions, one might consider that these arteries may be highly innervated with pressure-sensitive nociceptors. Other arteries that branch off the maxillary do not elicit similar pain patterns along their distributions. Therefore, it may be safe to assume the others are not that well innervated. The "vascular headaches" will last until Nature finally manages to satisfy the needs of the temporalis muscle, get adequate circulation through the superficial temporal artery, and "even everything out a little," i.e., take the "pressure" off. Given half a

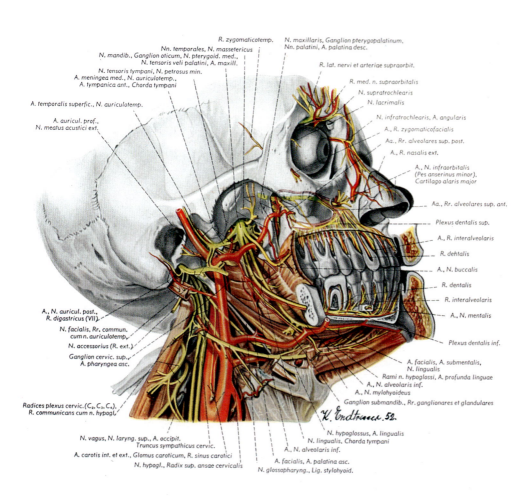

R. zygomaticotemp.
N. maxillaris, Ganglion pterygopalatinum,
Nn. temporales, N. massetericus
Nn. palatini, A. palatina desc.
N. mandib., Ganglion oticum, N. pterygoid. med.,
N. tensoris veli palatini, A. maxill.
R. lat. nervi et arteriae supraorbit.
N. tensoris tympani, N. petrosus min.
A. meningea med., N. auriculotemp.,
A. tympanica ant., Chorda tympani
R. med. n. supraorbitalis
N. supratrochlearis
A. temporalis superfic., N. auriculotemp.
N. lacrimalis
A. auricul. prof.,
N. meatus acustici ext.
N. infratrochlearis, A. angularis
A., R. zygomaticofacialis
Aa., Rr. alveolares sup. post.
A., R. nasalis ext.
A., N. infraorbitalis
(Pes anserinus minor),
Cartilago alaris major
Aa., Rr. alveolares sup. ant.
Plexus dentalis sup.
A., R. interalveolaris
R. dentalis
A., N. buccalis
R. dentalis
R. interalveolaris
A., N. auricul. post.,
R. digastricus (VII).
A., N. mentalis
N. facialis, Rr. commun.
cum n. auriculotemp.
N. accessorius (R. ext.)
Plexus dentalis inf.
Ganglion cervic. sup.,
A. pharyngea asc.
A. facialis, A. submentalis,
N. lingualis
Rami n. hypoglossi, A. profunda linguae
A., N. alveolaris inf.
A., N. mylohyoideus
Ganglion submandib., Rr. ganglionares et glandulares
Radices plexus cervic. (C₂, C₃, C₄),
R. communicans cum n. hypogl,
N. vagus, N. laryng. sup., A. occipit.
N. hypoglossus, A. lingualis
Truncus sympathicus cervic.
N. lingualis, Chorda tympani
A., N. alveolaris inf.
A. carotis int. et ext., Glomus caroticum, R. sinus carotici
N. hypogl., Radix sup. ansae cervicalis
A. facialis, A. palatina asc.
N. glossopharyng., Lig. stylohyoid.

Figure 3–21   Arteries and nerves of the jaw and deep layer of the face. The ramus of the mandible and deep muscles of mastication have been removed. The middle meningeal artery and arteries of the orbital cavity complex are directly linked to the external corotid via the maxillary artery. (Latin nomenclature is used in this illustration.) (From Pernkopf E: *Atlas of Topographical and Applied Human Anatomy*, vol 1. *Head and Neck.* Munich, Urban & Schwarzenberg, 1963, p 148. Used by permission.)

chance, Nature is ever willing to try to mend where mending is needed. The pain patterns of migraine, sinus, and vascular headaches are explained by the theory of carotid pressure redistribution. What makes the theory attract so much attention is that treatments of the FJO type that reposition the condyle down and forward in the fossa, thereby eliminating condylar pressure on the retrodiscal bilaminar tissues, also eliminate the classic symptoms of these types of headaches with a high percentage of success that is nothing short of alarming. After having observed such a high degree of success in eliminating the pain of these types of intense frontal, ocular, supraorbital, and temporal migrainelike headaches that appear in conjunction with functionally displaced condyles, there has emerged a certian body of avant-garde TMJ clinicians who have concluded that a true migraine or even other types of vascular distension headaches are extremely rare. Some are even honestly questioning whether there is such a thing or whether all such headaches of this type are merely varying manifestations of the classic TMJ-initiated–type headaches. In this case, the clinical techniques observed have generated a theory, instead of a theory generating an observable technique. Other systemic etiological agents may also be capable of generating classic migraine-type headaches. But the diagnosis of atypical migraine is often incorrectly used by physicians when in fact the true cause of the patient's symptoms is an improperly seated condyle!

Other symptoms associated with the patient with classic TMJ problems may also be accounted for by the theories of disrupted vascular function due to pressure. The causes of tinnitus, or buzzing, ringing, or hissing in the ears are poorly understood. Yet the anterior tympanic artery passes through the posterior fossa area of the joint at the tympanosquamous fissure, through which it passes in order to reach the tympanum. The deep auricular artery is another artery that serves the inner ear, and it arises from the maxillary branch of the external carotid close to its trunk. It follows the branch of the auriculotemporal nerve as it courses through the posterior joint space. It travels between the cartilage and bone of the acoustic meatus and supplies not only the skin of the meatus but also the outer surface of the eardrum. Restriction of circulation of these delicate but important arteries to the inner ear structures no doubt has an effect on the types of auricular symptoms the patients report.

Figure 3–22 Oblique lateral view of the arteries and nerves of the orbital complex after removal of the orbital roof. (Latin nomenclature is used in this illustration.) (From Pernkopf E: *Atlas of Topographical and Applied Human Anatomy*, vol 1. *Head and Neck*. Munich, Urban & Schwarzenberg, 1963, p 184. Used by permission.)

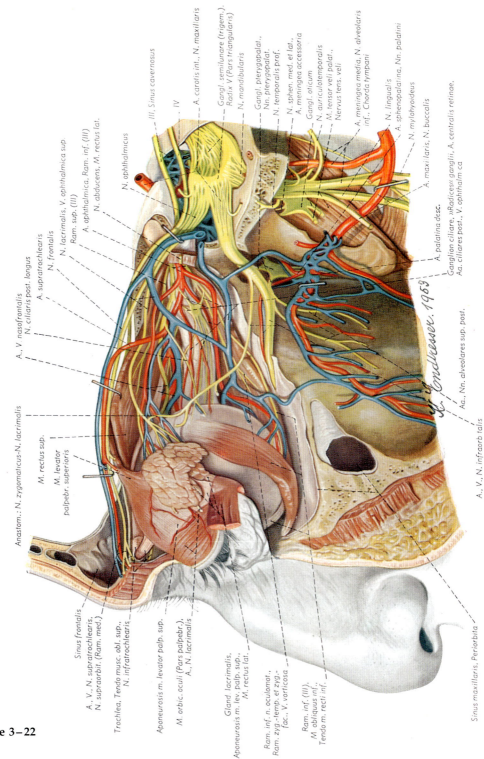

Anastom.: N. zygomaticus-N. lacrimalis

A., V. nasofrontalis

M. rectus sup.

N. ciliaris post. longus

A. supratrochlearis

M. levator
palpebr. superioris

N. frontalis

III, Sinus cavernosus

N. lacrimalis, V. ophthalmica sup.

Ram. sup. (III)

A. ophthalmica, Ram. inf. (III)

N. abducens, M. rectus lat.

IV

A. carotis int., N. maxillaris

Gangl. semilunare (trigem.),
Radix V (Pars triangularis)

N. mandibularis

Gangl. pterygopalat.,
Nn. pterygopalat.

N. temporalis prof.

N. sphen. med. et lat.

A. meningea accessoria

Gangl. oticum

N. auriculotemporalis

M. tensor veli palat.

Nervus tens. veli

A. meningea media, N. alveolaris
inf., Chorda tympani

N. lingualis

A. sphenopalatina, Nn. palatini

N. mylohyoideus

A. maxillaris, N. buccalis

N. ophthalmicus

A. palatina desc.

Ganglion ciliare, »Radices« ganglii, A. centralis retinae,
Aa. ciliares post., V. ophthalm ca

Aa. Nn. alveolares sup. post.

A., V., N. infraorb talis

Sinus frontalis

A., V., N. supratrochlearis,
N. supraorbit. (Ram. med.)

N. infratrochlearis

Trochlea, Tendo musc. obl. sup.,
N. infratrochlearis

Aponeurosis m. levator palp. sup.

M. orbic. oculi (Pars palpebr.),
A., N. lacrimalis

Gland. lacrimalis,

Aponeurosis m. lev. palp. sup.,
M. rectus lat.

Ram. inf. n. oculomot.,
Ram. zyg.-temp. et zyg.-
fac., V. vorticosa

Ram. inf. (III),
M. obliquus inf.,
Tendo m. recti inf.

Sinus maxillaris, Periorbita

Figure 3–22

THE NEURAL DEMYELINATION THEORY

Pain may also be referred from an originating site to a more distant site due to neurological dysfunction. It is a commonly observed phenomenon. Every dentist has had occasion to examine a patient who complains of a severe toothache in a lower molar only to find that the lower molar is fine but that the upper molar is in fact the one with a periapical abscess due to a necrotic pulp. Such circumstances have always been explained in terms of "signals getting crossed on the way to the brain" such that the patient actually perceives the pain in the lower tooth when it actually has its origin in the upper. This was attributed to the "primitiveness" of certain pain receptor sites for the dental area deep within the CNS. Well, primitiveness may not have as much to do with it as viruses.[130-135] Once

---

Figure 3–23 The right infratemporal fossa and TMJ. **(A)** After removal of the temporalis muscle, the zygomatic arch, the masseter muscle, and part of the mandible. **(B)** After removal of the lateral pterygoid muscle. **(C)** After removal of the mandible with the adjacent part of the neck. **(D)** From above, after removal of part of the middle cranial fossa. 1 = deep temporal nerve; 2 = deep temporal artery; 3 = upper head of lateral pterygoid; 4 = maxillary nerve; 5 = posterior superior alveolar nerve; 6 = posterior superior alveolar artery; 7 = infratemporal surface of maxilla; 8 = buccinator; 9 = buccal nerve; 10 = medial pterygoid; 11 = lingual nerve; 12 = inferior alveolar nerve; 13 = inferior alveolar artery; 14 = nerve to mylohyoid; 15 = lower head of lateral pterygoid; 16 = maxillary artery; 17 = masseteric nerve; 18 = articular disc of TMJ; 19 = capsule of TMJ; 20 = nerve to medial pterygoid; 21 = lateral pterygoid plate; 22 = chorda tympani; 23 = middle meningeal artery; 24 = accessory meningeal artery; 25 = mandibular nerve; 26 = nerve to lateral pterygoid; 27 = auriculotemporal nerve; 28 = tensor veli palatini; 29 = levator veli palatini; 30 = pharyngobasilar fascia; 31 = ascending palatine artery; 32 = superior constrictor of pharynx; 33 = pterygomandibular raphe; 34 = parotid duct; 35 = mucoperiosteum of mandible; 36 = submandibular ganglion; 37 = styloglossus; 38 = submandibular duct; 39 = hypoglossal nerve; 40 = mylohyoid; 41 = tendon of digastric; 42 = hyoid bone; 43 = thyrohyoid and nerve; 44 = stylohyoid; 45 = facial artery; 46 = hyoglossus; 47 = stylohyoid ligament; 48 = lingual artery; 49 = stylopharyngeus and glossopharyngeal nerve; 50 = ascending pharyngeal artery; 51 = internal carotid artery; 52 = hypoglossal nerve hooking round occipital artery and sternocleidomastoid branch; 53 = internal jugular vein; 54 = styloid process; 55 = roots of auriculotemporal nerve; 56 = posterior part of orbit; 57 = frontal nerve; 58 = floor of lateral part of middle cranial fossa; 59 = temporalis; 60 = optic nerve; 61 = oculomotor nerve; 62 = ophthalmic nerve; 63 = sphenoidal sinus; 64 = trigeminal nerve and ganglion; 65 = petrous part of temporal bone; 66 = greater petrosal nerve. (From McMinn RMH, Hutchings RT, Logan BM: *Color Atlas of Head and Neck Anatomy*. Chicago, Year Book Medical Publishers, Inc, 1985, p 116. Used by permission.)

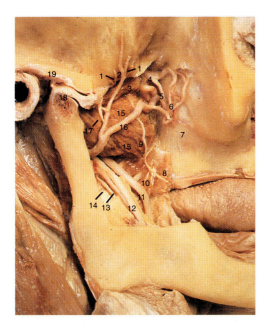

Figure 3–23(A)

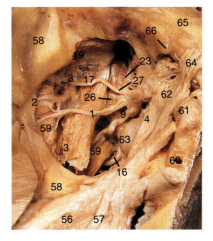

(B)

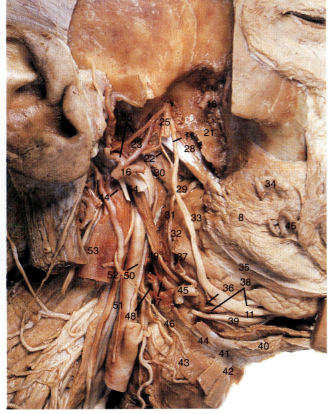

(C)

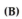

(D)

again, theory is relied upon to account for some of the symptomatology observed in the pain distribution patterns of the patient with classic TMJ problems.

The viruses responsible for herpes simplex (HSV-1) and varicella or herpes zoster are ubiquitous in nature. The herpes zoster virus is well known for its propensity to reproduce (travel) along posterior nerve trunks, the ganglia of the posterior nerve trunks, and the cerebral ganglia. This can result in the eruption of groups of small vesicles residing on an inflammatory base confluent with areas of dermis served by those receptive nerve trunks. The painful, swollen, macular eruptions of common herpes simplex in the area of the vermilion border of the lips are also often associated with periods of intensified stress, either physical or emotional.

In the early part of the 1980s some interesting advances were made in the knowledge of these common viruses. It was discovered that patients who suffered multiple herpetic infections showed EMG patterns indicative of occasional myospasm, fasciculation (small, localized areas of contraction of muscle tissue, visible through the dermis, that result from a spontaneous action of a number of fibers innervated by a single motor neuron), polyphasic motor potentials, as well as other signs of neuromuscular disruption. The investigators involved with these discoveries theorized that these signs and symptoms were suggestive of neural demyelination somewhere along the respective neural pathways involved. Viral demyelination often results in incomplete healing and repair of the demyelinized site. This, of course, can lead to improper signal transmissions or even cross-innervation as the electrical neural transmissions "jump" from one demyelinated neural pathway to another or even to normal, healthy, fully myelinated nerves. Eventual complete cessation of the nerve's ability to transmit impulses may also result. This can cause localized muscular atrophy of the innervated site if it occurs on a motor neuron. If viral demyelination occurs along sensory neurons, it is easy to conceive how a stimulus originating in one nerve, say the auriculotemporal, could "jump the track" at a given neurological or ganglionic site and be transmitted to the brain via a different neural pathway. As a result it would be perceived by the patient as a vague pain arising in a different area. Other studies by otolaryngological investigators have stated that HSV-1 often affects the gasserian (trigeminal) ganglion, facial nerves, and other cranial nerves and ganglia. When the HSV-1 virus becomes active and spreads along a nerve trunk, demyelination results as a product of a variant form of autoimmune response. Just how demyelination affects the ability of a nerve to control and/or transmit an impulse is not totally understood. Motor impulse can be impaired. Sensory impulses may also be impaired or redirected and result in referred pain. More knowledge of what actually happens is needed. The great frequency of occurrences of noxious stimulation (irritation, trauma) to the auriculotemporal nerve produces a large number of impulses, which, due to connection fibers of the facial nerve

(VII) and the number of ganglia (relay stations) involved in impulse transmission, may enter the CNS receptor sites in a number of possible ways. One thing is clear: repeated clinical observation reveals that reducing these vast numbers of noxious stimulations by eliminating pressure on the auriculotemporal nerve through repositioning the offending condyle down and forward out of the bilaminar zone and reducing chronic edematous intracapsular inflammation (another form of pressure on the nerve) resolves a great many if not all the headache and myofascial-type pains, regardless of their distribution, in the vast majority of patients with common TMJ problems. If some of the TMJ-type pain symptoms are in fact due to neurological dysfunction affected by mechanical and hydraulic pressures on the auriculotemporal nerve by an excessively superior posterior displaced condyle, it appears that decompression of the nerve by condylar advancement techniques results in ultimate resolution of whatever the neurological component of those pains might be.

HOMEOSTATIC DYSFUNCTION

Functionally oriented TMJ problems, which account for an enormous percentage of all cases, are caused by the NRDM/SPDC phenomenon. There are many stages of the TMJ pain-dysfunction condition that range from mild to severe. The secondary or accessory etiological agents responsible for enhancing and accelerating the onset of the condition that the malocclusion initiates are multifactorial. The two singularly most important facets of the TMJ symptomatology, however, are *stress* and *structure*. By "structure" is meant the relationship of the functional occlusion to the full-occlusion status of the disc-condyle-fossa complex. Although the two both commonly play a role in the appearance of the signs and symptoms of TMJ pain-dysfunction, the more important of the two is undoubtedly structure. For even in the complete absence of excessive stress, improperly balanced structure may of itself compromise the physical status of the joint to the point where this alone may bring on the occurrence of TMJ symptoms. Yet on the other hand, if the structure is ideal, as Nature intended, the patient at least has a chance of being symptom free under chronic periods of various forms of stress. And if symptoms of tired or sore muscles of mastication do occasionally appear in a structurally (and that also means occlusally) balanced individual as a result of overfunction, bruxism, etc., they are usually far less severe and of shorter duration. But once stress in any of its forms accumulates to a sufficient level of intensity and duration and combines with an imbalanced orthopedic and/or orthodontic structure, symptoms of TMJ pain-dysfunction, are bound to rise to the surface. The malocclusion (mechanical stress) ignites the TMJ fire, and all the other forms of stress—emotional, psychological, physiological, chemical, etc.—fan the flames.

It is not the purpose of this text to fully define or discuss the medical implications of stress and its effects on the TMJ other than by way of a review to remind the reader that it is a formidable force to be reckoned with and that knowledge of its forms and effects are important to a well-rounded approach to TMJ treatment. The very meaning of the term *stress* is ambiguous and may stand for many different things in different situations. Unless its specific meaning is clearly identified for the purposes of the respective discussion at hand, its interpretation can be misleading and lead to confusion and misunderstanding. This of course makes it a natural to fit right in with the rest of the vague and ambiguous terms used to describe the TMJ condition. But with a little clarification of its semantic meaning, a great deal of headway can be made in understanding the TMJ condition's physiological meaning. An improperly operating and/or painful TMJ is of itself a stressor to the body. The intimate relationship between stress and disease has long been common knowledge. Ever since the publication of the works of men like Hans Selye, whose landmark experiments using white rats led him to develop his theories of the "general adaptation syndrome," medical science has been aware of the direct chemical, physiological, and ultimately pathological relationship between untoward stress and the physical breakdown of the host. Stated simply, the human body is designed for stress. It is designed to adapt to stresses of all types on all levels. Stress in appropriate amounts is actually healthy for the body. However, when the accumulation of stress, in any one or a combination of its various forms, becomes great enough over a sufficiently adequate amount of time so as to push the host past the limits of his natural ability to compensate or properly *adapt*, physical degeneration ensues, often in the form that may be referred to as "disease." Thus the stress becomes pathological. Yet this pathological nature is more a matter of degree than of kind. Stress comes in many forms.

First there is physical or structural stress. This type of stress is the result of the biomechanical workings of the body itself. Exercise is a physical stressor. Only when such a physical stressor is carried to extremes does it become a form of pathological stress. An example would be strained or damaged muscles or ligaments of athletes, the appearance of blood in the urine of marathon runners, etc. A common aching back or sore shoulder is also an example of a symptomatic result of an excessive physical stress, but one from which the body may easily recover. Acute physical stress presents one type of picture, but chronic low-grade structural stress of an insidious nature presents quite another. Such a low-grade, yet chronic physical stressor might be represented by an occupational stress such as the type of improper stooping dentists are prone to do, the obvious physical problems of a mailman with one leg slightly longer than the other, or more specifically with respect to the subject at hand, an improper occlusion causing malalignment of the jaws during function. In such examples, chronicity sometimes proves more important than intensity.

Another form of stress to which the body is forced to adapt is chemical stress. Extremely complicated mechanisms within the body operate perpetually to keep the chemical environment of the entire system, even down to the intracellular level, balanced and buffered in the proper chemical homeostatic manner. The long list of commonly known metabolic disturbances that can cause havoc in the body bears ample testimony to the importance of maintaining a proper physiological chemistry. Diabetes mellitus is one of the most glaring examples. Chemical stressing of the body is an area we have a good deal of control over. Newly "rediscovered" by medical science, the process by which *we* influence the chemical or internal environments of our body in the form of diet and nutrition control has recently become very popular with physicians, other members of the health care profession, as well as with the general laity itself, as a brief excursion into any common bookstore will readily divulge.

It would be impossible to discuss the significance of proper nutrition in the brief space available here. But there can be no doubt as to its importance in maintaining proper health, especially to those individuals involved in the high-pressure, accelerated, stress-filled American life-style; this is even more so for those suffering from stress-aggravated TMJ pain-dysfunction symptoms. Briefly, the American diet may easily be nutritionally unsound if, for a given individual, it is canted in favor of high amounts of refined sugars (as opposed to the much more acceptable and less physiologically stressful naturally occurring sugars as in fresh fruits). The high degree of refined sugars in processed foods and low fiber content along with excessive amounts of stimulants (caffeine) and/or depressants (alcohol) can result in a diet that serves to act as a *chronic low-grade stressor*. Often one will observe that the more stress an individual is under (especially one who does not control his nutrition properly), the more prone that individual is to maintaining a diet high in the "quick fix" commodities of highly refined sugars, caffeine, and alcohol, not to mention smoking thrown in for good measure, although this particular habit is somewhat less prevalent now than in the past. The treating clinician need not be a nutritional expert or a health food "fanatic" but merely should inquire as to the customary dietary habits of the patient with TMJ problems, and if an obvious predisposition exists toward a considerably excessive usage of these elements, to which the patients will obligingly confess if questioned properly, the clinician may consider counseling the patient to a reduction of these elements as a means of reducing the overall stress load that must be adapted to and absorbed by the body. Some individuals seem to be more sensitive than others to dietary abuses. Some patients will surprisingly show a "sensitivity" to particular foods, some of which may be normally quite innocuous, such as milk, corn, dairy products (which turns out to be a bigger offender than formerly thought), or other items generally accepted as wholesome. Simple nutritional "experiments" may be undertaken by the patient at the advice of the treating clinician to determine whether certain foodstuffs or dietary regimens are inten-sifying either the stress load they are bearing or the frequency and/or intensity of the undesirable symptoms themselves. But there can be no doubt that dietary abuse in the form of ingestion of inappropriate amounts of refined sugars, caffeine, processed foods, alcohol, and to-bacco definitely exacerbate or intensify, maybe not the signs, but surely the symptoms of the attending TMJ pain-dysfunction–type headaches or other myofascial pains. The biochemical process of the homeostatic mech-anism of the mammalian species evolved naturally over hundreds of mil-lions of years. During that time, it was confronted with very few choco-late cupcakes or dry martinis. For eons, a ripe banana was most likely its biggest thrill!

Yet still another important form of stress that plays a critical role in the initiation of myofascial and TMJ symptoms is that of psychological and/or emotional stress. The effects of the emotions on the body are well known to all because we have all experienced them. Emotions are a part of daily life, and their effects are the result of naturally occurring neural and hormonal processes. The reddened face of embarrassment or anger, the perspiration and "sweaty palms" of stressful social interactions, the palpatating heart and dry mouth of a final examination, tax audit, or even the sight of a big buck coming through the woods on opening day of deer season are all perfectly natural emotional events. Yet, by their very na-ture, they are relatively brief in their scientifically measurable physiologi-cal effects on the body. A far more serious form of mental stress is the chronic, more insidious problem of psychological stress. The excessive mental strain of serious problems and tensions in the patient's work envi-ronment or personal life can have a great bearing on the physical well-being of the individual. Even a cursory review of these interrelationships would be nearly impossible in the space provided here. However, an im-portant inroad to gaining a groundwork understanding of the physiolog-ical significance of both mental and physiological stress and its relation-ship to the adaptive capacities of the body in general and the function of the TMJ and its musculature in specific may be obtained by a consider-ation of the commonly known and time-honored theories of the general adaptation syndrome of Hans Selye.[136–146]

After years of studying the effects of experimentally induced physi-cal stress on white rats and after clinically observing the effects of various forms of stress on patients at the University of Montreal, Selye devel-oped, among other theories, the concept of the general adaptation syn-drome (GAS) and the "local adaptation syndrome" (LAS). Selye notes that the word stress was at first defined as the "nonspecific response of the body to a demand." Stressing the entire body nonspecifically (by any of the aforementioned types of stress) produced a physiologically repeat-able set of general chemical and neural responses such as adrenal gland activation, diminution of lymphatic and reticuloendothelial activities, increased gastric acidity and digestive function alterations, loss of body weight, and a host of other less specific chemical and physical changes in the body that always appeared together (in varying degrees depending on the stress type and its intensity and duration) as a manifest group of reactions. This generalized, nonspecific, physiologically measurable, and repeatable response of the body to stressors was what Selye meant by GAS.

Alternately, when tissues are locally and acutely stressed as in trauma, infection, or other localized noxious stimuli, there also appeared in turn a *localized* tissue reaction in the form of inflammation and other localized tissue responses that Selye labeled the LAS.

He also points out that the two types of naturally occurring adaptive responses to stress, the GAS and the LAS, are chemically and neurologically interconnected and work hand in hand. What he refers to as "chemical alarm signals" are sent out by locally stressed tissues as a result of the LAS being activated by the noxious stimuli. These "signals" reach the CNS via the blood stream (or sometimes directly through the peripheral nervous system as in histamine or bradykinin release) and stimulate the control centers in the CNS to initiate the responses of the GAS by means of activation of the endocrine system, especially the pituitary and adrenal glands. These endocrine glands in turn produce, among others, two very important adaptive hormones, adrenocorticotropic hormone (ACTH), and adrenaline. This remotely induced, CNS governed neural response to stimulate hormonal production is an effort of the body to produce *adaptive* hormones to help the body through its period of undue stress, a stress that often might be in the form of common wear and tear. Thus the generalized nonspecific response of the GAS is activated for, supportive of, and stimulated by the localized response, the LAS.

Selye goes on to conveniently lump the adaptive hormones into two main categories: the anti-inflammatory adaptive hormones (glucocorticoids) such as ACTH, cortisone, and cortisol and the proinflammatory adaptive hormones (mineralocorticoids) such as somatotropic hormone (STH), aldosterone, and desoxycorticosterone (DOC). The aforementioned anti-inflammatory group inhibits excessive defensive physiological reactions, whereas the second category mentioned, the proinflammatory group, as the name implies, stimulates the defensive reactions of the body such as the process of common tissue inflammation.

Further, these processes may be either sensitized or exhausted by other hormones (especially epinephrine and thyroid hormones), nervous reactions, diet, and the tissue's memories of previous exposure to stress (like the chronic structural stress of a malocclusion in an individual who might also suffer from chronic bruxism).

Upon careful reflection, the role of the GAS/LAS adaptive phenomenon in the overall picture of TMJ problems becomes clear. Simply stated, chronic irritation and stressing of local tissues, such as the TMJ and its supporting musculature, from such chronic stressors as the aforementioned skeletal and/or dental malocclusion that is worsened by bruxism, causes localized tissue damage in the joint and therefore elicits a chronic LAS response in the TMJ area. This in turn stimulates a chronic GAS response throughout the whole body. The receptor tissues of the body become less sensitive to the repetitive low-grade stimulation of the various neural and hormonal adaptive reactions. The source of these adaptive stimuli may also become fatigued, and when greater periods of stress intermittently occur, the body (especially one "getting on in years") is less capable of fully adapting or compensating to the accumulations of what has now become no longer "healthy" but more correctly "pathological" stress. As a result, untoward responses result. These untoward responses for the patient with functionally induced TMJ arthrosis most often occur in the form of chronic headache, TMJ pain-dysfunction, myofascial pain, other homeostatic irregularities, and a whole host of other symptoms associated with chronic "TMJ syndrome"!

This may be at first a little confusing, but it bears out in the observance of the pretreatment and posttreatment anamnesis of patients who have been suffering from functionally induced TMJ problems. A pretreatment history of such patients commonly reveals not only a history of TMJ pain-dysfunction, headache, and neck pain but also various degrees of indigestion, irregularity, complaints of cold hands and feet (especially in females), stomach or bowel gas, excessive menstrual cramping or even menstrual irregularity, poor sleep, fatigue, or a general lack of energy. Upon correction of the joint problems, reversal of less nutritionally correct eating habits to a more appropriate and well-balanced diet, and the use of other forms of "stress relief," it is surprising how many of these systemic pretreatment symptoms diminish or disappear altogether.

The Selye theories state and support with enormous amounts of clinical evidence that chronic low-grade sympathomimetic, "fight-or-flight" responses elicited by the body due to the chronic stimulation of the GAS (which is a result of the accumulation of many forms of stress including the TMJ's own LAS) causes perpetual low-level amounts of stress adaptation hormones such as adrenaline to be produced by the body. Receptor hyposensitivity or exhaustion to such agents can lead to many of the above generalized symptoms, especially those concerned with circulation and digestion. Eliminating the noxious and excessive untoward stress to the body represented by an imbalanced, painful, and dysfunctioning TMJ will greatly aid that body in the reduction of the amount of stimulation of the specific LAS, which in turn results in less activity of the nonspecific GAS, which again in turn leaves the body stronger, "fresher," and more able to adapt to more acceptable stressors of daily life with a general all-around system that is not as depleted, desensitized, or exhausted.

The irony in all this is the vicious cycle represented by the phenomenon of bruxism. Briefly, bruxism is one of the body's ways of dealing with accumulated structural stress. Some feel it results from mental stress; others strongly feel that superior posterior condylar displacement off the disc is the ultimate triggering mechanism. It is theorized that the body is trying to "grind" its own anterior incisal or other occlusal interferences out of the way to free up the mandibular arc of closure and hence aid in decompressing the joint. Yet the more an individual is stressed by his own malocclusion as well as various other stressors to a level past the point where the body can successfully or easily adapt, the more this general adaptive phenomenon might be called into play, which depletes the body somewhat and leaves it all the more vulnerable to the effects of other subsequent improper or excessive stressors. This could easily in turn ironically lead to further bruxism! Patients with TMJ problems in an accelerated, high-tension life-style may characteristically skip breakfast in their hurry to race the clock to work, only to work physically and/or mentally hard all day and eat improperly (or not at all) along the way. They come home to a large meal requiring intense digestion, brux all night long on a skeletal and/or dental malocclusion robbing them of proper rest, wake up to repeat the process again the next day, and wonder why they often feel tired with frequent headaches and why their jaw muscles, ears, and temples are sore in the morning. The more they become stressed, the more both local and general symptoms increase, and the worse off they become. Yet, others seem to thrive on such stressful living and seem to adapt very well to it. What is the reason? One part of the answer might very well lie in the status of one of the body's greatest stress absorbers—the TMJ. The big question becomes whether the condyle rests properly on the disk during full-contact occlusion (bruxism) or improperly in the highly neurovascular bilaminar zone, with the disc "squished" forward ahead of it.

One will also observe that during periods of intense emotional, psychological, or even physical stress, the adaptive stress-compensating mechanisms of the body are called upon to perform to the fullest, and the body sustains an impressive and accelerated level of performance and/or resilience. Yet once the crisis is passed, the body, now somewhat depleted, seems to only then show the consequences of such "full-throttle" performance. Once the general adaptive mechanisms cease to exert their influence, the system seems to physiologically "let down" in a state of weakened recuperation. End-organ exhaustion may result. Sickness, general types of malaise, or other types of heretofore-hidden homeostatic breakdowns rise to the surface and become manifest. This may also occur in modified localized forms, even before the crisis is past, due to simple exhaustion of the system. This would account for the sporadic and sudden onset of massive amounts of symptoms associated with classic migraine-type headaches, i.e., aura, photosensitivity, nausea, vomiting, and finally intense vascular-type headache pains. Nature tries to readjust to varying circumstances, but you can burn Her physiological candle at both ends for only so long.

Numerous texts abound that are written on different levels for both health care professionals and laymen that are filled with information on the role of proper nutrition in health and disease. They range from manuals of sound nutritional facts to tomes of out-and-out quackery. It is not our purpose to discuss this discipline here. Suffice it to say that patients with TMJ problems have enough of a stress load provided to them by their malocclusions without worsening the circumstances by means of dietary excesses of unneeded biochemically stressful items and/or nutritional deficiencies of much-needed essential items. One interesting and sometimes helpful dietary regimen promoted consists of what is referred to as a "basic diet experiment," as listed below. Essentially, what it entails is a trial period of from 5 to 10 days during which the patient totally abstains from what are thought to be biochemically stressful agents, i.e., refined sugars, caffeine, alcohol, and processed white flour items. This dietary regimen accentuates items such as the more naturally occurring sugars available in fresh fruits and whole grain and unprocessed, nonartificial, natural-type foodstuffs. If due to the anamnesis of the case the patient is suspected of being sensitive to dietary control, as a surprising number of them are, they may be placed on the basic diet experiment for 10 days prior to insertion of the splint to see whether this has any effect on the frequency of headache pain or myofascial discomfort or how they feel in general. The basic diet experiment advocates the complete elimination during the trial period of not only conventional household sugar out of the sugar bowl but also the hidden sugars in processed foods. Instruct patients to read labels, and if anything ending in "-ose" appears in the first four ingredients listed on the label, tell the patient to avoid it completely. At first this may seem nearly impossible, with all the refined sugars processed into the commercially produced American diet, but instruct patients that it is for their own good and that such a strict type of dietary abstinence is only for a period of 10 days prior to insertion of the splint. Stress the consumption of fresh and natural foods as much as possible. Also warn those who are sugar or caffeine "addicts," like those who drink 3 or 4 cans of cola or 12 cups of coffee with sugar per day (and you will be surprised at how many there are), that they may experience headaches or nervousness about the second or third day of complete abstinence as the body actually goes through a short period of minor forms of common withdrawal from what is actually a slight chemical dependency. They may intensely crave these things for a day or so, but fortunately such cravings pass quickly. If after 10 days of faithful adherence to such a diet the patients note improvement in how they feel, they are then aware of the relationship of nutrition to their particular levels of stress and what it may do for them. Instruct them that it is desirable to maintain the "diet" at about the 80% to 90% level of what they have just experienced because this will be a great help in reducing at least the chemical stress load on the body. This also allows the patient and clinician to determine what percentage of the myofascial problem, if any, is related purely to dietary factors (or more correctly abuses) prior to splint insertion. If the basic diet experiment and the splint therapy are instituted simultaneously, such differentiations cannot be made. This also makes clear to both clinicians and patients alike that the occlusion cannot be blamed for everything. Then, when the treatment is complete, if the patient persists in dietary abuses after once knowing he has proved for himself that he is the type susceptible to such factors, any recurring occasional problems of muscle soreness, bruxism, etc., are his own responsibility and cannot be blamed on the clinician, although this does not obviate reexamination to determine whether new or undetected occlusal disharmonies are present.

Many Americans, especially those in accelerated, stress-filled lifestyles, tend to quite often eat what is convenient for them, not necessarily what is good for them. Pain and dysfunction are a sign of at least some form of bodily breakdown. Maybe part of the problem is related to the nature of the fuel the body is forced to run on!

Just why some patients who have been treated successfully for functionally induced TMJ problems and have been nutritionally "cleaned up" will suffer a "hangover-type" headache the morning after eating a chocolate sundae is unknown. Yet it is surprising how sensitive some patients are to such things as chocolate, caffeine, red wines, the fusel oils of champagne, etc. Although the mechanisms of "food allergy" headaches is uncertain, two clinical observations have been made with great certainty. First, such things do exist, but there is currently no way, other than the aforementioned experimental abstinence methods, of telling which patient will be sensitive and which will not. Nor is there any way of telling which foods or beverages will be the offending agents. The aforementioned items of refined sugars, caffeine, alcohol, and tobacco are common offenders. Second, patients can develop a form of tolerance and a mild form of "addiction" to such substances that makes total abstinence resemble a brief period of withdrawal after which the cravings cease but reexposure to the offending agent may elicit a more intense response than usual. It is as if the body has lost its adaptive ability to cope with such biochemical insults.

Other stressors besides nutritional abuses can upset the homeostatic balance of patients and contribute to their particular picture of TMJ symptomatology. If the distal-driving occlusion ignites the TMJ fire and other nutritional, emotional, and physiological stressors fan the flames, then the additional intensifying stressors represented by the periodic fluctuations of estrogen and progesterone attendant to the female menstrual cycle can turn it into a blast furnace. The physiological and emotional changes experienced by women as a result of the menstrual cycle are clearly a source of stress to their entire homeostatic system. This is a commonly observed circumstance to which any postpubertal female will readily attest. It will be observed that the vast majority of patients presenting for TMJ treatment will be female in ratios far beyond the time-honored 4 to 1. Current estimates are more like 8 to 1 or greater. The details of the exact physiological interactions of this mechanism with the level of intensity of TMJ symptoms is unknown, but overriding generalizations can be made. Females who have gone through puberty simply do not hold up well under the circumstances brought on by the typical TMJ condition. Their resilience against the problems that a functionally induced TMJ arthrosis represents clearly seem to be less than that of men. But there is no difference in how they respond to treatment. Eliminate condylar displacement into the posterior joint space at full occlusion, and male or female, the patient will experience relief of their TMJ-related symptoms. This in turn will leave the body more fit to manage the other physiological problems it must face in a day.

GENERAL SYSTEMIC DYSFUNCTIONS

At this point it would be best to remind the reader that the purpose of this text is to discuss the etiology, diagnosis, and treatment of the malocclusion-initiated, functionally oriented TMJ arthrosis. The chief area of concern for both patient and clinician in these areas is the cardinal symptom of the condition, i.e., pain. It is most commonly a headache-type pain but can manifest itself in a variety of fashions and in a variety of anatomical regions in the maxillofacial complex. It can be exacerbated, modified, and intensified by stress. But a superiorly posteriorly displaced condyle is not the only thing that can give the patient varying manifestations of cephalalgia. Although it is by far the leading cause, there are other much less frequently observed conditions of a general systemic nature that the clinician should keep in mind that may cause headache symptoms in the complete absence of a true TMJ problem of a functional nature.

The following paragraphs list some of the more commonly known diseases and conditions that may produce myofascial or cephalalgic-type pains.

Neurological diseases can not only produce pain, but they are often associated with disruption of motor and/or sensory actions of the affected peripheral nerves or areas of the CNS.

Trigeminal neuralgia is characterized by paroxysmal pain of a sudden, sharp, lancinating nature that is precipitated by various stimuli. Sometimes it only requires touching a certain trigger area on the surface of the skin to incite the reaction. However, the pain is only of brief duration and follows the distribution of one of the branches of the trigeminal nerve. Facial grimace (or tic, hence the name tic douloureux) also is associated with this condition. Glossopharyngeal neuralgia is a similar condition that affects the glossopharyngeal nerve distribution. Another neuralgia, sphenopalatine neuralgia, has been reported to cause "cluster" headaches.

Neuroma, or a tumor of the nerve itself, of the various cranial nerves may also occur. The acoustic neuroma is one of the most common. However, it is benign.

Meningioma involves the tissue that wraps the brain and spinal cord. They are most common in the midline of the brain, but they can be anywhere on the meningeal tissue. Most are benign and cause cephalalgia-type pains because of the traction and stretching they induce on the meninges and/or dura. The pain actually originates in the dura because the brain itself has no sensory innervation.

Miscellaneous neoplasms of any sort may metastasize to the brain. Tumor-type cephalalgic pain is usually gradual in onset, it is steady and unremitting, and it reaches a crescendo over a period of months.

Epidermoid (sebaceous) cysts can cause traction-type headache pain. They commonly occur in males on the back of the scalp and neck at the hairline.

Lymphomas of the Hodgkin's type or non-Hodgkin's type, which are tumors of the lymphatic system, can cause pressure headaches when the sinuses are affected.

Malignant otitis externa is not an actual malignancy but a recurring infection of the external ear canal. It is a very aggressive infection, almost like an osteomyelitis, that is very difficult to treat. A variety of other otic infections may also occur that can cause pain in the auricular and TMJ area, such as serous otitis or otitis media.

Other more common causes of cephalalgia are paranasal sinus infections, which never cause pain in the nasal sinus itself but rather refer pain to the surrounding areas; menstrual irregularities; viral encephalitis; hyperthyroidism; hypoglycemia due to diabetes mellitus; fad diets; eating disorders such as anorexia nervosa; and side reactions from common medications, one of the most common offenders of which are birth control pills.

VARIOUS TYPES OF TMJ ARTHRITIDES

The main focus of attention the FJO approach addresses in the TMJ theater of arthritides is on that type of joint arthritis and/or disarticulation that we have been discussing whereby occlusal and/or orthopedic imbalances anteriorly in the jaws during the functional generation of the forces of occlusion result in a disharmonious or abnormal functioning posteriorly of the TMJ and its associated musculature. We have seen how this process alone may result in tooth pain, jaw pain, tinnitus, endless varieties of headache, and myofascial pain of a chronic or acute nature along with actual joint pain and dysfunction. We have also seen that there is often attending intracapsular tissue changes that can lead to full-scale degeneration of bony and cartilaginous tissues. Yet, in addition to this main subject of what is essentially a traumatic TMJ-type arthritis of a functionally oriented nature, it would serve well to briefly review the other types of pathology that may exist either alone or in conjunction with the above that are capable of producing a similar symptomatic picture or most likely confusing, compounding, and intensifying it further.

Osteoarthritis

Before specifically discussing the details of the different manifestations of osteoarthritis, it would be handy to consider a brief overview of the common characteristics this group of conditions all exhibit in general. More correctly referred to as degenerative arthritis, osteoarthritis is a chronic condition, insidious in onset, that represents the effects of time and use on the joint tissues of the body. Hence, this type is also commonly thought of as simple "wear-and-tear" arthritis. It may easily result from the natural transition along the degenerative pathway from the common functionally traumatic TMJ arthritic process mentioned above. Avascular necrosis may represent an important link in the general degenerative pathway the joint may follow from functionally oriented traumatic arthritis to chronic osteoarthritis. Some feel that the host resistance level is a major determinant as to whether or not chronic traumatic functional pain-dysfunction–type TMJ arthritis will eventually develop into what may be defined as osteoarthritis. Others feel that although this may or may not be a factor, the extent of the malocclusion and its ability to distal-drive the mandibular arc of closure, i.e., the severity of the malocclusion and the attending NRDM/SPDC phenomenon (or lack thereof), act as its own limiting factors as to whether or not this transition will take place. However, one thing by definition is sure. Chronic localized trauma to the joint itself has been established as a prime etiological agent in the development of these types of conditions. Symptomatically with respect to the TMJ, these two types, chronic functionally induced arthritis and osteoarthritis, appear nearly identical. The more advanced osteoarthritic form of the condition, however, more clearly presents definitive osseous changes that may be either directly observable clinically or detected by means of radiography. One difference between the two by definition is that chronic degenerative osteoarthritis is associated with a lack of acute inflammation of the joint, or at least a more muted form of it. However, there are important exceptions to this as we shall see later. But this lack of intense inflammation could easily result from Nature sort of reaching a homeostatic equilibrium between the remaining available joint space at hand and the needs of the opposing surfaces of that joint space for the healing and nutritive sustenance of the available circulation. In osteoarthritic manifestations, as the intervening cartilage is gradually eroded away by chronic abuse or wear and tear, the joint space between the articulating bony surfaces characteristically gets smaller, and the bones seem to "drift" closer to one another until in the specific case of the TMJ the intra-articular cartilage and/or its posterior attachment is completely destroyed and the opposing articulating osseous elements finally make contact, bone on bone. Without the normal cushion of fibrocartilage in the form of an intra-articular disc between them to protect their articular surfaces, the interfacing bones suffer osseous breakdown, at which point osteoarthritic remodeling results. Both the articular cartilage and the bony articular surfaces of the joint degenerate. As a result, the articular surfaces of the bones present a roughened or irregular border radiographically. Eburnation may also be present, which is the process whereby the denuded surface of the bone becomes condensed or hardened and gives it the characteristic "ivory-like" appearance. Sometimes the edges of the cartilage covering the articular surface of the bone survive the degenerative process (due to better blood supply around the periphery) and become somewhat calcified to produce the "lipping" that is also characteristically seen on the head of the condyle in advanced forms of the condition. The abuses of wear and tear may have the condylar head worn flat. Synovial membranes, at first chronically inflamed, may also break down or on occasion may lose small ragged portions that remain in the synovial space where they may form cartilagenous-type foreign bodies or calcifications known as "joint mice." Oddly, it has been observed clinically that there seems to be no direct correlation between the degree of bony changes and the severity of the symptoms! Correct treatment to remove the source of traumatic function to the joint relieves the patient's symptoms, but the osseous changes in the articular portions of the bone remain as if immutable. It has been pointed out that the difference between chronic traumatic TMJ arthritis and osteoarthritis is more a matter of degree than of type with respect to the TMJ. The two in all likelihood merely represent various manifestations of the same degenerative process.

More specifically, osteoarthritis is sometimes referred to as degenerative or hypertrophic osteoarthrosis in an effort to emphasize the hypertrophic changes exhibited by the cartilage and bone of the involved joint. It is a condition ubiquitous in Nature and something from which we all will most likely suffer in one form or another as we advance in years. One paradoxical attribute often noted concerning osteoarthritis is that most patients only experience minimal pain and stiffness of the affected joint. However, a small percentage of less fortunate patients may experience severe symptoms. Another seeming contradiction is that there is no inflammatory component associated with the condition. This may be accounted for by the equilibrium of Nature's attempts at healing the injured site as previously alluded to, and such an effort would be enhanced by the fact that as the condylar surface is resorbed due to the remodeling that takes place, the posterior joint space necessarily gains volume by default. It's as if the condyles "melt down" under pressure until an equilibrium is reached between the demands of the tissue and the availability of pressure-free joint space. At this point things seem to "cool down" within the joint, and the characteristic inflammation associated with more acute situations disappears. This also brings to light another point of semantic confusion. The noninflammatory degeneration of an articular cartilage is correctly referred to as an arthrosis. The term *arthritis* implies active and reasonably intense localized inflammation. Thus the notion of a chronic degenerative osteoarthritis of the TMJ starts to take on a slightly more vague and contradictory meaning, but then again, in the field of TMJ semantics, it's in good terminological company.

Another point to bear in mind is that inflammation within the joint is most often a product of the functional abuse it must be forced to endure. Inflammation within the TMJ capsule can wax and wane with the amount of bruxism the joint experiences. Therefore, use of either the "-itis" or "-osis" suffix is more a matter of the patient's present symptomatic condition and thus is subject to some fluctuation.

Three basic types of osteoarthritis are defined as per the type of joints in which the condition occurs. The first type is characterized by the formation of knobby enlargements of the joints of the fingers, referred to as Heberden's nodes. These usually appear over a period of years. The condition is not usually acutely painful, is more prevalent in females than in males, and tends to be familial. It can, however, occur in an acutely painful form that causes painful swelling to appear over a period of 3 to 4 weeks. It is usually confined to only one finger or joint. This acute form of the condition usually runs its course in 1 to 2 weeks and is self-limiting, although it can be recurrent.

The second type of osteoarthrosis occurs in the spine and is the simple result of the accumulation of wear over the years. As the intravertebral discs wear, the joint space narrows, and the spine shortens. The condition is not of itself painful and is one of the factors responsible for the loss of total body height in old age.

The third form of osteoarthrosis is associated with weight-bearing joints. It is this type that serves as the classic model of osteoarthritis and is the category to which the TMJ, as a stress-bearing joint, belongs. This type of osteoarthritis/arthrosis manifests itself in the TMJ in three basic types, all of which involve some sort of effort by Nature to adapt to the demands of the individual members concerned with the situation. They are the following.

Regressive remodeling   This first form of degenerative remodeling is the most common process observed under the category of osteoarthritic changes within the TMJ. Not only do the joint spaces appear narrower, a common observation associated with earlier forms of the TMJ condylar displacement condition, but the condyle also exhibits flattening or other forms of irregularities over its articular surface. Over a period of time, degenerative remodeling always implies the presence of sclerotic bone in the area where the original articular outline has been lost. Chronic synovitis often accompanies this stage of degeneration due to irritation of these tissues. The synovial membranes may also thicken due to their irritation. Modern studies with magnetic resonance imaging techniques have shown that these areas of sclerotic bone are not confined to the articular surface but exhibit a "soaking-in" effect, and pathological osseous alterations may be seen to extend well down into the condylar head and neck in more severe cases. Of course, as might be surmised, joint sounds of the crepitus variety are also commonly present during joint movements, as are a whole raft of other signs and symptoms traditionally associated with advanced forms of TMJ arthritic degeneration: limited range of motion, irregular or deviated mandibular opening and closing movements, pain in the actual joint area during loading (as in masticating coarse foods), pain upon external palpation of the joint, cephalalgia, cervicalgia, myofascial pains of the classic TMJ type, and even vertigo and facial muscle spasm problems. As an advanced form of TMJ degeneration, the osteoarthritis/arthrosis of the joint is all but invariably the end stages of a process that began with a malocclusion-initiated NRDM/SPDC phenomenon, i.e., attending anterior disc displacement; reciprocal clicking; occasional periods of clinically closed-lock, limited-opening situations; and traditional TMJ-type headache, neck ache, and myofascial pains. With an exacerbation of intracapsular inflammation present as a result of a period of intensified bruxism, reduced host resistance, or other such abuses, the condition may be referred to as a degenerative osteoarthritis. When things are a bit "cooler" intracapsularly due to the diminished edema and inflammation that result from Nature's attempts to cope, it may be addressed as an osteoarthrosis. Either way, it's the end of the line for a joint that once was fine and whole and worked well until something in the occlusion started forcing the mandibular arc of closure back too far and lit the fuse.

Peripheral remodeling   Sometimes referred to as circumferential remodeling, this second type of TMJ osteoarthritis/arthrosis peripheral on remodeling consists of shortening of the top of the condylar head's convex capitular surface such that it appears to be flattened. The edges of the condyle are lipped in a fashion that gives the condyle a mushroomed appearance. This mushrooming of the edge of the condyle's articular facet is due to the remodeling activity that takes place there. As previously stated, most anteriorly displaced discs are displaced both anteriorly and medially. This implies degeneration of the connective tissues at the lateral pole, such as the lateral collateral ligament. The peripheral bone at the edge of the condylar articular facet adjacent to the edges of the area of capitular resorption and the area of disc degeneration at the lateral pole proliferates and grows into this area, thus producing the characteristic mushroom-shaped lipping. It gives an outline to the condylar head that lets one imagine the condyle as a high-speed projectile that struck the target—fossa—with enough velocity to peel back its edges and flatten its head similar to a bullet mushrooming on impact. Peripheral remodeling can also occur at the medial pole but may only be detected via anteroposterior radiographic views. As with other forms of osteoarthritic degeneration, the remodeling is a product of Nature trying to deal with the reduced functional joint space.

Progressive remodeling   As the name implies the third type of osteoarthritis known as progressive remodeling represents the opposite of regressive remodeling. In this manifestation, bone does not "melt away," but rather "spikes up," for progressive remodeling is associated with osteophyte formation. This can occur on the condylar and/or eminential articular surfaces. This is almost invariably associated with discal or posterior lamina perforation. Pain and joint sounds upon motion are commonly associated with osteophyte formation. They often appear as sharp little bumps or spicules on the condyle or articular surface of the eminence directly adjacent to the area of the perforation. It is again associated with excessive encroachment of the condylar head into the posterior joint space.

Rheumatoid Arthritis

This disorder is of systemic origins, and the etiology remains as yet unknown. In times past under the aegis of the theory of focal infection, it was once erroneously thought that rheumatoid arthritis resulted from streptococcal infections of the teeth and tonsils. As a result of that theory innumerable abscessed teeth and infected tonsils were removed in an effort to eliminate the "foci" of infection and stem the tide of the joint diseases. Now the prime etiological factor is believed to be of an autoimmune response disparity. Insidious in onset, although it may be acute in children (Still's disease), it usually affects the smaller joints of the body, i.e., fingers and toes, with TMJ involvement appearing in only about 10%

Figure 3–24   Rheumatoid arthritis of the TMJ. Fewer than 0.1% of all patients with TMJ problems are rheumatoid arthritis patients. **(A)** Cephalometric radiograph of a 12-year-old girl with bilateral rheumatoid arthritis of the TMJs. **(B)** Cephalogram of the same patient at 16 years of age. **(C)** Cephalometric tracing of A. **(D)** Cephalometric tracing of B. As the condyles resorb due to the rheumatoid arthritic process, note how the mandibular plane angle increases and an anterior open bite develops due to loss of posterior vertical support as a result of reduced condylar height. **(E)** Radiographs of condyles of the same patient at 16 years of age. Note the diminutive condylar size and ragged "moth-eaten" appearance. **(F)** Another case of rheumatoid arthritis of the TMJs in a 12-year-old girl. Again note the condylar distortion, resorption, and ragged appearance. (Courtesy of Dr. Jack Marteney, Tucson.)

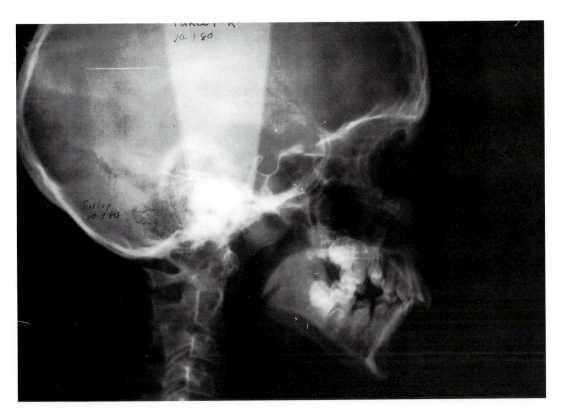

Figure 3–24(A)

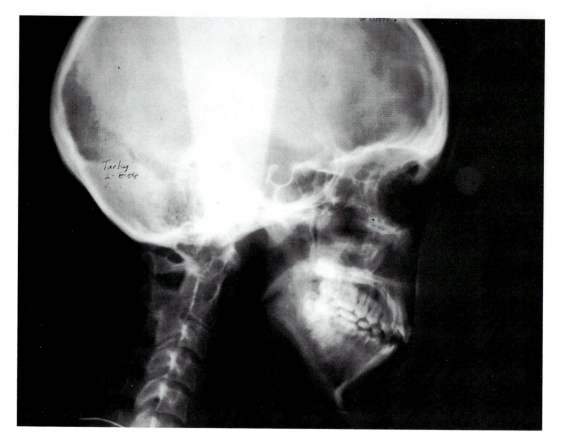

(B)

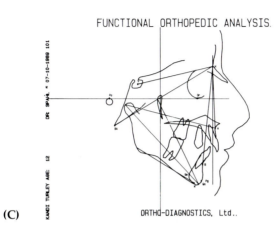

(C)

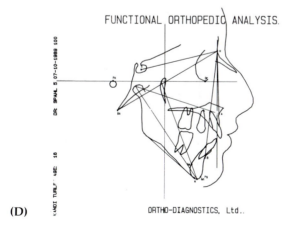

(D)

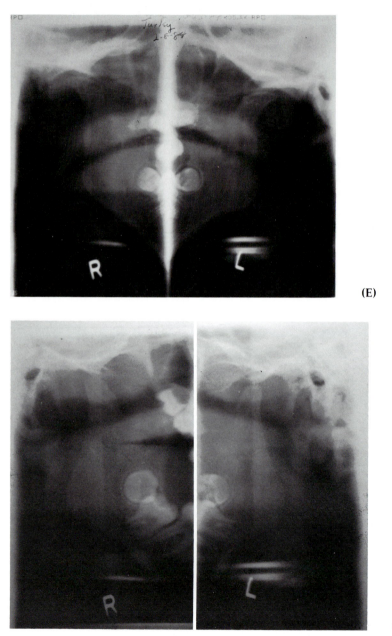

(E)

(F)

of the patients with systemic rheumatoid arthritis. Although the disorder is characteristic in its exacerbations and remissions, the joint changes are permanent. The most common sites of occurrence, the joints of the fingers or toes, characteristically swell, deform, and take on what is called a "doughy" feel. The synovial membranes seem to "attack and destroy" the intra-articular cartilage and adjacent bone and are so particularly affected as to cause some to suggest that the disease might be more correctly referred to as "synovioarthritis" to contrast it to the previously mentioned osteoarthritis. In the later stages of the disorder the appearance of the swollen synovial membranes around the affected joints, the appearance in some cases of subcutaneous nodules (usually on the forearm dorsal surface similar to those of rheumatic fever), the general history of a gradual onset starting with morning stiffness, and the sporadic nature of the occurrence of the painful symptoms make for an easy clinical diagnosis. The synovial membranes are oddly the culprits in this type of arthritis. By a mechanism not clearly understood, as the membranes invade and erode the joint cartilage itself as well as the articular bone, the joint space characteristically appears to widen as the opposing bones of the affected joint seem to radiographically drift away from one another and the space fills with a "doughy" type of scar tissue. Should such a type of arthritis be present in a TMJ in the complete absence of a posteriorly displaced condyle and no other structural imbalances and/or occlusal interferences contributing to that particular joint's arthritis, treatment should be deferred to the appropriate medical authorities for systemic management. But such patients should be carefully examined to ensure that functional disharmonies are not compounding the problem by adding noxious stimuli of the chronic traumatic arthritis type to an already medically compromised joint. Suspicions of early stages of the rheumatoid type of disorder resulting from the anamnesis of the case should also induce medical evaluation and confirmation of the existence of the systemic condition through appropriate laboratory tests. However, not every patient with rheumatoid arthritis will degenerate to the state of complete joint crippling. A large percentage of these patients go on to full remission, whereas only a lesser percentage continue on to the more crippling forms of the advanced stages of the disease.

Part of the reason for this is that, like the osteoarthritis/arthrosis variety, rheumatoid arthritis manifests itself in various levels of involvement. The mildest form is monocyclic rheumatoid arthritis, which lasts for only several months, is self-limiting, and leaves no permanent form of structural damage or disability in the joint after remission. A more advanced level of involvement is referred to as polycyclic rheumatoid, which is the same as the monocyclic type other than it recurs on a periodic basis. There will be long periods of remission interrupted by sporadic exacerbations of the condition with little or no long-term structural damage or disability remaining in the joint. The most advanced level of involvement and, unfortunately for the general populace of patients, the most common is the chronic rheumatoid variety. Differential diagnosis of this type is usually predicated upon the presence of rheumatoid factor in the blood sample and the duration of the symptoms, i.e., symptoms that have been present on a consistent basis for a year or longer.

Another aspect that is similar to osteoarthritis/arthrosis is that rheumatoid arthritis goes through a series of stages in the process of joint degeneration. In the TMJ it has a predictible sequence of manifestations. The first is the edema phase, which is characterized by intracapsular edema and posterior capsulitis. As might be expected, pressure in a rearward direction on the mandible causes a sharp pain in the joint, whereas the patient may protrude the jaw with relative impunity. The soft-tissue swelling around the joint in unison with the intracapsular edema present can make normal functional occlusion of the teeth so painful that the patients complain of not being able to close their back teeth together. This may be accompanied by a limited range of jaw opening and/or deviation to one side. One thing about rheumatoid arthritis is definitely different from osteoarthritis: characteristically, once the condition starts to attack and dissolve bone, the joint spaces start getting larger, not smaller. The second level of rheumatoid arthritic involvement of the TMJ is the granulation phase. Here gross remodeling has seriously deformed the original outline of the condylar head. The outline of the fossa also suffers bony degeneration and as a result appears to widen out its arc. This also adds to the impression that the bones are drifting apart. It has been noted that the appearance of the condyle at this stage of degeneration resembles the necrosis seen in joints after steroid injection directly into the joint. (This particular treatment modality is of course contraindicated for patients with TMJ problems.) The next phase is a more advanced manifestation of the granulation phase. Here the joint space seems inordinately enlarged as both the condyle and fossa suffer advanced bony erosion. The final phase is the osteoarthritic phase of rheumatoid arthritis and is characterized by collapse of the joint, hence compression of the joint space once again, advanced degenerative remodeling, and acute pain. The unfortunate patients who suffer from rheumatoid arthritis in conjunction with a distal-driving malocclusion require a teamwork approach to treatment and a carefully monitored liaison between the dental and medical practitioner.

Gout

Gouty arthritis is mentioned here as a reminder that a careful history is important to proper diagnosis. It is seldom that one will observe this condition affecting the TMJ as the joints of the extremities are usually affected, most often being those of the foot. The old name for this disease, "podagra," comes from the Greek roots *pod* for "foot" and *agra* for "attack." Associated throughout history with men of genius and "rich living," gout is almost exclusive to males and results from deposits in the affected joints of overabundant amounts of uric acid. These deposits can form gouty tophi in the joints of the fingers that cause these joints to swell and appear identical to those of rheumatoid arthritis. Again, such conditions are in the realm of general medicine, but patients should be carefully screened for possible concomitant joint disharmonies of dental origins.

Miscellaneous

TMJ arthritidies may also be a result of a host of various other acute or subacute etiological agents. Systemic symptoms along with a careful history and clinical examinations utilizing appropriate radiographs will help determine whether the actual signs and symptoms of true functionally caused traumatic TMJ arthritis are present. Obviously nothing would be more confusing to the diagnostician than a functionally induced localized TMJ pain-dysfunction problem that is complicated, intensified, and/or camouflaged by a generalized systemic malady of some sort. Difficult TMJ management cases evidenced by attending complaints of generalized body, joint, or muscle aches, pains, and/or weakness, unusual pain patterns, general malaise, unusual psychological patterns or signs of severe episodes of clinical depression require expert, comprehensive medical evaluation that include—but are not limited to—tests for blood dyscrasias, hormone imbalances (especially thyroid), dietary deficiencies and even autoimmune conditions (i.e., lupus erythematosus).

Nonarticular Rheumatism

One of the newly "rediscovered" areas of concern that can be categorized under the general heading of homeostatic dysfunctions is that whole raft of muscle, joint, and ligament pain conditions lumped under the evasive term of nonarticular rheumatism. The term *rheumatism* is of ancient origins, yet in modern-day usage it has numerous vague meanings, which of course makes it right at home in the TMJ theater of operations. Its most distant etymological root is the Greek word *rheuma*, meaning a "watery or catarrhal discharge." Rheumatism is used in our times to denote, among other things, any of a number of unexplained or poorly understood aches and pains of the muscles, ligaments, and joints of the body. This category of conditions is also referred to in a number of terms: soft-tissue rheumatism, fibrositis, myositis, anxiety neurosis, and depressive reaction. These disorders are broadly divided into two main types, generalized conditions and localized or regional conditions. Over 100 variations of the condition are included under the category of nonarticular rheumatism, but 2, fibromyalgia and fibrositis, are of noteworthy interest to the TMJ clinician due to their commonly observed propensity to intensify and/or augment the myofascial symptoms experienced by the patient with typical TMJ problems. The two things these conditions all have in common is that, first, they "set up" the muscles of the TMJ patient, thereby making them more sensitive to the type of abuse distal-driving malocclusions are capable of administering, and second, the vast majority of these soft-tissue rheumatism-type disorders are readily resolved by proper nutrition, rest, healthy exercise, and generally supportive efforts at regaining homeostatic balance, i.e., stress reduction in all the forms in which stress assaults the body: physical, chemical, emotional, psychological, and environmental.

Fibromyalgia has been defined as a generalized syndrome of muscle skeletal aches, pains, and stiffness of periodic and fluctuating occurrence. These symptoms must occur over a period of time lasting longer than 90 days and in three or more anatomical locations. The patient may perceive a subjective swelling in these areas that might not necessarily be observable by the clinician. The condition is aggravated by stress, lack of proper rest, excessive exercise, overexertion or overwork, cold damp weather, and general fatigue. What is disconcerting to the diagnostician concerning this condition is that it occurs in the complete absence of any other physical, radiographic, neurological, or laboratory finding (except of course for the possibility of a superiorly posteriorly displaced condyle in the joint). This condition may even be present in the complete absence of any TMJ findings. Along with areas of consistent tenderness and the propensity for the condition to be exacerbated by dietary excesses (sugar, caffeine, "junk foods," etc.) and other forms of stress, the appearance of periodic headache-type symptoms has also been noted.

Fibrositis is a closely related condition and another form of soft-tissue rheumatism that is characterized by vague aches and dull pains over large areas of the body. It too is characterized by disturbed sleep patterns, and in addition, morning stiffness is observed. The distinguishing characteristic of this particular condition is that there is a focal tenderness in approximately 14 specific anatomical locations including the clavicular area, suprapectoral area, frontal subiliac crest area, posterior cervical and trapezoidal regions, base of the spine, elbow, gluteal area, and the popliteal fossa. It is strongly felt that muscle tonus alteration plays a serious role here (as with many of the other nonarticular rheumatism-type conditions). As previously stated, muscle tonus exists in resting muscles to keep the muscles in a state of taut readiness for contraction and, as a result, also imparts a certain tension on its tendons at either end. Excessive muscle tonus or excessive muscular contraction that is not resolved and counteracted by deep relaxation during sleep can result in a perpetual form of tension on these tendons that produces pain. In the maxillo-facial complex these pains can result from muscles that are already com-promised by a distal-driving malocclusion and further compromised by poor nutrition, dietary abuses, host homeostatic imbalance due to stress, and the big thing—bruxism! Such tension-related headaches of this type coming from a maxillofacial complex with a compromised TMJ (the initial fire) have been referred to by some as myofascial pain-dysfunction syn-drome. Fibrositis is the equivalent muscle component of this notion that erupts in other areas. Patients with fibrositis will complain of exquisitely sensitive, highly defined trigger point areas that may actually be palpated by the well-experienced diagnostician. They appear as small gelatinous tender or tight spots in the muscle. The sleep disturbance symptoms these patients exhibit show electroencephalogram readings similar to those found in sleep deprivation studies. Muscles are overworked, over-tensed, and "overtonused," if you will, without the benefit of what the poet refers to as "balmy sleep, Nature's sweet restorer." This is due to stress and general homeostatic imbalance. Some authorities characterize the typical patient with fibrositis as not only having the 14 focal areas of tenderness but also as being the aggressive, competitive, A-type person-ality female who perceives that she is under a great deal of stress; is both-ered by menstrual irregularities, excessive cramping, or general premen-strual syndrome–type problems; is in poor physical condition (from an athletic standpoint); is overworked and underrested; is prone to highly refined sugar, caffeine, alcohol, tobacco, and "junk food" abuses in her diet; and is generally nutritionally "bankrupt." None of this helps the TMJ that has a superiorly posteriorly displaced condyle in it at full occlu-sion. It is a vicious cycle of each condition worsening the other. Each acts as a physiological drain on the body to lessen its ability to deal with the other. Such relationships represent more fanning of the occlusion-ignited TMJ flames.

One thing that is remarkable about fibromyalgia, fibromyositis, and the whole family of nonarticular rheumatism–type problems that they represent and that may occur in conjunction with a bona fide distal displacement–type TMJ problem is that once the condyle is correctly re-positioned down and forward in the fossa by proper FJO techniques and the patient is additionally given a modicum of the most basic homeostatic support in the form of proper nutrition, rest, and stress reduction, it is amazing how many of these problems resolve themselves without any other major forms of treatment. The TMJ at times seems to be the focal point. Once corrected, the headaches, the muscle aches in the neck and back, the vague pains, the stiffness and fatigue, the disturbed sleep, and many other bothersome systemic-type problems of a stressed individual seem to subside. If treatment is interrupted due to a lost splint or appli-ance, not only do the localized TMJ symptoms return, the attending sys-temic symptoms of the soft-tissue rheumatism types that were present at the beginning of treatment also return. For the patient suffering from functionally induced TMJ problems, putting the condyle in the right place, down and forward in the joint, isn't everything; but it's the main thing. It is a commonsense procedure, and when followed by other simple commonsense procedures of general systemic support, such treatment leaves Nature in the best position to rebalance many of the homeostatic mechanisms on Her own that have gone awry due to the initial fire set in the TMJ by the NRDM/SPDC phenomenon. It also places treatment for this vicious cycle of interrelated problems well within the domain of any clinician familiar with FJO methodology. For such a clinician not only has the ability to properly reposition the condyle in balanced functional occlusion, but in so doing thereby also enlists the services of a most powerful partner with respect to addressing complicated systemic homeostatic problems, Nature Herself.

SUMMARY

Many vague and nondescript signs, symptoms, and systemic irregularities accompany the stressed individual with a functionally oriented TMJ problem. They are Nature's reaction to the initial focal point of the TMJ insult. Such an insult represents a figurative leak in the physiological dike needed to keep the whole homeostatic scene running well under stress. Once that initial focal point of insult is remedied, Nature can in turn resolve most of these reactive problems. It is not a matter of a multifactored, multicompartmentalized disease or series of diseases with many different mysterious etiological agents. It is not a matter of long, drawn-out lists of conditions and causative factors. It is not a matter of manditory team approach and consensus diagnosis. True, the exceptional cases will always exist. They of course turn out to be quite rare. That is why they are exceptional. However, in the vast majority of cases, the functionally initiated TMJ problem of the average patient is a matter of many varied signs and symptoms that are the effects of but one chief initiating focal etiological cause. Trouble starts when the balance of the whole system is disrupted by a distal-driving occlusion initiating the NRDM/SPDC phenomenon: neuromuscular reflexive displacement of the mandible causing superior posterior displacement of the condyle.

"Condemn the fault,
and not the actor of it."

William Shakespeare
Measure for Measure *Act II, scene ii*

References

1. Ochoa JL, Torebjork HE: Pain from skin and muscle (abstract). *Pain Suppl* 1981; 1:887.
2. Torebjork HE, Ochoa JL: Specific sensations evoked by activity in single identified sensory units in man. *Acta Physiol Scand* 1980; 110:445–447.
3. Bonica JJ: Neurophysiologic and pathologic aspects of acute and chronic pain. *Arch Surg* 1977; 112:750–761.
4. Melzack R: *The Puzzle of Pain*. New York, Basic Books, Inc, Publishers, 1973.
5. Campbell J: Distribution and treatment of pain in temporomandibular arthroses. *Br Dent J* 1958; 105:393–402.
6. Bell WE: *Orofacial Pains,* ed 3. Chicago, Year Book Medical Publishers, Inc, 1985.
7. Travell J: Temporomandibular joint pain referred from the head and neck. *J Prosthet Dent* 1960; 10:745–763.
8. Williams HL, Elkins EC: Myalgia of the head. *Arch Phys Ther* 1942; 23:14–22.
9. Brodie AG: Anatomy and physiology of the head and neck musculature. *Am J Orthod* 1950; 36:831–844.
10. Fonder AC: The Dental Physician. Rock Falls, Ill, Medical-Dental Arts, 1985, pp 105–115.
11. Travell J: Myofacial trigger points: A clinical view, in Bonica JJ (ed): *Advances in Pain Research and Therapy,* vol 1. New York, Raven Press, 1976, pp 919–926.
12. Inman VT, Saunders JB: Referred pain from skeletal structures, *J Nerv Ment Dis* 1944; 99:650–667.
13. Kendall HO, Kendall FP, Wadsworth GE: *Muscles, Testing and Function,* ed 2. Baltimore, Williams & Wilkins, 1971.
14. Simons DG: Muscle pain syndromes—Parts I, II. *Am J Phys Med* 1975; 54:289–311; 1976; 55:15–42.
15. Travell J, Bigelow NH: Referred somatic pain does not follow a simple segmental pattern (abstract). *Fed Proc* 1946; 5:106.

16. Travell J, Rinzler SH: The myofacial genesis of pain. *Postgrad Med* 1952; 11:425–434.
17. Travell J: Mechanical headache. *Headache* 1967; 7:23–29.
18. Kellgren JH: A preliminary account of referred pains arising from muscle. *Br Med J* 1938; 1:325–337.
19. Kellgren JH: Observations on referred pain arising from muscle. *Clin Sci* 1938; 3:175–190.
20. Berges PU: Myofascial pain syndromes. *Postgrad Med* 1973; 53:161–168.
21. Bonica JJ: Management of myofascial pain syndromes in general practice. *JAMA* 1957; 164:732–738.
22. Cooper AL: Trigger point injection: Its place in physical medicine. *Arch Phys Med* 1961; 42:704–709.
23. Kraus H: *Clinical Treatment of Back and Neck Pain.* New York, McGraw-Hill International Book Co, 1970, pp 95, 107.
24. Bates T, Grunwaldt E: Myofascial pain in childhood. *J Pediatr* 1958; 53:198–209.
25. Gorrell RL: Troublesome ankle disorders and what to do about them. *Consultant* 1976; 16:64–69.
26. Gutstein M: Common rheumatism and physiotherapy. *Br J Phys Med* 1946; 3:46–50.
27. Sinclair DC: The remote reference of pain around the skin. *Brain* 1949; 72:364–372.
28. Sola AE, Rodenberger ML, Gettys BB: Incidence of hypersensitive areas in shoulder muscles. *Am J Phys Med* 1955; 34:585–590.
29. Trommer PR, Gellman MB: Trigger point syndrome. *Rheumatism* 1952; 8:67–72.
30. MacDonald AJR: Abnormally tender muscle regions and associated painful movements. *Pain* 1980; 8:197–205.
31. de Valera E, Raftery H: Lower abdominal and pelvic pain in women, in Bonica JJ (ed): *Advances in Pain Research and Therapy,* vol 1. New York, Raven Press, 1976, pp 935–936.
32. Dittrich RJ: Low-back pain—referred pain from the deep somatic structure of the back. *Lancet* 1963; 7:63–68.
33. Hackett GS: *Ligament and Tendon Relaxation Treated by Prototherapy,* ed 3. Springfield, Ill, Charles C Thomas Publishers, 1958, pp 27–36.
34. Kellgren JH: Deep pain sensibility. *Lancet* 1949; 1:943–949.
35. Melzack R, Wall PD: Pain mechanisms, a new theory. *Science* 1965; 150:971–979.
36. Wall PD: The gate control theory of pain mechanisms: A reexamination and restatement. *Brain* 1978; 101:1–14.
37. Kraus H: The use of surface anesthesia for the treatment of painful motion. *JAMA* 1941; 116:2582–2587.
38. Picaza J, et al: Pain supression by peripheral nerve stimulation. *Surg Neurol* 1975; 4:105–114.
39. Liboff AR, Rinaldi RA (eds): Electrically mediated growth mechanism in living systems. *Ann N Y Acad Sci* 1974; 238:1–593.
40. Sternbach RA, Ignelzi RJ, Deems LM, et al: Transcutaneous electrical analgesia: A follow-up analysis. *Pain* 1976; 2:35–41.
41. Long DM, Hagfors N: Electrical stimulation in the nervous system: The cur-

rent status of electrical stimulation of the nervous system for the relief of pain. *Pain* 1975; 1:109–123.

42. Kane K, Taub A: A history of local electrical analgesia. *Pain* 1975; 1:125–138.

43. Ignelzi RJ, Atkinson JH: Pain and its modulation: Part 2—efferent mechanisms. *Neurosurgery* 1980; 6:584–590.

44. Almay BGL, Johansson F, Von Knorring L, et al: Endorphins in psychogenic pain syndromes. *Pain* 1978; 5:153–162.

45. Terenius L: Endorphins in chronic pain, in Bonica JJ, Liebeskind JC, Albe-Fessard DG (eds): *Advances in Pain Research and Therapy,* vol 3. New York, Raven Press, 1979, pp 459–471.

46. Perl ER: Sensitization of nociceptors and its relation to sensation, in Bonica JJ, Albe-Fessard DG (eds): *Advances in Pain Research and Therapy,* vol 1. New York, Raven Press, 1976, pp 17–28.

47. Good MG: The role of skeletal muscles in the pathogenesis of diseases. *Acta Med Scand* 1950; 138:285–292.

48. Melzale R: Relation of myofascial trigger points to acupuncture and mechanisms of pain. *Arch Phys Med Rehabil* 1981; 62:114–117.

49. Milne RJ, Foreman RD, Giesler CJ Jr, et al: Convergence of cutaneous and pelvic visceral nociceptive inputs on to primate spinothalamic neurons. *Pain* 1981; 11:163–183.

50. Ruch TC: Pathophysiology of pain, in Ruch TC, Patton HD (eds): *Physiology and Biophysics,* ed 19. Philadelphia, WB Saunders Co, 1965, pp 357, 358.

51. Sinclair DC, Weddell G, Feindel WH: Referred pain and associated phenomena. *Brain* 1948; 71:184–211.

52. Weiss S, Davis D: The significance of the afferent impulses from the skin in the mechanisms of visceral, pain, skin infiltration as a useful therapeutic measure. *Am J Med Sci* 1928; 176:517–536.

53. Greene CS: Myofascial pain-dysfunction syndrome: The evolution of concepts, in Sornat BG, Taskin DM (eds): *The Temporomandibular Joint.* Springfield, Ill, Charles C. Thomas Publishers, 1980.

54. Posselt U: *Physiology of Occlusion and Rehabilitation.* Philadelphia, FA Davis Co Publishers, 1962, p 88.

55. Hankey GT: Discussion: Affections of the temporomandibular joint. *Proc R Soc Med* 1956; 49:983–994.

56. Lindblom G: Disorders of the temporomandibular joint. *Acta Odont Scand* 1953; 11:61–85.

57. Staz J: The treatment of disturbances of the temporomandibular articulation. *Off J Dent Assoc S Afr* 1951; 6:314–335.

58. Soderberg F: Malokklusion-arthoses—otalgie. *Acta Otolaryngol Suppl (Scand)* 1950; 95:85–98.

59. Walsh JP: Temporomandibular arthritis, mandibular displacement and facial pain. *Off J Dent Assoc S Afr* 1950; 5:430–436.

60. Sicher H: Temporomandibular articulation in mandibular overclosure. *J Am Dent Assoc* 1948; 36:131–139.

61. Hansson T, Nilner M: A study of the occurrence of symptoms of diseases of the temporomandibular joint masticatory musculature and related structures. *J Oral Rehabil* 1975; 2:313–324.

62. McCarty W: Diagnosis and treatment of internal derangement of the articular disc and mandibular condyle, in Solberg WK, Clark GT (eds): *Temporo-*

mandibular Joint Problems, Chicago, Quintessence Publishing Co, 1980, pp 145–168.

63. McNeill C, Danzig WM, Farrar WB, et al: Craniomandibular (TMJ) disorders—the state of the art. *J Prosthet Dent* 1980; 44:334–337.

64. Mikhail M, Rosen H: History and etiology of myofascial pain-dysfunction syndrome. *J Prosthet Dent* 1980; 44:338–444.

65. Schwartz LL: *Disorders of the Temporomandibular Joint.* Philadelphia, WB Saunders Co, 1959.

66. Weinberg LA: Role of condylar position in TMJ dysfunction-pain syndrome. *J Prosthet Dent* 1979; 41:636–643.

67. Gelb H: *Clinical Management of Head, Neck and TMJ Pain and Dysfunction.* Philadelphia, WB Saunders Co, 1985, p 109.

68. Agerberg G, Carlsson GE: Functional disorders of the masticatory system. 1. Distribution of symptoms according to age and sex as judged from investigation by questionnaire, *Acta Odont Scand* 1972; 30:597–613.

69. Rohlin M, Westesson P, Eriksson L: The correlation of temporomandibular joint sounds with joint morphology in fifty-five autopsy specimens. *J Oral Maxillofac Surg* 1985; 44:194–200.

70. Gross A, Gale EN: A prevalence study of the clinical signs associated with mandibular dysfunction. *J Am Dent Assoc* 1983; 107:932–936.

71. Farrar WB, McCarty WL: The TMJ dilemma. *J Ala Dent Assoc* 1979; 63:19–21.

72. Westesson P: Double contrast arthrography and internal derangement of the temporomandibular joint. *Swed Dent J Suppl* 1982; 13.

73. Solberg WK: Epidemiology, incidence and prevalence of temporomandibular disorders: A review, in *The President's Commission on Examination, Diagnosis and Management of Temporomandibular Disorders.* Chicago, American Dental Association, 1983, pp 30–39.

74. Bush FM, Butler JH, Abbott DM: The relationship of TMJ clicking to palpable facial pain. *J Craniomandib Prac* 1983; 1:43–47.

75. Rees LA: Structure and function of the mandibular joint, *Br Dent J* 1954; 96:125–133.

76. Toller PA: Opaque arthrography of the temporomandibular joint. *Int J Oral Surg* 1974; 3:17–28.

77. Blackwood HJJ: Pathology of the temporomandibular joint. *J Am Dent Assoc* 1969; 79:118–124.

78. Moffett BC, Johnson LC, McCabe JB, et al: Articular remodeling in the adult human temporomandibular joint. *Am J Anat* 1964; 115:119–141.

79. Moss ML: The functional matrix, in Kraus BS, Reidel R (eds): *Vistas in Orthodontics.* Philadelphia, Lea & Febiger, 1962.

80. Moss ML: The primacy of functional matrices in orofacial growth. *Practitioner* 1968; 19:65–73.

81. Moss ML, Rankow R: The role of the functional matrix in mandibular growth. *Angle Orthod* 1968; 38:95–103.

82. Moss ML, Salentijn L: The primary role of functional matrices in facial growth. *Am J Orthod* 1969; 55:566–577.

83. Needham DM: Biochemistry of muscle, in Bourne GH (ed): *The Structure and Function of Muscle,* ed 2, vol 3. New York, Academic Press, Inc, 1973, p 377.

84. Yemm R, Berry DC: Passive control in mandibular rest position. *J Prosthet Dent* 1969; 22:30–36.

85. Manns A, Miralles R, Palazzi C: EMG bite force and elongation of the masseter muscle under isometric voluntary contractions and variations of vertical dimension. *J Prosthet Dent* 1979; 42:674–682.
86. Hellsing G: Functional adaptation to changes in vertical dimension. *J Prosthet Dent* 1984; 52:867–870.
87. Schulhof RJ, Engle GA: Results of class II functional appliance treatment. *JCO* 1982; 16:587–599.
88. McNamara JA Jr, Connelly TG, McBridge MC: Histological studies of temporomandibular joint adaptations, in *Determinants of Mandibular Form and Growth*, Monograph 4, Craniofacial Growth Series. Ann Arbor, Center for Human Growth and Development, University of Michigan, 1975, pp 209–277.
89. McNamara JA Jr: Quantitative analysis of temporomandibular joint adaptations to protrusive function. *Am J Orthod* 1979; 76:593–611.
90. McNamara JA Jr: Functional determinants of craniofacial size and shape. *Eur J Orthod* 1980; 2:131–159.
91. McNamara JA Jr: Dentofacial adaptations in adult patients following functional regulator therapy. *Am J Orthod* 1984; 85:57–71.
92. Elgoyhen JC, Moyers RE, McNamara JA Jr, et al: Craniofacial adaptations to protrusive function in young rhesus monkeys. *Am J Orthod* 1972; 62:469–480.
93. Graber TM, Neumann B: Functional jaw orthopedics: The changes of a concept, in *Removable Orthodontic Appliances*. Philadelphia, WB Saunders Co, 1975, pp 118–132.
94. Witt E: Muscular physiological investigations into the effects of bi-maxillary appliances. *Trans Eur Orthod Soc* 1973; 49:448–450.
95. Stockli PW, Willert HG: Tissue response in the temporomandibular joint resulting from an anterior displacement of the mandible. *Am J Orthod* 1971; 60:142–155.
96. Reey RW, Eastwood A: The passive activator: Case selection, treatment response and corrective mechanics. *Am J Orthod* 1978; 73:378–409.
97. Petrovic AG, Stutzmann J, Oudet C: Control processes in postnatal growth of the condylar cartilage of the mandible, in McNamara AJ Jr (ed): *Determinants of Mandibular Form and Growth*, Monograph 4, Craniofacial Growth Series. Ann Arbor, Center for Human Growth and Development, University of Michigan, 1975, pp 101–153.
98. Petrovic AG: Control of postnatal growth of secondary cartilages by mechanisms regulating occlusion. *Trans Eur Orthod Soc* 1974; 44:69–75.
99. Moss JP: An investigation of muscle activity of patients with class II, division 1 malocclusion and changes during treatment. *Trans Eur Orthod Soc* 1975; 51:87–101.
100. Freeland TD: Muscle function during treatment with functional regulator. *Angle Orthod* 1979; 49:247–258.
101. Ahlgren J: Early and late electromyographic response to treatment with activators. *Am J Orthod* 1978; 74:88–93.
102. Ahlin J, White GE, Tsamtsouris A, et al: *Maxillofacial Orthopedics: A Clinical Approach for the Growing Child*. Chicago, Quintessence Publishing Co, 1984, pp 77–80.

103. Bell WE: *Temporomandibular Disorders: Classification-Diagnosis-Management.* Chicago, Year Book Medical Publishers, Inc, 1982, pp 66–67.

104. Kobuta K, Masegi T: Muscle spindle supply to human jaw muscle. *J Dent Res* 1977; 56:901–909.

105. Mohl ND: Neuromuscular mechanisms in mandibular function. *Dent Clin North Am* 1978; 22:63–71.

106. Bechtol CO: Muscle physiology, in *The American Academy of Orthopedic Surgeons: International Course Lectures,* vol 5. St Louis, CV Mosby Co, 1948.

107. McNamara JA Jr: The independent functions of the two heads of the lateral pterygoid muscle. *Am J Anat* 1973; 138:197–205.

108. Lipke DP, Gay T, Gross BD, et al: An electromyographic study of the human lateral pterygoid muscle (abstract 713). *J Dent Res* 1977; 56:230.

109. Mahan PE, Wilkinson TM, Gibbs CH, et al: Superior and inferior bellies of the lateral pterygoid muscle EMG activity of basic jaw positions. *J Prosthet Dent* 1983; 50:710–718.

110. Gibbs CH, Mahan PE, Wilkinson TM, et al: EMG activity of the superior belly of the lateral pterygoid muscle in relation to other jaw muscles. *J Prosthet Dent* 1984; 51:691–702.

111. Wilkinson TM: The relationship between the disk and the lateral pterygoid muscle in the human temporomandibular joint. *J Prosthet Dent* 1988; 60:715–724.

112. Willis RD, DiCosimo CJ: The absence of proprioceptive nerve endings in the human periodontal ligament: The role of periodontal mechanoreceptors in the reflex control of mastication. *Oral Surg* 1939; 48:108–111.

113. Sessle BJ, Schmidt A: Effects of controlled tooth stimulation on jaw muscle activity in man. *Arch Oral Biol* 1972; 17:1597–1607.

114. Hannam AG, Matthews B, Yemm R: Receptors involved in the response of the masseter muscle to tooth contact in man. *Arch Oral Biol* 1970; 15:17–24.

115. Ahlgren J: The silent period in the EMG of the jaw muscles during mastication and its relationship to tooth contact. *Acta Odont Scand* 1969; 27:219–227.

116. Bell WE: Nonsurgical management of the pain-dysfunction syndrome. *J Am Dent Assoc* 1969; 79:161–170.

117. Bonica JJ: Myofascial syndromes with trigger mechanism, in Bonica JJ (ed): *The Management of Pain.* Philadelphia, Lea & Febiger, 1953, pp 1150–1151.

118. Brown BR: Diagnosis and therapy of common myofascial syndromes. *JAMA* 1978; 239:646–648.

119. Cailliet R: *Soft Tissue Pain and Disability.* Philadelphia, FA Davis Co Publishers, 1977, pp 32–35.

120. Gillette HE: Office management of musculoskeletal pain, *Texas State J Med* 1966; 62:47–53.

121. D'ambrosia RD: *Musculoskeletal Disorders: Regional Examination and Differential Diagnosis.* Philadelphia, JB Lippincott, 1977, p 332.

122. Laskin DM: Etiology of the pain dysfunction syndrome. *J Am Dent Assoc* 1969; 79:147–153.

123. Pace JB: Commonly overlooked pain syndromes responsive to simple therapy. *Postgrad Med* 1975; 58:107–113.

124. Reynolds MD: Myofascial trigger point syndromes in the practice of rheumatology. *Arch Phys Med Rehabil* 1981; 62:111–114.

125. Swezey RL, Spiegel TM: Evaluation and treatment of local musculoskeletal disorders in elderly patients. *Geriatrics* 1979; 34:56–75.

126. Travell J: Identification of myofascial trigger point syndromes: A case of a typical facial neuralgia. *Arch Phys Med Rehabil* 1981; 62:100–106.

127. Adams RD: *Diseases of Muscle: A Study in Pathology,* ed 3. Hagerstown, Md, Harper & Row Publishers, Inc, 1975, pp 280–291, 316, 317.

128. Schmalbruch H: Contracture knots in normal and diseased muscle fibers. *Brain* 1973; 96:637–640.

129. Awad EA: Interstitial myofibrositis: Hypothesis of the mechanism. *Arch Phys Med* 1973; 54:440–453.

130. Adour KK: Acute temporomandibular joint pain-dysfunction syndrome, neurotologic and electromyographic study. *Am J Otolaryngol* 1981; 2:114–122.

131. Adour KK: Costen's syndrome revisited; craniopolyganglionitis as a form of temporomandibular joint pain-dysfunction syndrome. Presented at the American Equilibration Society, Chicago, 1982.

132. Adour KK: Bell's palsy: A complete expression of acute benign polyneuritis. *Prim Care* 1975; 2:717–733.

133. Adour KK: The true nature of Bell's palsy: An analysis of 1,000 consecutive patients. *Laryngoscope* 1978; 88:787–801.

134. Stein R, Tonning FM: Acute peripheral facial palsy. *Arch Otolaryngol* 1973; 98:187–190.

135. DeVriese PP: Facial paralysis in cephalic herpes zoster. *Am Otol Rhinol Laryngol* 1968; 77:1101–1119.

136. Selye H: *The Stress of Life,* ed 2. New York, McGraw-Hill International Book Co, 1970.

137. Selye H: The General-Adaptation Syndrome. *Annu Rev Med* 1951; 2:327–343.

138. Selye H: Induction of topical resistance to acute tissue injury. *Surg Clin North Am* 1953; 33:1417–1444.

139. Selye H: The influence of STH, ACTH, and cortisone upon resistance to infection. *Can Med Assoc J* 1951; 64:489–494.

140. Selye H: On the mechanism through which hydrocortisone affects the resistance of tissue to injury. *JAMA* 1953; 152:1207–1213.

141. Selye H: Sketch for a unified theory of medicine *Int Rec Med* 1954; 167:181–204.

142. Selye H: *The Story of the Adaptation Syndrome.* Montreal, Acta, Inc, 1952.

143. Selye H: *Stress.* Montreal, Acta, Inc, 1950.

144. Selye H: Stress and Disease. *Science* 1955; 122:625–631.

145. Selye H: What is stress? *Metabolism* 1956; 5:525–530.

146. Selye H: *Stress Without Distress.* Philadelphia, JB Lippincott, 1974.

CHAPTER 4
Through the Looking Glass

DIAGNOSIS

Any reasonable attempt at treating a condition that is as multisymp-tomatic as temporomandibular joint (TMJ) arthrosis is predicated upon a proper diagnosis. We would be under great duress to construct a program of effective therapeutic measures capable of resecuring the biological health and balanced function of the TMJ without first determining the nature of the biomechanical, physiological, and pathological problems afflicting it. We simply can't fix it until we first know what's wrong with it. The problem in the past is that it has been very difficult to peer into the innermost recesses of the TMJ to see what is bothering it. This inaccessibility to the naked eye has led TMJ investigators to turn to other methods of visualizing the joint. Radiology was the first and obvious choice. However, the earliest attempts at obtaining radiographs of the TMJ were hampered by problems of overlapping osseous anatomy, a lack of definition of target images, and a general uncertainty as to just how to correctly interpret the images that were obtained. There seemed to be an obsession among early investigators with trying to focus in on the intra-articular disc, as if it were the chief agent of concern. Yet accompanying this fascination with this little fibrocartilagenous portion of the joint was a disheartening acceptance that the disc would never be seen on a radiograph due to its lack of radiopacity. The simplest, most economical, and most practical radiographic devices, as well as the images they produced, were panned by the world of academia as being of no value to "disc-concerned" clinicians and researchers. Only the expensive, institution-oriented radiographic devices that produced sophisticated images (and enormous price tags) were touted to be worthy of a condition so perplexing as "TMJ syndrome." Team approaches enlisting numerous subspecialties of both dentistry and medicine were espoused as the only proper way to hunt for clues as to what might be causing the patient's myofascial headache pain and joint dysfunction. It could then best be determined which of the allied fields of the healing arts should be called upon to institute treatments. Interestingly, very few treatment plans in those times called for orthodontics! Numerous electronic gadgets were devised and employed to provide diagnostic information concerning things like the amount of electrical activity the muscles produced, the kinds of joint sounds that were generated, what kind of temperature patterns the respective anatomy involved produced, or what the concentrations of certain chemicals were in the patient's blood, urine, synovial fluid, and hair. Examination procedures were promoted that involved progressively longer appointment times with steadily increasing amounts of paperwork, history taking, and record keeping. And not only were therapeutic methods becoming ever more increasingly involved and varied, but the diagnostic procedures that spawned them were themselves becoming more complex. The diagnosis and treatment of common TMJ problems seemed to be drifting farther and farther away from the realm of the common practitioner. Seeing into the true heart of the TMJ problem seemed to be a vision that might never be practically realized. According to some, such was the developing trend of the times, or at least they thought it should have been. But all that has changed.

The purpose of the procedure involved in examining a TMJ is to effectively and efficiently obtain the necessary information that will allow the practitioner to determine the nature and extent of the TMJ problem and construct a reasonable treatment plan designed to address the needs made evident by such information. The differential aspects of a diagnosis should also be given paramount attention to decipher those problems that are of a true functionally oriented nature as opposed to those that lie within other allied realms of the health care disciplines. Fortunately, this is not difficult. A proper TMJ diagnostic examination procedure may be divided into three main areas: the history and anamnesis; the clinical examination; and the radiographic or, now more correctly, "imaging" procedures. Each subdivision is critical to a complete and confirmed diagnosis of a TMJ pain-dysfunction condition.

HISTORY AND ANAMNESIS

A carefully recorded and detailed medical and dental history is an important part of any attempt at diagnosis of a TMJ problem.[1, 2] It is especially important in the differential diagnosis between common problems of a functionally generated nature vs. the much less frequently seen problems that can mimic common TMJ symptoms of headache or facial pains but rather are of a general systemic origin. The "history" involves the medical and dental record of the patient. It consists of past diagnoses, observations, and treatments. It implies things that the patient has been informed of in the past by medical or dental personnel. Information pertaining to things like results of laboratory tests, types of allergies present, condition of the circulatory or endocrine systems, types of medical or dental diseases the patient might have contracted, etc., fall into the category of a history. The "anamnesis" of the patient with respect to his TMJ problem involves something a bit different but very important to the final diagnosis. The term *anamnesis* is pure Greek and it means "recollection" or "the faculty of memory." It consists of the patient's recollection of the pattern of previous occurrence of signs or symptoms, sensations, psychological or emotional moods, reactions, or other personal observations of the patients themselves. It also includes dates or times of occurrence, precipitating factors, if any, and what the patient's general view of the problem is from his own point of view. The importance of recording the patient's anamnesis in his own words cannot be overly stressed. By carefully asking the proper questions and recording a brief summary of the patient's answers, the clinician shows concern and compassion. Such questioning also elicits information from patients that they might be a bit too embarrassed to divulge. Often one will hear, "You know, Doc, this may sound crazy, but I hear a popping sound in my ears when I chew," or "I know this sounds silly, but when I grit my back teeth I hear a hissing sound deep in my ear." Often careful exploration of the patient's anamnesis will give important clues to the severity of the TMJ condition, possible precipitating or exacerbating factors, or the general level of resistance to the condition as a whole. It is the anamnesis, the patient's own observation and opinion of how the condition has affected him in the past, that produces something of utmost importance to both the patient and the treating clinician—the chief complaint! It is usually what compels the patient to seek treatment and should be the first thing recorded in the patient's chart by the diagnostician. It should also be plainly recorded in the patient's own words, bad grammar and all, for it is this yardstick that will be used by the patient (and even the practitioner as well) to measure the success or failure of the subsequent treatments employed to address the case. Technical terms may be used later. Initially, it is the patient's right to register what signs and/or symptoms bother him the most. It is to this end that future treatments should be oriented. The most common complaint by far will be those of headache, neck ache, myofascial pains, or general soreness or tiredness of the masticatory musculature. Patients should simply be asked to describe their perception of their problem in their own words. It is amazing how many times these words offer enormous insights to the overall problem when one interprets them in light of what we now know about TMJ function and dysfunction. What is also amazing is how in some instances these words will almost tell the clinician just how to treat the case.

The most often heard complaint of the patient with TMJ problems is that of pain, although sometimes the reciprocal clicking of an anteromedially displaced disc is so profound that it causes the patient to seek treatment unaware that the headaches are intimately related to the TMJs.[3-9] The headache-type pain, or cephalalgia, is very often accompanied by neck ache and upper shoulder pain, or cervicalgia, although again many patients do not associate cervicalgia with their jaw joints or a functional joint noise they are aware of. These pains or myalgias are often the result of the activity of overshortened muscles that must overwork to compensate for another chief finding associated with patients with TMJ conditions, a lack of posterior vertical dimension of the occlusion. This condition posteriorly is worsened by a distal-deflecting form of anterior incisal interference further forward in the malocclusion. Continued use of these muscles that are foreshortened and fatigued will cause pain. Patients will sometimes develop their own forms of limited ranges of motion to avoid the painful stretching of these abused and sensitive muscles. Patients, if asked, may even complain of mid to lower back pains. Another frequent observation in patients with "classic" TMJ problems is the occurrence of intense retroorbital and/or occipital-type headache pains.

While interviewing patients to seek the past medical and dental history, remind the patients not to diagnose themselves. Often one will hear "Oh yes, Doctor, I get headaches, but I have a sinus problem," or "I get headaches, but I have allergies." When questioning patients on these issues, it is handy to use the interrogation principles commonly used by trial lawyers: the what, where, why, and when method. "Tell me about your headaches. What are your symptoms? Where does it hurt? How does it hurt? When does it hurt? What makes it hurt more? What seems to precipitate an attack? How long does it last? What makes you feel better? What medicines do you take for it? How often do you take them? How well do they work? What other symptoms do you feel? Why do you think this is occurring?" The last question is more important than it might first appear. Many patients have been to numerous health care providers of various types or may have had a number of previously rendered treatments by the time they arrive in the office of a TMJ-oriented dental practitioner. Some have been given false diagnoses such as "migraine" or "stress." Some have been given no diagnosis, which is even worse, for this can be a source of "cancer phobia" because some will fear they have a brain tumor of some sort. It may even cause some patients to question their own sanity. Some will have been told rather coldly by frustrated and exasperated medical officers of some sort, "Lady, it's all in your head." Little do such diagnosticians know how right they are!

CLINICAL EXAMINATION

Once the history and anamnesis have been recorded, the clinician may proceed from the area of recording the chief complaint and the patient's perceptions of the problem to that of determining his own opinions of the type and level of involvement of the patient's condition via direct *clinical* examination. As a matter of definition, the direct clinical examination is concerned with those signs and symptoms that may be observed and recorded by the clinician directly from the patient without the aid of major forms of diagnostic modalities and as such does not include the imaging portion of the entire diagnostic procedure. Therefore, the direct clinical evaluation of the patient involves four basic procedures: (1) palpation to identify the anatomical origins of pain, (2) auscultation of the joint during function to determine the presence of joint sounds, (3) range of motion measurements of the mandible, and (4) analysis of the occlusion. These procedures are quick and relatively easy to perform and provide a great deal of reliable and basic data concerning the status of not only the patient's TMJs but also the entire masticatory mechanism that operates them. This information is then ultimately analyzed in conjunction with the various forms of images of the joint that might be subsequently produced.

Palpation

The lateral portions of the joint and most of the muscles of mastication are accessible to direct manual palpation by the examining clinician. Those muscles that are inaccessible to direct palpation may be examined indirectly through functional manipulation. The muscles of mastication must often overwork in an inefficient manner in malocclusions, which results in the condyle being driven too far up and back at full occlusion. An indication such abuse has taken place will be manifest by muscles that are sore to palpation. The pain may result from a variety of factors, but they will be sore nonetheless. And muscles in a healthy, balanced, well-functioning maxillofacial complex simply should not be sore to reasonable amounts of direct manual palpation. Muscle tenderness is indicative of some level of fatigue and/or trauma that is usually directly proportional to the duration and level of intensity of the insult. This can result from sim-

Figure 4–1　Auscultation and palpation of the TMJs during function. **(A)** Start at the fully closed intercuspal position. **(B)** Then have the patient slowly open to the maximum range of opening and then slowly close again to full occlusion. The joints may be palpated in similar fashion with the clinician's fingertips over the joint area.

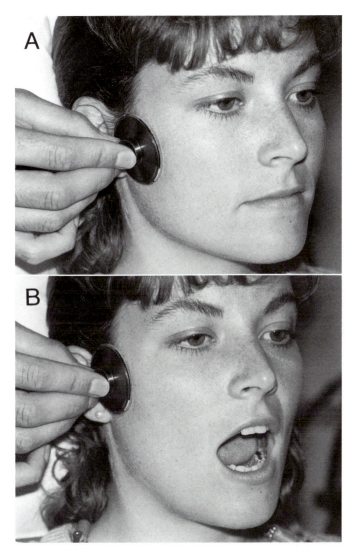

Figure 4–1

ple mechanisms, such as lactic acidosis, or more advanced mechanisms, such as muscle splinting, trigger point irritation, or referred pain. When pain occurs, Nature is trying to tell us something. In more ways than one, being a good diagnostician involves the art of being a good listener.

The joint itself may be palpated both directly and via functional manipulation. Direct external palpation may consist of two types. First, the clinician may palpate directly over the lateral aspect of the joint. This should be done in both the closed and opened positions. When the mouth is opened wide, a depression is felt by the examiner that represents an enlarged superior and posterior joint space resulting from the condyle having translated down and forward in the act of opening. It should be noted whether there is pain elicited due to firm but gentle digital pressure over this area. If so, it may be a true arthralgia from the joint, or it may be a form of myalgia from the posterior deep fibers of a tender masseter muscle, which covers a portion of the anterior joint capsule in this area. The second method of palpating the joint involves placing the tips of the little fingers in the external auditory meatus in the open-mouth position. This allows digital pressure to be placed on the retrodiscal bilaminar areas. Using only the first method may allow for a bias to enter due to muscle tenderness from the masseter, but if both methods elicit pain from the joint, it is strongly indicative of a true chronic TMJ capsular pain. However, this is not necessarily to be equated with an acute or exacerbated form of the condition. The bilaminar or retrodiscal tissues of most every patient with functionally oriented TMJ problems are chronically traumatized to some degree and therefore sensitive. But in the more intense forms of the condition, in acute exacerbations due to increased periods of bruxism, etc., or in true acute situations due to trauma, the chronic retrodiscitis of the bilaminar zone may escalate to a capsulitis. In this condition, the pain will increase upon full-force interdigitation of the teeth in habitual occlusion (i.e., condyles up and back), but the pain in the joint will decrease or cease altogether if forceful occlusion is effected with the condyle located more down and forward in the fossa as in the instance of biting on a cotton roll. The former increases mechanical pressure and therefore pain on the inflammation-sensitized capsular and retrodiscal tissues, whereas the latter decreases intracapsular and retrodiscal pressure and therefore pain. Sensitivity of the bilaminar zone of the joint may also be tested via functional manipulation by applying manual pressure to the chin and forcibly attempting to close the mandible in what has been referred to in the past as the ligamentous centric relation. This may only distort already-damaged temporomandibular ligaments in neuromuscular reflexive displacement of the mandible causing superior posterior displacement of the condyle (NRDM/SPDC)-type cases, but it also applies direct condylar pressure to retrodiscal tissues. Closing the mandible for the patient in such a manner may elicit true arthralgic pain from the joint, and its presence is almost always indicative of at least some degree of posterior capsulitis. Such manipulation may also induce tinnitus-type sensations in the ear of the patient with a biofunctionally compromised joint.

Another important finding that may be detectable by means of direct external digital palpation is the presence of reciprocal clicking. Some forms of clicking are "soft" enough to require stethoscopic auscultation in order to determine their presence. However, if a robust click is present upon opening, the examiner can often detect it by placing his fingertips over the condylar area while the patient is at the fully clenched position of maximum habitual dental occlusion and having the patient open widely and close back to that fully closed position in a slow repeated fashion. The opening click will most usually be the more profound of the two. The closing click may be greatly diminished or even totally imperceptible to the tactile sensations of digital palpation. Nevertheless, if an opening click is present, at least conceptually if not biomechanically, the reciprocal closing equivalent must necessarily be present by default. In some instances the clicking may be so profound, especially in the opening motion, as to be audible to the examiner from a speaking distance or even "from across the room." Patients are often aware of their own reciprocal clicking when it is of the more profound variety and express consternation that it causes them embarrassment while eating. Derision from siblings or other family members who observe them and self-consciousness in front of friends and others in social situations is usually the source of this complaint.

Another enlightening observation is the clinical elimination of this type of clicking almost instantly due to the phenomenon of engaging the "as if" position. When clicking is present due to a superiorly posteriorly displaced condyle and an anteromedially displaced disc, the examiner may instruct the patient to slide their mandible forward in an incisal end-to-end position or farther. Instruct the patient to mimic biting off a thread with their front teeth. This would place the mandible in a more forward position anteroposteriorly. It also pulls the condyle down and forward in the joint. This represents an approximation of the position the mandible would assume after the completion of mandibular advancement and posterior vertical increasing procedures accomplished with functional jaw orthopedic (FJO) techniques. It is "as if" the mandible has already been advanced, "as if" it were more anteriorly located than it actually is. This "as if" position may cause the condyle to slide past the heel of the disc back onto the concave underside of the disc, a process referred to as disc reduction. If this happens, the patient may then open and close to that exact end-to-end (or farther) position without allowing the mandible to go back at any time during the exercise, and as a result the condyle stays on the disc during repeated opening and closing to the "as if" position. Such an exercise may cause the joint to click once upon opening the first time after advancing the mandible to the incisal end-to-end position or farther.

If this occurs, it is usually due to the fact that the heel may be so thick, the posterior attachment so distorted, and collateral ligaments so elongated that the condylar head merely pushes the disc ahead of it as the mandible is advanced to the more anterior starting position of the exercise. However, once the first opening cycle takes place from the more advanced "as if" beginning position, the condyle hops back onto the disc and stays there since the closing cycle only returns the mandible to the orthopedically more advanced incisal end-to-end position instead of going all the way up and back (too far) to the fully retruded position dictated by the occlusion and insufficient posterior vertical. In either of the two previously described scenarios of employing the "as if" position of "artificial mandibular advancement," if the clicking disappears, it shows that not only is mandibular advancement necessary, not only is the condyle being forced too far superiorly and posteriorly at full occlusion, not only is the disc being anteromedially displaced, but also, and this is encouraging, the disc is recapturable! Posterior mandibular, hence condylar, displacement is the problem; mandibular advancement with FJO is the solution.

Another scenario that is possible is that there is reciprocal clicking confined to one side due to a malocclusion-directed shift in the mandibular arc of closure to that same side. In such cases, advance the mandible so as to align the orthopedic midlines. (This is a condylar alignment designation, not an arch-to-arch dental midline alignment, which may be entirely different). In other words, advancing to the "as if" incisal end-to-end position or farther while at the same time slightly moving the mandible laterally to the contralateral side usually approximates orthopedic midline alignment. Dental and labial frenum midlines often coincide with orthopedic midlines, although not necessarily, hence they may also be used as a guide for advancement and midline correction to the "as if" position for the exercise. Once accomplished, if the patient can open widely and close again to the corrected advanced incisal position without allowing the mandible to close any farther back and the clicking disappears on the ipsilateral side, it shows that the mandible is in a state of retrusion at full occlusion and that not only is advancement necessary to correct it but that the advancement must be greater on the ipsilateral side to account for the midline shift of the entire mandible to that side upon full closure.

Another beneficial procedure for the sake of patients' education as to the nature of their problem is to use the "as if" exercise to demonstrate to patients the need for mandibular advancement by having them perform the exercise while feeling their joints with their own fingers. First, have them feel the joints in the habitual full-occlusion starting-point translation cycle so that they feel what happens when the joint clicks if they are not already aware of the presence of the clicking. Then have them slide their lower jaw forward to the corrected "as if" position, repeat the opening and closing cycle from that advanced starting position, and note how smoothly and quietly their joints operate. That is what Nature intended. That will be your future therapeutic goal. When the joints do operate that way, after advancement therapy, not only will the noise be a thing of the past, but so will be the related symptoms of the headache, neck ache, and myofascial pains.

Palpation of the muscles of mastication and recording of the levels of sensitivity exhibited by them have long been a traditional part of a comprehensive TMJ examination.[11-14] The tendency over the years seems to have been to palpate increasing numbers of muscles and registering the amount of pain elicited in subjective scales of 1 to 5, with 1 representing slight discomfort and 5 representing an exquisitely sensitive or painful response. The amount of detail engendered during this phase of the examination is a product of the clinician's discretion. However, the status of such main muscles as the temporalis, masseter, medial and lateral pterygoids, digastrics, sternocleidomastoids, and the trapezius muscles with respect to sensitivity to direct digital palpation or indirect functional stimulation should definitely be recorded. The distinction between even only two levels of discomfort, as in mild or severe, is usually adequate. Masticatory muscles invariably exhibit some degree of sensitivity or soreness to palpation in functionally oriented TMJ problems. Yet, because of what we now know about muscles and how and why they exhibit various types of pain, it becomes easier to appreciate why the TMJ symptomatic picture can be so varied. A number of basic tenets of muscle function and dysfunction must be kept in mind.

The soreness and stiffness of common exertion and overuse of a muscle that occur the next day are usually attributed to the accumulation of metabolic products, especially lactic acids, within the muscle tissue. This causes discomfort at both rest and in function. This is different from muscle splinting, which exhibits no discomfort at rest but only in function. It has its origins in the central nervous system (CNS) and represents a hypertonicity of a muscle that acts as a protective mechanism. Nature is beginning to send signals that it wants the threatened part or area stabilized, i.e., left alone, so that necessary biological repairs might be completed. The pain of contracture of muscles involved in muscle splinting is designed to act as the deterrent to further contracture, therefore a deterrent to further movement of the injured part or area. It is often accompanied by a sense of loss of strength in that muscle. There is usually no major structural dysfunction involved. If muscle splinting is perpetuated due to chronicity of the insult, it leads to muscle spasm. This definitely interferes with function and is theorized as being one of the chief contributing agents in the formation of trigger points. If allowed to degenerate even further, chronic muscle spasm and certain other pathological agents can lead to myofibrotic changes and localized muscle contracture known as myositis. This is believed to be due to the formation of cicatricial tissue in the muscle, a sophisticated histological form of scarring. The resultant contracture associated with such advanced states of muscle abuse responds only fairly to attempts at mild continuous traction techniques aimed at lengthening the muscle. But there are other consequences that result from things like long-term muscle abuse, repeated muscle splinting, and recurrent spasms associated with functional TMJ problems. The chronicity of such problems allows the stage to be set for the emergence of the secondary effects of chronic deep pain. It is these secondary effects that caused the early investigators to feel that there were many separate types of TMJ problems, intracapsular and extracapsular, with many types of etiological agents culpable. Disc derangements and condylar displacements were thought to be of one type. Muscle pains and dysfunctions were thought to be another. The secondary effects of chronic deep pain as seen in the patient with typical TMJ problems can account for such misinterpretation by virtue of their ability to affect muscles in a series of strange ways. The collective term used to describe this phenomenon is *CNS excitatory effects*, and it consists of such phenomena as referred pain, trigger point formation, secondary hyperalgesia, and cycling myospasm. One thing they all have in common *symptomatically* is that they all involve muscles. One thing they all have in common *etiologically* is that they all require a chronic, relatively uninterrupted source of deep pain. The appearance of these effects is in direct proportion to the level of severity and chronicity of the insult.

Referred pain, sometimes called heterotropic pain, requires a synaptic circuit with the CNS. Once the initial pain impulse "jumps the neurological track," it is perceived as originating at another site, usually on the same nerve trunk as the true pain source, although not necessarily. Stimulation of the primary site in such situations elicits pain in not only that site but also in the secondary site. Stimulation of the secondary site will not produce pain at either location. Neither will injection with anesthetic stop pain if administered only to the secondary site. But anesthetizing the primary source not only eliminates pain at that source but also in the secondary site, which is perfectly logical.

As previously noted, a trigger point in a muscle is a focus of hyperirritability that is sensitive or painful to palpation or other forms of compression and, if sufficiently hypersensitive, not only results in pain at that specific locus but also may give rise to referred plain at other sites or even referred autonomic phenomena and distortion of proprioception. Trigger points may be active or latent. Like secondary hyperalgesia, trigger points may persist even after the main source of deep pain input (in this case the TMJ-muscle complex) has been rectified, for as long as a year or two past the end of successful treatment of the initial problem. Active trigger points are a source of pain for the patient on a periodic basis. Latent trigger points are those that the patient is unaware of and are related to a previously occurring source of injury or deep pain several years previously. They may persist on a chronic basis and become exacerbated by overuse of the muscle, reactivation of the initial injury, or other forms of abuse to cause muscle pain, stiffness, and weakness. Trigger points are even common in children. It is believed that the number of active trigger points increases through adulthood only to taper off and become latent in old age to then burden the patient with muscle and joint stiffness. The normal electromyographic (EMG) activity of trigger point areas indicates that they are not foci of muscle spasm activity.[15–17] Yet they can induce myospastic activity in a muscle if they are provocated.[18] This is why the painful overstretching of severely involved muscles of mastication in a TMJ patient with functional appliances like the Bionator or Orthopedic Corrector I or active plates with occlusal coverings that are too thick occasionally results in spasms of the elevator muscles. Provocation of the trigger points in the associated musculature by overstretching can induce protective myospastic activity.

The object, however, in palpating the muscles of mastication of the patient with TMJ problems is to provide documentation of whether or not they are sore and, if so, to what general degree. They may be tender due to simple muscle splinting or periodic spasm. They may be sore due to trigger point irritability at the primary foci. They may be sore due to referred pain from trigger points, neurological misconnections, or other central nervous system excitatory effects we as yet do not even understand that result from chronic muscle, ligament, and joint deep-pain input. They may be sore simply because they have been forced to perpetually deliver the mandible too far superiorly and posteriorly against the whole design intent of the entire joint-muscle complex, in the process impinging on some of their own nerves and constricting some of their own blood supply. They are most likely sore due to a combination of all of these factors. Regardless of what the causes may be, we are only interested for the present in recording whether or not they are sensitive to palpation and, if so, to what extent. If they are in fact sensitive or painful, it represents a major finding in the process of determining the diagnosis. For if things were right with the condyle-fossa-disc relationship, they shouldn't be.

The *masseter* muscle may be palpated directly at its origins, belly, and insertion simultaneously both intraorally and extraorally with the thumb and index finger. The origin is often sensitive, as is the belly, in patients who suffer a lack of sufficient posterior vertical dimension of occlusion or if they experience chronic clenching or bruxism. Active trigger points in the masseter can cause pain in the muscle itself and restriction of movement. Unilateral tinnitus may also be encountered as a result of activated trigger points in the masseter's deep portion that refer motor unit activity to the stapedius muscle. Trigger points in the masseter muscle may also refer pain ipsilaterally to the mandible, gingivae, molars, and paranasal sinus area. Trigger points may be activated in this muscle to make it sore due to bruxism, occlusal interferences, or emotional stress,

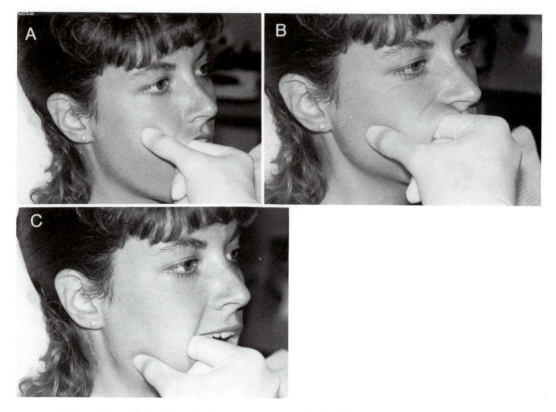

Figure 4–2   Palpation of the masseter muscle. **(A)** Origin at the base of the zygomatic arch; **(B)** belly of the muscle; **(C)** insertion of the muscle at the lower border of the mandible.

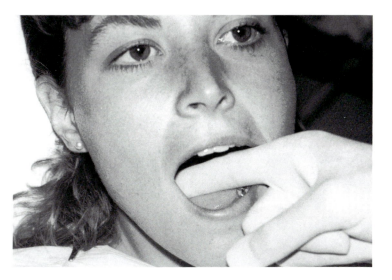

Figure 4–3   Palpation of the medial pterygoid.

especially if the mandible must be overretruded due to an insufficient posterior vertical dimension of occlusion. Although this muscle is commonly sore to palpation in patients with TMJ problems, the pain elicited must be distinguished from pains that might have their origin in the parotid gland due to local infection or a sialolith.

The *medial (internal) pterygoid* muscle, which in turn works on the inside of the ramus, is the synergistic companion to the masseter muscle, which works on the outside. It is often the most sensitive of the elevator muscles of mastication that are accessible to direct digital palpation.[19–22] It is easily palpated by the examiner by running the index finger distally along the base of the myohyoid ridge in the floor of the mouth until the depressions of the pterygomandibular raphe area below the third molar area is felt. Then, finger pressure directed laterally toward the ramus along the inferior border and back toward the gonial region will usually elicit a painful response in most patients with TMJ problems. Activated trigger points in the medial pterygoid, one of the three main muscles of the mandible, as might be expected, can restrict jaw opening. Pain upon jaw opening would be indicative of simple muscle splinting. If pain is present upon opening and the amount of opening is also restricted somewhat, it could be due to trigger point activation, early stages of myospastic activity, or combinations of both. Trigger point activation in the medial pterygoid can also give rise to referred pains in the tongue and back of the throat. They can also result in pain referred deep into the ear and into the TMJ itself. Because of its proximity to the tensor veli palatini muscle, which must impinge on the medial pterygoid in order to perform its func-

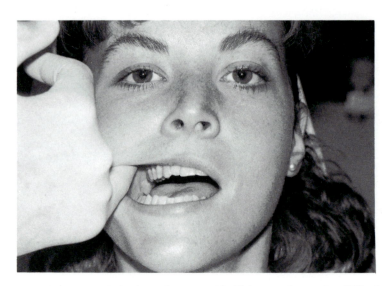

Figure 4–4   Palpation of the lateral pterygoid. This muscle can be difficult to reach. It may be palpated somewhat indirectly by having the patient open his or her mouth part way and move it as far laterally to the ipsilateral side as possible. The examiner then slides a finger along the superior buccal sulcus area to the hamular notch region and then presses up and inward. In patients with functionally induced TMJ problems this muscle area is invariably sensitive.

tion of dilation of the eustachian tube, muscle splinting or early forms of myospasms of the medial pterygoid, which cause it to stiffen up enough that the diminutive tensor veli palatini cannot overcome such resistance, can result in the inability of that tensor muscle to properly keep the tube patent, thus causing a sensation of stuffiness in the ears (barohypoacusis). The usual noxious stimuli can activate or exacerbate trigger points in the medial pterygoid, i.e., bruxism, emotional stress, wide jaw opening, and certain nutritional factors. Just why the medial pterygoid is almost invariably more sensitive to palpation than is its counterpart, the masseter, is unknown, but this is a common clinical finding.

Another interesting finding is that on occasion the lingual nerve courses through the medial pterygoid instead of around it. High levels of muscle splinting or myospastic activity in the medial pterygoid muscle have been reported to manifest themselves in individuals whose lingual nerves happen to course through this muscle as a tingling, burning or even painful sensation in the tongue on the ipsilateral side.[23] These sensations have also been reported to subside once a splint is inserted and/or proper mandibular repositioning techniques as used in FJO-type therapies are instituted. Pressure on the lingual nerve entrapped in the bracing or spastic medial pterygoid is considered the most likely cause. A distal-driving malocclusion forcing the condyle to seat too far up and back in the fossa also forces this important closing muscle to work against its design intent. When muscles are forced to do that, various levels of pain and stiffness are the only way they can protect themselves.

The *lateral pterygoids* should most likely be thought of as three muscles with the common surname of pterygoid but with the individual names of inferior, superior, and "roof of superior." The inferior head or belly acts antagonistically to the other two.[24, 25] The superior belly should be thought of as two muscles for the simple reason that, in posterior condylar/anterior disc displacement situations common to most functionally induced TMJ problems, the muscle may be simultaneously overstretched on its inferior portion and foreshortened on its superior (roof) portion, thereby allowing for myostatic contracture due to the manner in which it is now known to attach to the condyle and anterior portion of the joint's capsular ligament.[26] The lateral pterygoids may be evaluated indirectly through functional manipulation. Pain elicited by wide opening, clenching, or protrusion of the mandible against resistance but not elicited by biting on cotton rolls, tongue blades, or splints in which the acrylic occlusal coverings are not too thick (2.0 mm or less on average) is indicative of inferior lateral pterygoid muscle pain. Pain that is elicited when biting on thin objects or by merely clenching but that is not elicited by wide opening or opening against resistance is indicative of pain from the superior head. As previously stated, controversy exists as to whether or not the inferior portion of the lateral pterygoids may be palpated digitally.[27-30] One thing is certain: of all areas palpated, medially and posteriorly directed digital pressure from the examiner's little finger in the hamular notch area over the area of the pterygoid plexus is the one diagnostic procedure that elicits the most painful response in most patients with TMJ problems.[31-34] Correspondingly, posterior superior condylar displacement stretches the lateral pterygoid in the complete opposite direction of its design intent. Trigger points in these muscles can refer pain to the TMJ itself, the maxillary sinus, and the retro-orbital area.[35] This offers yet another possible explanation for the commonly registered complaint of many patients with TMJ problems of headache pains in the retro-orbital or supraorbital area. These are often mistakenly attributed to sinus problems, allergy, or even that threadbare diagnostic whipping boy, migraine.

The *temporalis* is easily accessible to direct palpation externally on the side of the head except for its insertion at the coronoid process, which is accessible to palpation intraorally if the patient opens to about the midway point. As previously described, the temporalis is designed more for control than power. It is like three separate muscles with three separate actions by virtue of the fanlike distribution of its fibers. The largest portion of the muscle is composed of anterior fibers that run primarily in a vertical direction and are responsible for elevating the mandible. The less robust middle third of the muscle has fibers running obliquely and is responsible for a combined retraction- and elevation-type motion of the mandible. The posterior third is composed of an even smaller number of fibers that run in an almost horizontal direction. These fibers are responsible for retraction of the mandible and perform yeoman service in mandibular retrusion–type cases. In conjunction with components of other muscles, they must work diligently to retract the mandible enough to pull the condyle up and back off the disc since they directly oppose the action of the fibers of lateral pterygoids, which attach to the condylar head and neck. One of the interesting aspects of this muscle in patients with TMJ problems is that trigger points that form in the muscle in chronic TMJ abuse situations can refer phantom sensations of hypersensitivity to heat, cold, and even percussion to any one of the maxillary teeth! Intense or chronic bruxism can activate such trigger points, and many a patient has been told that their recently sensitized, periodontally healthy, caries-free upper teeth were responding that way because "extra stress causes lots of grinding on them during sleep." Occlusal irregularities and insufficient posterior vertical dimension of occlusion will also activate trigger points in the temporalis. Once again, trigger points in this muscle can refer headache-type pains to the back of the head and the supraorbital and retro-orbital areas.[36-39] Thus one more mechanism is added to the long list of reasons that TMJ symptoms can be manifest as headaches in the occipital and eye areas. This unfortunate muscle is also saddled with the complication of having its main arterial supply source, the superficial temporal artery, course right through the posterior joint space. Here it is subject to occlusion of its lumen by nearly 90% during full occlusion in superior posterior condylar displacement situations. It is also subject to the far more pernicious problems of pressure from edema in these areas due to the increased synovial hydraulic pressures attendant to the more acute or severe intracapsular inflammatory processes. The waxing and waning of such edema with the severity of abuse rendered to the joint due to bruxism, hard chewing, clenching, etc., plays havoc with the circulation to this muscle, which is calling for more blood due to the extra work it must do to help close the mandible in such a retrusive state. Overwork a muscle and then don't feed it properly: Nature doesn't like that.

In order to facilitate palpation of this muscle the operator may place the fingertips on the periphery of the origins of the muscle along the gen-

---

Figure 4–5   Palpation of the temporalis.
Figure 4–6   Palpation of the digastric.

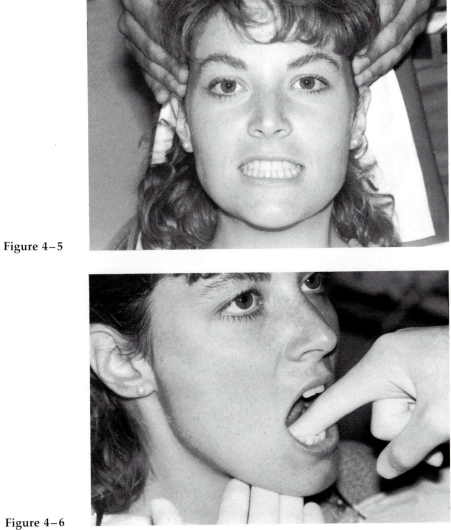

Figure 4-5

Figure 4-6

eral area of the parietotemporal suture and ask the patient to moderately clench his teeth together in a pulsating fashion. This will make the borders of this muscle stand out clearly to tactile sensations. Then gently but firmly rubbing this muscle in small circular motions with the fingertips will divulge any muscle sensitivity in any of its three main areas.

The *anterior belly of the digastric* muscle is another muscle that assists with the arduous task of excessive retrusion of the mandible in distal-driving types of malocclusion situations in patients with TMJ conditions. Its design intent makes it quite inefficient at this, but it participates nonetheless. It also is one of the muscles with a high incidence of sensitivity to palpation in functional TMJ problems. It may be palpated by placing the index finger in the floor of the mouth, placing the thumb of the same hand against the inferior border of the mandible externally, and then pressing the thumb up and inward. Firm pressure in this manner will push the anterior belly of the digastric up into the sublingual space where it may be pressed between the thumb and forefinger. It is often quite sensitive in patients with TMJ problems. Chronic mandibular retrusive situations, as in Class II, Division 2, deep-bite malocclusions, can result in myostatic contracture of this little muscle. Trigger points in this anterior belly can refer pain to the lower incisors. As might be expected, bruxism can activate trigger points in the anterior digastric, but mouth breathing is also a possible source of trigger point activation!

The *cervical musculature* is often a site of recurrent pains for many patients with TMJ problems. This is due to the posture these patients often exhibit. It has been shown that about 70% of patients with Class II malocclusions hold their head forward on their spine by about 10 degrees.[40] Since the human head represents a 10- to 12-lb weight, this forward, inclined, chronic head posture places a strain on the girdle of cervical musculature that must keep the head perched atop the single atlas vertebra, CI. Sometimes the cervicalgia will be the chief complaint and outweigh any other myofascial or headache-type pains. Often they have caused the patient to seek chiropractic treatments, which may offer some temporary relief for the neck and even TMJ pain. But these symptoms of neck pains,

---

Figure 4–7 Cervical musculature. As may be seen from these illustrations, a great variety of musculature is employed in bracing the head and neck. Plenty of areas for trigger point formation due to the chronic abuse of a forward head posture that is often observed in TMJ patients with skeletally retruded mandibles. **(A)** Frontal view; **(B)** left lateral view. (Color code: blue, brachial musculature; red, ventrolateral musculature; green, musculature of the shoulder girdle; yellow, somatic dorsal musculature.) Latin nomenclature is used. (From Pernkopf E: *Atlas of Topographical and Applied Human Anatomy*, vol 1. *Head and Neck*. Munich, Urban & Schwarzenberg, 1963, pp 216, 217. Used by permission.)

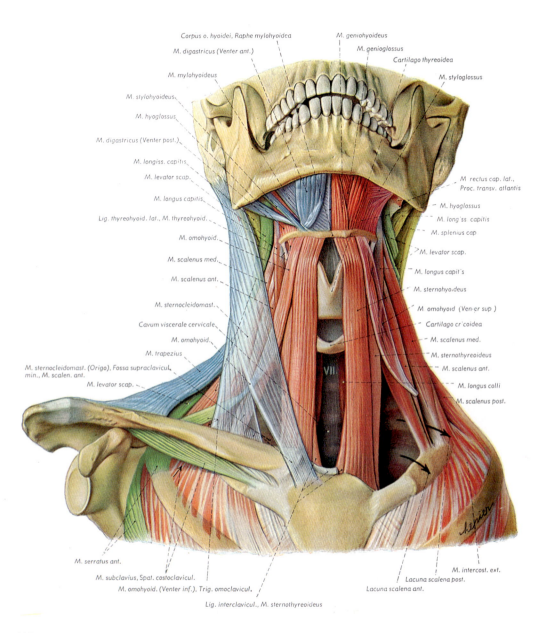

Corpus o. hyoidei, Raphe mylohyoidea
M. geniohyoideus
M. digastricus (Venter ant.)
M. genioglossus
Cartilago thyreoidea
M. mylohyoideus
M. styloglossus
M. stylohyoideus
M. hyoglossus
M. digastricus (Venter post.)
M. longiss. capitis
M. levator scap.
M rectus cap. lat., Proc. transv. atlantis
M. longus capitis
M. hyoglossus
Lig. thyreohyoid. lat., M. thyreohyoid.
M. long'ss capitis
M. omohyoid.
M. splenius cap
M. scalenus med.
M. levator scap.
M. scalenus ant.
M. longus capit's
M. sternohyoideus
M. sternocleidomast.
M omohyoid (Ven·er sup)
Cavum viscerale cervicale
Cartilago cricoidea
M. omohyoid.
M. scalenus med.
M. trapezius
M. sternothyreoideus
M. sternocleidomast. (Origo), Fossa supraclavicul. min., M. scalen. ant.
M. scalenus ant.
M. levator scap.
M. longus colli
M. scalenus post.
M. serratus ant.
M. intercost. ext.
M. subclavius, Spat. costoclavicul.
Lacuna scalena post.
M. omohyoid. (Venter inf.), Trig. omoclavicul.
Lacuna scalena ant.
Lig. interclavicul., M. sternothyreoideus

VII

(A)

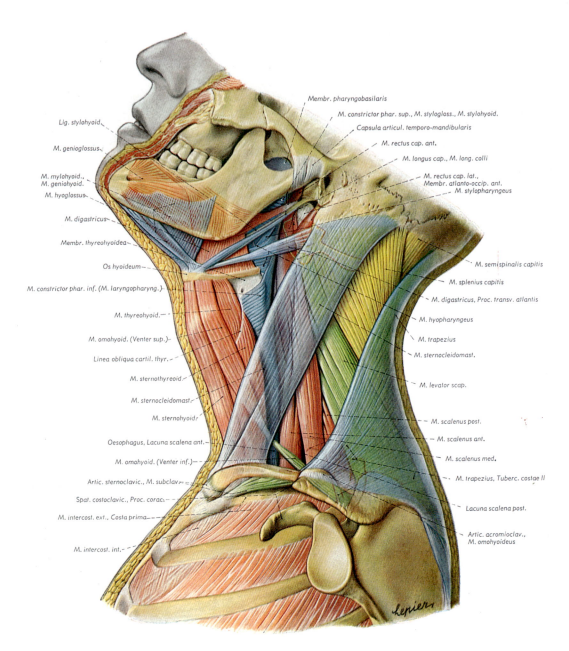

Membr. pharyngobasilaris

M. constrictor phar. sup., M. stylogloss., M. stylohyoid.

Capsula articul. temporo-mandibularis

M. rectus cap. ant.

M. longus cap., M. long. colli

M. rectus cap. lat.,
Membr. atlanto-occip. ant.

M. stylopharyngeus

Lig. stylohyoid

M. genioglossus

M. mylohyoid.,
M. geniohyoid.

M. hyoglossus

M. digastricus

Membr. thyreohyoidea

Os hyoideum

M. constrictor phar. inf. (M. laryngopharyng.)

M. thyreohyoid.

M. omohyoid. (Venter sup.)

Linea obliqua cartil. thyr.

M. sternothyreoid

M. sternocleidomast.

M. sternohyoid

Oesophagus, Lacuna scalena ant.

M. omohyoid. (Venter inf.)

Artic. sternoclavic., M. subclav.

Spat. costoclavic., Proc. corac.

M. intercost. ext., Costa prima

M. intercost. int.

M. semispinalis capitis

M. splenius capitis

M. digastricus, Proc. transv. atlantis

M. hyopharyngeus

M. trapezius

M. sternocleidomast.

M. levator scap.

M. scalenus post.

M. scalenus ant.

M. scalenus med.

M. trapezius, Tuberc. costae II

Lacuna scalena post.

Artic. acromioclav.,
M. omohyoideus

Lepier

(B)

usually distributed along the course of the upper parts of the trapezius muscle, usually return due to the failure of chiropractic adjustments to eliminate the functional imbalance in the TMJs that is in turn due to the effects of malocclusion. It has been theorized that the forward head posture is the result of Nature's effort to enlarge an airway that may be somewhat constricted due to visceral impingement attendant on mandibular retrusion, Pierre Robin's old concept. Many factors may be responsible, but it has been universally observed by clinicians that an extremely high percentage of TMJ patients with attending muscular-generated cervicalgia experience relief of these pains once the original TMJ orthopedic imbalance has been corrected.

Which muscles of the cervical girdle the examiner palpates is a matter of the individual clinician's own knowledge, skills, and personal preferences. However, the two most often involved are the two most accessible, the trapezius and the sternocleidomastoid. The former is quite often sore to palpation in patients with TMJ problems.

Stress and Bruxism: An Old Glove Turned Inside Out

There has been an exciting new viewpoint proposed concerning the role of stress and bruxism in the patient with TMJ problems. A part of this new theory is a new opinion as to what actually acts as the primary etiological agent for bruxism. However, in order to better appreciate the significance and appeal of this theory, a clear understanding of former theories on these issues is imperative. They are the old standard chess pieces of stress, posture, bruxism, and occlusal disharmonies of the TMJ chess board. But in the new viewpoint they have been slightly rearranged and, as a result, represent an entire new game plan by virtue of their theoretical "repositioning" on the board.

It has long been observed that both emotional tension and chronic psychological stress and anxiety are intimately connected with the level of severity of the TMJ symptomatic picture. When mental stresses are increased, symptoms of headache and other myofascial pains have been observed to increase. The psychological stressors seem particularly culpable in this regard due to the fact that they often represent a chronic low-grade (and sometimes not so low grade) stressor that has been shown to have a relation to increased muscle agitation, myogenous types of pains, and various forms of dysfunctions of the muscle splinting-myospasm variety.[41-50] The masseters are known to be one of the first to exhibit splinting, increased contraction, or other signs of irritation when the patient experiences emotional and/or psychological stress. The emotional stressors are of a more acute nature. Their effects are more sudden, as is their dissipation. Hence, emotional effects may wax and wane periodically during a given time frame. The effects of combined emotional and psychological stress seem to be additive and operate a bit differently under somewhat of a threshold mechanism. When the accumulation of such stressors becomes greater than the body's ability to deal with it from a physiological standpoint, symptoms begin to appear. However, this has also been observed to occur in only certain patients. It is not a universal finding.

Occlusal interferences were thought by some to be one of the etiological components of some TMJ disorders.[51, 52] Others, noting that a discrepancy between centric relation and centric occlusion was shown to exist in 90% of the population, felt that occlusal disharmonies were not a major etiological factor.[53–56] It was observed that a "high spot" on a recently placed restoration might cause the tooth to be sore or hypersensitive to biting or to temperature, but such usually didn't reflect itself in the form of joint pain. It was also known that a certain number and type of occlusal interferences that occurred in the fully occluded position usually only resulted in tooth damage (excessive occlusal wear) or muscle effects. The muscles are known to have a certain range of adaptability, and occlusal interferences of specific varieties can cause changes in the habitual patterns of muscular movement of the jaw. This, of course, we now know forms the basis of the NRDM/SPDC phenomenon. Thus, the significance of the occlusal interference was for decades the object of controversial debate, but the direction in which it might cause the mandible to deflect to full occlusion was never thought of as a major etiological factor, at least not until more modern times. All that was conjectured was that occlusal disharmonies might result in associated muscle-oriented pain and dysfunction. Huge wear facets on artificial restorations or even natural teeth in asymptomatic patients had to be figuratively swept under the theoretical rug.

Bruxism on the other hand, in both its nocturnal and diurnal forms, was thought to be intimately related to emotional tension. It was debated that an occlusal interference might stimulate bruxism, but no evidence could be produced to support this theory, and as a result it received little support. It was shown that an occlusal prematurity had an inhibitory effect on elevator muscle activity anyway. Since most of the evidence of the times indicated that bruxism was a CNS-generated activity, emotional and psychological stress was considered the chief cause, and sore, painful, dysfunctioning musculature and even internal joint damage were thought to be the effects. Well, now it appears that only part of this observation is in fact what might actually be happening. A new theory based on extensive clinical observations has been proposed that looks at all this differently.

In a bold departure from traditional viewpoints, certain members of the "FJO camp" have observed and therefore proposed that it is not mental stress that is the exclusive etiological agent in initiating bruxism; rather, two other factors act as primary causes: function of the muscles of mastication at an improperly shortened length and irritation of the ner-

vous tissue of the bilaminar zone by a condyle that is superiorly and posteriorly displaced and riding off the disc![57] The bruxism is just as damaging to the joint structures and plays just as much havoc with the muscles,
but it is initiated by condylar displacement, not just stress. The bruxism
may be an effort of the body to "autoequilibrate" the distal-driving anterior incisal interferences out of its own mandibular-arc-of-closure's way.
This would account for the excessive incisal wear of lower anterior teeth
or the "cingulum ditching" seen on the lingual surfaces of upper anterior
teeth in many Class II, Division 2, deep-bite type of cases. As for how to
account for the increased incidence of associated TMJ symptoms of cephalalgia, cervicalgia, and myofascial pains associated with periods of increased mental stress, the new theory reaches back almost a half century
to call on the well-known findings of Canadian stress researcher Hans
Selye and his discoveries of the relationships of the general adaptation
syndrome (GAS) and the local adaptation syndrome (LAS).

It is well known that Selye was quite right in stating that stress in all
its forms can stimulate the body to engage general adaptive measures.
The manifestations of the adrenaline-driven "fight-or-flight" responses of
the sympathetic nervous system are an often-cited example. He has also
shown the relationship, previously discussed in this text, of the LAS to
activation the GAS. Now a chronically abused TMJ with a condyle riding
off the disc is a potent LAS entity in its own right. This is more than capable of stimulating GAS responses in the host. But that is not the main
issue with respect to stress. The role chronic mental stress plays in the big
picture is in its propensity to stimulate the GAS in a fashion that in effect
"sets up" the patient for the further abuses dished out by bruxism, itself
stimulated in turn by a condyle riding up in the bilaminar zone. Chronic
low-grade stimulation of the GAS can lead to weakening or exhaustion of
the system and desensitization of receptor target organs and mechanisms.
This in effect leaves entire portions of the body's physiological system
somewhat depleted of reserves that might be needed when other more
acute forms of physiological crises occur. Thus periodic episodes of intense stress exhaust the body's generalized adaptive and recovery systems prematurely, and they are therefore less resilient and less able to repair the localized injuries caused by the bruxism. The damage bruxism
represents then merely rises to the surface more readily. This causes the
mistaken notion that it was the increased stress that caused the increased
severity of symptoms, i.e., the "tension headache," when in fact it was
the body's inability, due to depletion of its own reserves, to heal the
abused muscles rapidly enough to recover from the perpetual effects of
the bruxism, that brings pain symptoms to the surface. The increased
muscle tonicity and other myogenic problems manifest during increased
periods of stress are a result of being physiologically "unattended to" by
the adaptive and repair mechanisms of the body because its physiological
reserves are depleted temporarily by a different form of insult. With less

recuperative strength available to help abused muscles and joint structures recover, the joint and musculature become an even greater LAS stressor in their own right. Simplistically, it may be thought of as a case where the body makes a steady effort to deal with a physiologically compromised TMJ but has less ability to do so at times, which in turn causes the joint and musculature to exacerbate symptoms in a call for more attention. That physiological attention is at times difficult for the body to render because increased periods of other extraneous forms of stress have depleted its adaptive reserves and left it (if you will be so indulgent as to forgive the play on words) quite simply "out of GAS!"

When the condyle is brought back down and forward into its proper place back on the disc, when the muscles of mastication may once again operate at their normal full nonforeshortened length, when the nerves of the auriculotemporal neurovascular bundle cease being irritated by condylar intrusion, bruxism stops! This has been observed on a regular basis. It has long been known that adequately increasing the vertical dimension of occlusion causes a calming effect on the overactivity of the elevator muscles of mastication. This is why, if properly executed, "mandibular stabilization prosthesis–type" splint techniques will reduce the EMG activity of closing muscles in bruxing situations. However, the vertical must be adequate, i.e., a splint constructed properly so as to bring the condyle far enough down and forward in the fossa so as to preclude condylar irritation of the bilaminar zone. And it is also commonly known that this effect will occur *only* when the splint is worn.

To clarify why patients who are stressed present the type of symptomatic picture they do, consider the following scenarios. First, a patient who is not suffering from a functionally induced TMJ arthrosis and who is not stressed will not exhibit classic TMJ symptoms of cephalalgia, cervicalgia, or myofascial pain. A patient whose TMJs are fine, i.e., condyle on the disc, will not experience headaches due to increased periods of stress either. Neither will they inordinately brux. A patient whose TMJs are compromised but who is fortunate enough to be relatively unstressed will have a common TMJ symptomatic picture with a certain modicum of headaches and myofascial discomforts proportional to the severity of condylar displacement. But in our worst-case scenario, a patient with a compromised TMJ due to a distal-driving malocclusion who is also stressed will experience an even greater level of severity of pain and discomfort because the stress represents a way of physiologically siphoning off the body's ability to deal with the abused muscles and joints that are made worse not only by function but also the self-initiated burdens of bruxism.

It is commonly observed in the treatment of these patients that after the retruded condyle has been corrected to its proper place back down and forward on the disc once again, symptoms subside even though the stress the patient experiences does not.[58–63] They will report that their pain symptoms are gone even though they still have the same work environment, the same home environment, the same boss, the same job, the same spouse, the same financial difficulties, the same personal problems, the same all-around stress! It is the vicious cycle of malocclusion/condyle off disc/muscle foreshortening/bruxism that is the etiological chain of events that allows the patient with TMJ problems to experience pain and dysfunction. Stress only intensifies the problem and leaves patients less resilient, less capable of dealing with the compromised stomatognathic system from which they suffer.

Auscultation

Although often the reciprocal clicking in patients with TMJ problems is so profound that it may be heard from a speaking distance and may be palpated easily with the fingers during opening and closing movements of the jaw, sometimes the clicking or other types of joint noises are so faint that they require the aid of a stethoscope to be heard. All joint sounds, regardless of the variety, should be of interest to the diagnostician, especially clicking. However, it must be remembered that occasionally a nonpathological click may be present. If it exists and is detected by the operator and if the patient is completely free of any other signs or symptoms such as headaches, tenderness of the muscles of mastication to palpation, etc., the patient should be informed of it, and it should be duly recorded in the patient's chart. Placing the patient on periodic recall to continue observation of the joints over a long period of time is then justified. However, it must be remembered that functionally induced TMJ arthrosis is a progressive condition and clicking may often be the harbinger of unpleasant things to come. If the clicking is "soft" enough to require detection with a stethoscope, be certain that the patient begins the translation motion from the fully occluded and clenched position. The earlier the click may be heard in the opening cycle, the greater the chances of fully recapturing the disc with mandibular advancement procedures. But remember, reduction of the joint is not the primary treatment goal but rather reduction of the pain.

Crepitus is the sound of bone rubbing on bone. It implies a perforation in either the posterior attachment or in the intra-articular disc. Most perforations occur in the posterior lamina, as true discal perforations are relatively rare. The detection of crepitus, or a sound like sandpaper rubbing against sandpaper, that is due to a perforation will usually be confirmed by a properly oriented transcranial radiograph or tomogram in which the condylar head is seen to obliterate some portion of the superior and/or anterior joint space. It would appear that the anterior or superior portion of the condylar head is in flush contact with a portion of the roof of the fossa or articular eminence at the full-occlusion position. Crepitus due to perforations of the disc or posterior attachment is always a sign of an advanced level of degeneration within the joint. Yet conventional FJO principles of treatment still apply and fortunately as a result obviate the need for plication-type surgery in such instances. It has now been shown that once condylar decompression techniques of the FJO variety are implemented, and mandibles are permanently advanced, scar tissue forms in the area of the perforation in the posterior attachment.

This scar tissue then acts as a makeshift "pseudo-disc" upon which the condyle then functions. The permanently anteriorly displaced original disc disintegrates somewhat in its "jammed forward" deranged position in the anterior recess of the capsular cavity, thus allowing an acceptable modicum of condylar translation to take place once again. This improves what would formerly have been somewhat limited ranges of opening for such a case.

Range-of-Motion Measurements

Important diagnostic information relative to the condition of the muscles and the status of the disc-condyle assembly can be obtained from range-of-motion measurements. Two types of motions are measured, the maximum interincisal opening, measured in millimeters between the incisal edges of the upper and lower anterior teeth, and the lateral excursive movement. This measurement is registered as the horizontal distance between the midlines of the upper and lower centrals with the lower jaw in its maximum state of lateral excursion.

The maximum interincisal opening can reveal a number of things. In a normal healthy adult male, the maximum range should be from 45 to 58 mm or more. Healthy adult females should reach 45 to 50 mm or more. Children beyond 6 years of age should be able to open 40 mm or more. Therefore, an interincisal opening of less than 40 mm is indicative of restricted range of opening, regardless of the patient's age. As previously alluded to, the muscles, the joint capsule, and the intracapsular structures themselves all have the ability under certain circumstances to limit the maximum range of opening. Hence limitation of opening is divided into three categories of problems, extracapsular, capsular, and intracapsular.

Extracapsular limitation of opening is due to muscles that are rebelling against their normal work range due to some form of abuse that is being meted out to either to themselves or to nearby structures. This most often takes the form of protective CNS excitatory effects such as the increased tonus and painful resistance to movement (contracture) due to muscle splinting or even the more advanced form of such phenomena, frank myospasm. When such bilateral myogenic problems are confined to the elevator muscles, the resistance to reaching the former full stretch length due to splinting or myospasm limits the range of opening, but

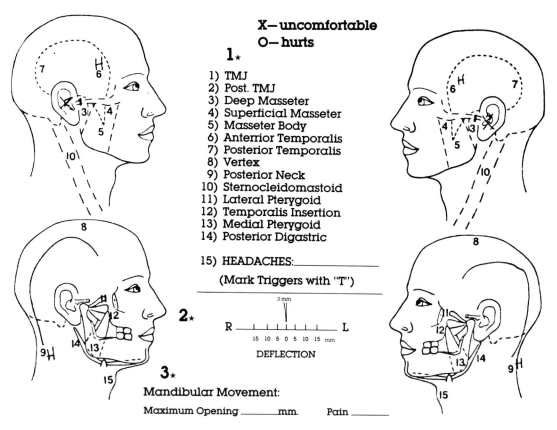

X— uncomfortable
O— hurts

1★

1) TMJ
2) Post. TMJ
3) Deep Masseter
4) Superficial Masseter
5) Masseter Body
6) Anterior Temporalis
7) Posterior Temporalis
8) Vertex
9) Posterior Neck
10) Sternocleidomastoid
11) Lateral Pterygoid
12) Temporalis Insertion
13) Medial Pterygoid
14) Posterior Digastric

15) HEADACHES:_____

(Mark Triggers with "T")

3 mm

R ⊢⊢⊢⊢⊢⊢⊢⊢⊢ L
   15 10 5 0 5 10 15 mm

DEFLECTION

2★

3★

Mandibular Movement:

Maximum Opening _____mm.   Pain _____

Figure 4–8   Sample of a muscle chart included in the examination forms used by Dr. John Witzig.

since the lateral pterygoids are not involved, the straight protrusive motion without opening and the lateral excursive movements are not limited. It must be noted here that limitation of lateral excursion can be a result of not only a splinted or spastic lateral pterygoid but also an anterior displacement of the disc. Therefore, if lateral excursion is at its full normal range, it may be assumed that not only are the contralateral lateral pterygoids reasonably sound but also the condyle is on the disc on the contralateral side. (This will be discussed in more detail shortly.) Once the maximum range of opening dips below 40 mm, the elevator muscles of mastication are starting to rebel and cramp in their protective muscle splinting process. Taken to its physiological conclusion, the range of opening can gradually lessen as the muscle splinting worsens and reaches its climax in a limited range of opening of only several millimeters as the elevator muscles have reached a state of frank myospasm. As the jaw is opened to its maximum, albeit limited, range due to the splinted muscles' resistance to stretch, further forced opening past the point of limitation elicits pain from the elevator muscles. Mastication also elicits a painful response from muscles in such a state.

Muscle dysfunction may also result in deflection of the mandible if the muscular splinting or spastic problems are confined to one side in unilateral myogenic problems. A deflection to the affected or unaffected side can occur depending on the muscle or muscles involved. Deflection is defined as a gradual and continuous displacement of the mandibular midline throughout the entire range of movement. (This is to be differentiated from a mandibular deviation, which consists of a brief displacement of the mandibular midline with its return to the center by completion of the opening movement. Deviation is due to a discal interference.) The direction to which the muscular deflection forces the midline during opening is also informative as to just which muscles might be involved. If the medial pterygoid muscle on one side is splinted, foreshortened, or cramped, it will cause the condyle on the same side to translate toward the unaffected side and therefore a resultant midline shift to the *unaffected* side. This is of course only true if the medial pterygoid is the *only muscle*

Figure 4–9   Measurement of lateral excursive movement. Midlines are aligned with the mandible slightly protruded so as to facilitate visualization. **(A)** Then the furthest extent of lateral excursion of the mandible is measured in millimeters from the midline of the upper central incisors to the midline of the lower central incisors. It should range from 10 to 15 mm. **(B)** When the condyle is riding off the back edge of the disc at full occlusion, it jams the disc ahead and medially to it when the mandible is moved laterally to the contralateral side. This limits the lateral excursive measurement to the contralateral side to about 7 to 9 mm or less. (Part B Courtesy of Dr. John Witzig.)

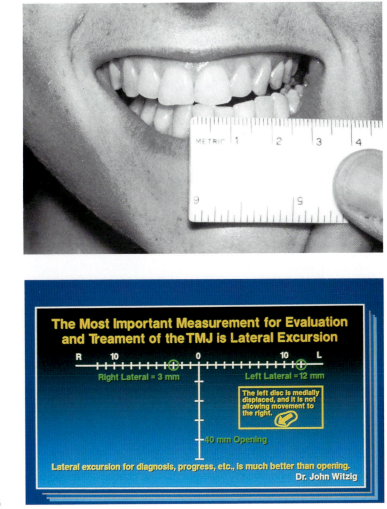

Figure 4–9(A)

(B)

involved. Conversely, if the masseter and temporalis muscles are cramped or otherwise restricted on one side, a more common scenario, the range of motion on that same side, will of course be limited. But it will not be limited on the opposite side since this is a deflection scenario and therefore by necessity unilateral. Hence, the mandible on the unaffected side has a full range of motion. Therefore, an opening procedure would deflect the midline to the affected side. Deflection that is purely muscular due to unilateral cramping may be differentiated from deflection due to a unilateral intracapsular problem by observing the extent of the lateral excursion possible. Deflection that is due strictly to muscles on the affected side will also exhibit a normal range of lateral excursion (12 to 15 mm). Also straight protrusion is unaffected. Deflection that is intracapsular in nature will result in a deflection to the affected (ipsilateral) side but a restricted lateral excursive movement toward the unaffected (contralateral) side.

Capsular restrictions of mandibular ranges of motion are not common. They result from shrinkage of the capsular ligament that surrounds the disc-condyle-fossa assembly. This may occur as a result of inflammatory diseases, fibrotic changes due to surgery, the use of sclerosing agents, or adhesions (another form of intracapsular scarring resulting from chronic abuse). Capsular restriction of movement would result in limitation of translation of the condyle on the affected side. This limitation is obvious in all the condylar excursions, each of which is affected to the same relative degree. The maximum range of interincisal opening may hover in the 25- to 28-mm range. Should an actual capsulitis be present, pain will increase if the teeth are clenched firmly at habitual occlusion, but it will decrease or even disappear while biting on cotton rolls. Also, firm pressure on the mandible in a posterior direction will elicit pain from the joint.

Intracapsular restriction of motion implies an anteromedially displaced disc in the classic "clinical closed-lock" state of nonreduction. The perpetually displaced disc acts to obstruct the translation of the condyle down and forward. The condyle is up and back off the posterior heel of the disc and in the initial attempts at opening cannot renegotiate the disc. Hence the disc is jammed ahead of the condyle as if crumpled or balled up into a fibrocartilagenous obstruction. Therefore, the opening motion, what there is of it, is almost exclusively confined to the rotation phase only and expresses an interincisal opening in the range of 25 to 27 mm. Not only is the opening movement restricted, but the straight protrusive and lateral excursive movements are also restricted. If the problem is unilateral, the mandibular midline is deflected at the point of discal obstruction to the same (ipsilateral) side while lateral excursion to the opposite unaffected (contralateral) side is restricted. Lateral excursive movements to the ipsilateral side are not restricted because the ipsilateral condyle rotates about a vertical axis on the posterior attachment just as if it were on a disc, except with a lot more damage.

Of course, there is nothing to preclude a combination of these circumstances occurring simultaneously in an advanced state of TMJ involvement. Opening may be restricted in some fashion due to intracapsular problems such as jamming of the disc ahead of the condyle. It may be worsened by cramped or splinted muscles, which would exhibit a painful response to forced attempts at stretching them past their spasm-foreshortened limits of length. Nature is using all its protective mechanisms in an effort to stem the tide of abuse being administered to the musculature and especially the retrodiscal bilaminar zone by a condyle that is being driven too far superiorly and posteriorly by the NRDM/SPDC phenomenon. Such a state represents figuratively a physiological cry for help and an attempt at complete shutdown until repairs can be made. The dental profession has always tried to help out in this process a little. Fortunately, the time has now finally come when we can help a lot.

A very important range-of-motion measurement is that of the linear horizontal distance representing the lateral excursive movement. It is measured as the horizontal distance in millimeters between the midlines of the upper and lower central incisors when the patient is executing the maximum state of lateral excursive movement their joints will allow. This simple measurement is an excellent indicator of the presence of an anteriorly displaced disc. The normal range of lateral excursion should be 12 to 15 mm. Anything less than 10 mm is considered a sign of a joint that is dysfunctioning. A 3- to 5-mm lateral excursive measurement is a definite sign of an anteromedially displaced disc.

Let us construct a hypothetical example of a case where a mandible is suffering from a severe orthopedic midline shift in the full-occlusion position such that the left condyle is superiorly and posteriorly displaced with a resultant anteromedially displaced disc but the right disc-condyle-fossa relationship is perfectly normal. In the left lateral excursive movement, the left condyle rotates about its vertical axis (twists) as the body of the mandible shifts to the left. The right disc-condyle assembly must translate down the articular eminence of the right joint, and as it does, it also moves ever so slightly in a medial direction also. Motion in this plane is of course quickly limited by the medial wall of the glenoid fossa. The fact that the right condyle is *on* the disc is what permits this entire action to take place. Note that as the left condyle merely twists about its vertical axis, it may easily do so whether it is on the disc (which in this example it is not) or riding on the posterior bilaminar attachments due to its superior posterior displacement and the anteromedial displacement of the left disc. In the right lateral excursive movement, something quite different happens. In the right excursive movement, the right condyle twists about its vertical axis, and the left condyle should translate down the left eminential slope. But the disc is already displaced anteromedially ahead of the condyle. As the right lateral excursive movement is initiated, the left condyle attempts to move down and slightly medially in the left fossa. But it is soon jammed against the anteromedially displaced disc, which halts the condyle's translation, and the lateral excursive movement is stopped short. Thus an abbreviated lateral excursive measurement is a sign of a rather severely involved joint and a rather severely anteromedially displaced disc. However, a full range of lateral excursive motion may occur if the anteromedial displacement is not severe because the condyle quickly negotiates the disc early in the translatory cycle and therefore, once on the disc, may complete the necessary translation to effect the full lateral movement. The clicking present during normal opening and closing movements usually indicates that the disc is anteromedially displaced. The limitations of the lateral excursive movement *confirm* that the disc on the contralateral side is anteromedially displaced.

IMAGING THE JOINT

Prior to the age when imaging the joint has become a highly refined procedure, many diagnoses and treatment plans were effected for patients with functionally oriented TMJ problems on very primitive or poorly defined radiographic images or even no images at all! The history/anamnesis and clinical examination for myofascial pain and reciprocal clicking are two very important members of the basic triad of diagnostic procedures involved in rendering a modern-day diagnosis of TMJ pain-dysfunction conditions. They form what is referred to as the clinical diagnosis of the condition. This has long been the mainstay of TMJ therapeutics. Fortunately, we may now augment that clinical diagnosis with joint images produced by means of a variety of techniques and methodologies. The methods involved range from radiographs produced with conventional x-rays all the way to images that are an astounding result of the most discrete and sophisticated forms of atomic energy. Being that joint function is so important and since that implies proper movement of the component parts, the human TMJ has been imaged in a wide variety of positions of function that range from fully closed positions (a position of paramount interest to modern-day TMJ clinicians), through all the various phases of translation, all the way to the fully opened position. It has also been imaged from a variety of aspects: lateral, inferior, frontal, and endless angular variants of the same.

The problems that first confronted the early investigators who attempted to image the joint were legion. First, there was the age-old problem of trying to project a three-dimensional object, and a rather anatomically complex three-dimensional object at that, onto a two-dimensional surface. The rounded dome and lateral wall of the glenoid fossa and the mediolaterally flattened jelly bean–type shape of the condylar head are objects stereoscopically prone to a variety of silhouette projections as a result of such a process. Superimposition of extraneous osseous structures was a major problem and precluded direct lateral projections because one joint would resultantly be superimposed upon the other, thus obscuring almost all details. Another problem that frustrated the early investigators who were all but obsessed with the condition of soft tissues within the joint, especially the intra-articular disc, was that only the actual subarticular bone could be seen on the conventional radiograph. The dense fibrous articular tissues of the condylar head and articular eminence as well as the all-important disc remained unseen. When conditions within the joint had degenerated enough to result in changes in the contours of the subarticular bone itself, it could not only be seen (if angulations of the x-ray beam were correct), but it could also be assumed that changes in the unseen articular surfaces had preceded it. Although the space between portions of the outline of the condyle and the outline of the fossa and eminence could be seen, more concern was originally expressed, unfortunately, over the status of the unseen tissues of the anterior joint space than over those that were much more important from a clinical standpoint in the posterior joint space.

Conventional radiography of the joint has been refined into three basic types of projections. An image produced by a beam traveling laterally through the joint area from below the midface in an upward direction is called a transpharyngeal view. An image produced by a beam traveling laterally through the joint from above the midface and downward is termed a transcranial view. These methods allow the main target beam to bypass the proximal joint closest to the x-ray source by passing under or over it in order to project the image of the more distant joint on the opposite side of the head onto the film. A projection that results from the beam passing from the front of the face from anterior to posterior through the joint with the mouth open so the condyle comes into view from behind the more forwardly superimposed structures is referred to as a transorbital view.

Tomography represents the next level up in sophistication of joint imaging by conventional radiographic x-ray–type energy sources. In the tomographic technique, the x-ray source and the film move in a mechanical fashion precalculated to purposefully blur the structures on either side of a given target depth. It is the radiographic equivalent of taking a slice out of a given depth of target area and focusing the x-ray beam in such a way that only the area within that particular slice is projected clearly on the film. Computers are employed to manage tomographic-type data to produce even more sophisticated images. The pinnacle of high technology is currently represented by nuclear magnetic resonance imaging (MRI), which employs a computer-interpreted radio signal produced by the atoms of the target area as a result of being placed and energized in rapidly oscillating magnetic fields. Both soft tissues as well as hard tissues and even things like inflammatory fluids appear in such images.

In an effort to be practical for the rank-and-file practitioners, a number of criteria have emerged by which the value of particular imaging procedures are judged. The methods would hopefully involve equipment the common practitioner may both afford and operate easily. It should produce images that are well defined and as free as possible from superimposition of extraneous structure. It should also produce relatively little distortion. The techniques should be standardized enough to permit superimposition of serial films for before and after comparisons of the joints of the same individual involved in treatment. It should also permit viewing of the joint in any of its positions from full occlusion to full opening. And finally, the technique should be adaptable enough to accommodate the variance in condylar shape and angulation to the sagittal plane to permit sharp images to be obtained of the condyle and fossa regardless of their individual angular polarity.

TMJ investigators have made every effort to seek the best way of obtaining truly revealing images of the TMJ that would give trustworthy evidence of the nature of the patient's joint problem. They have gone to great lengths to construct just the right sort of figurative looking glass that would enable them to "peep through the blanket of the dark" and view what up until now has been one of Nature's mysterious little places. But now the initial concern for the disc, although still important, has been replaced in the opinion of the more avant-garde TMJ clinicians by a concern for something even more important. As a result, just what they are now looking for, how they interpret what they see, and the manner in which they produce the images of what they want to see will no doubt for some traditional TMJ clinicians turn out to be something of a surprise.

"I will sit down now,
but the time will come
when you will hear from me."

English Prime Minister Benjamin Disraeli
First Speech, House of Commons
7 December 1837

Transcranial Radiography

The location of the TMJ at the base of the skull where it is surrounded by a great deal of anatomy has made acquiring a clearly defined nondistorted radiograph a difficult task. A straight lateral view would of course superimpose one side of the head over the other and therefore one joint over the other and obliterate the important detail for which the radiograph was originally taken. Therefore, techniques were developed whereby the central x-ray beam was aimed obliquely at one joint in such a way that it bypasses the other. This preserves the delicate detail of the projected image from obliteration due to superimposition of the opposite joint. However, there were still a number of problems that confronted early investigators of the transcranial TMJ radiographic technique. Although sometimes films would provide a clear view of the condyle and an outline of the fossa and joint spaces, other times they would not. This was a result of the wide range of variance in joints with respect to the angulation of the mediolateral pole of the condylar head with respect to the central beam. As might be imagined, this resulted in a great deal of controversy over the value of the transcranial radiograph as a diagnostic tool. Some felt it was capable of producing excellent results but was merely extremely technique sensitive.[64-78] Others thought it was completely worthless as far as providing assessment of condyle-to-fossa relationships.[79-83] Some felt it was valuable because it provided important information relative to the condition of the subarticular bone.[84] Others thought it was of little if any value because it could not reveal the position or status of the intra-articular disc,[85] an entity that was the prime center of attention in earlier days. This controversy might still be valid except for two important considerations. First, modern-day TMJ clinicians appreciate the value of knowledge of the status of the disc and subarticular bone, but their chief concern has now become the amount of joint space, particularly the superior and posterior joint space between the condylar head and dome and posterior wall of the fossa. For this is the dwelling place of the auriculotemporal neurovascular bundle, the superficial temporal artery, and the other highly innervated tissues of the bilaminar zone. Second, observing these spaces clearly on a transcranial film is predicated on aligning the central beam of the x-ray head parallel to the mediolateral polar axis of the condylar head. This is now easily done by means of the use of proper head-holding equipment and the pilot film, i.e., the submental vertex view. Thus the transcranial radiograph, after having suffered a highly controversial and somewhat dubious debut, has reemerged as the cornerstone of TMJ radiographic technique. Controversy still exists in this area. However, it is not over the quality of the image or amount of distortion present in the film but rather how to interpret what it means.

In order to obtain a transcranial film with as little distortion as possible, the position of the patient's head and the alignment of the tube become critical. The patient's Frankfort horizontal plane should be parallel to the floor, and the patient should be seated in an upright position. Variance of the patient's head from this standardized position will result in films with greater superimposition of structures and will preclude comparison of separate films of the same individual as in before and after treatment. The most common angulation of the central beam needed to produce good films turns out to be 20 degrees vertical angulation and from 20 to 24 degrees from the posterior. Original equipment designed by the Denar Corporation (Acurad 100) was preset at a 25-degree vertical angulation and a 10-degree anteroposterior angulation. Even if the patient would require a different anteroposterior angulation, this original equipment is still of great value for two main reasons. First, the patient's head may be adjusted in the head holder if need be by rotating it *toward* the film cassette slightly. This may be done by placing the ear rod of the side opposite the cassette posterior to the external auditory meatus. However, this is difficult to reproduce exactly in subsequent films. Second, even if the original settings of the device are not completely satisfactory, as long as the patient's Frankfort plane is kept parallel to the floor and as long as the head-holding device with its film cassette is kept parallel to the floor, pretreatment and posttreatment films may be compared for posterior joint space decompression in the full-occlusion position anyway. For then the amount of distortion on each radiograph becomes the same, and it all becomes relative. All that will happen if the central beam doesn't travel exactly down the mediolateral condylar polar axis is that the posterior and anterior joint spaces will appear slightly more constricted than they really are. It must be remembered that decisions to treat the patient by the downward and forward mandibular advancement techniques of FJO are based on the history, anamnesis, and clinical examination of the patient and only confirmed by radiography. Thus, if posterior joint space decompression becomes a treatment goal, comparison of even "uncorrected" before and after transcranial films will suffice.

More advanced equipment developed by Denar (Acurad 200) in 1974

Figure 4–10   The evolution of the transcranial radiographic technique. **(A)** In the Gillis technique the point of entry of the central ray is ½ in. in front and 2 in. above the external auditory meatus in a direction first parallel with then perpendicular to the angulation of occlusal plane (symbolized by long white lines parallel with and perpendicular to the occlusal plane in the middle drawing). **(B)** In the Grewcock technique, the central ray is aligned merely 2 in. above the external auditory meatus in a direction perpendicular to the angulation of the occlusal plane. **(C)** In the Lindblom technique the central ray is aimed ½ in. above and 2 in. *behind* the external auditory meatus in a direction first parallel with and then up perpendicular to that individual's particular occlusal plane. **(D)** In the McQueen technique the central ray is directed from a point just below the zygomatic arch and ¾ in. anterior to the posterior border of the ramus. **(E)** Commercially produced nonadjustable transcranial radiographic devices such as the Denar Acurad 100 use average fixed angulations similar to the Lindblom technique. The pencil symbolizes the direction of the central ray. More advanced equipment such as the Denar Acurad 200 are fully adjustable and designed for use with pilot films (submental vertex) to determine individual condylar polar axis angulations. **(F)** This illustration depicts the images projected on the transcranial film and the reason they appear as they do.

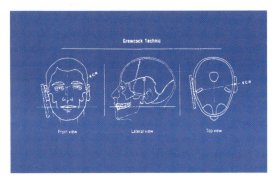

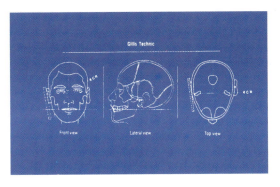

Figure 4–10(A)   (B)

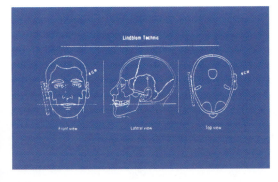

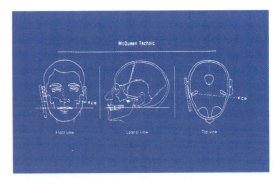

(C)   (D)

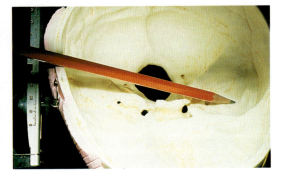

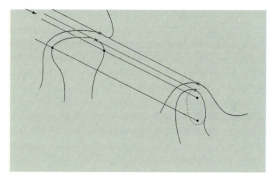

(E)   (F)

compensates for variance in the condylar polar axis by employing measurements from the submental vertex view. This view entails the use of the special head and x-ray tube-holding device designed for this purpose (Versatech),* which can be used with most conventional dental x-ray units. The object of this device is to aim the central beam directly up the sagittal plane from beneath the patient's head. This is accomplished by having the patient lean back in a small flexible chair and tip the head back to that Frankfort plane that is actually perpendicular to the floor. In this position an x-ray beam horizontal to the floor and directed up through the bottom of the patient's chin produces an image on a film in a cassette over the patient's crown (the cassette is perpendicular to the horizontal x-ray beam). This is the submental vertex view. It clearly displays the mediolateral condylar polar axis. A tracing is made of the midsagittal plane by merely observing the midpalatal suture. Then the respective condylar polar axis lines are drawn and extended to meet a perpendicular line to this midsagittal line. The angles between this perpendicular and the condylar axes are measured and recorded. The values of these angles then determine the settings used on the head-holding device used to take the transcranial film. Thus the angulation of the beam may be adjusted to match the condylar polar axes of any patient. For a large percentage of patients, the conventional angular settings as represented by the older

---

*As of October 1, 1990, this equipment was replaced by a more advanced model, the Acurad 300, which accomplishes the same thing.

Figure 4–11   Pilot film (submental vertex) used to determine condylar polarity. **(A)** Versatech x-ray head tube holding device used to obtain submental vertex as well as other cephalometric views. **(B)** Angulation of the patient, film cassette, and x-ray head used to produce submental vertex pilot films. **(C)** Submental vertex film. **(D)** Tracing of a submental vertex film. **(E)** The angulation line of the condylar poles (polar axis) forms an angle (curved arrows) to the midsagittal plane (line through the midpalatal suture) that is measured internally and then transferred to an adjustable transcranial radiographic unit (Acurad 200) to ensure that central beam is parallel to condylar axis for the best view of the posterior joint space in cases where the condylar polar angle varies extensively from the average, which is about 10 degrees. **(F)** The equipment used to generate the submental vertex film may also be used to generate other views of the condyles by changing tube holder settings and patient head angulation. An example is the common Townes view (patient's head down, mouth open, central beam 30 degrees to the film). Note how well both the medial and lateral poles of the condyles may be seen. **(G)** An interesting view that is also possible with the Denar Versatech is the transorbital view (patient's head turned 20 degrees to the central beam, film cassette behind the patient's head). **(H)** Transorbital radiograph landmarks.

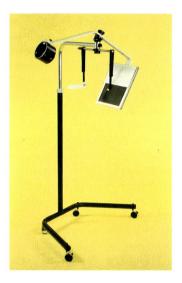

Figure 4–11(A)   (B)

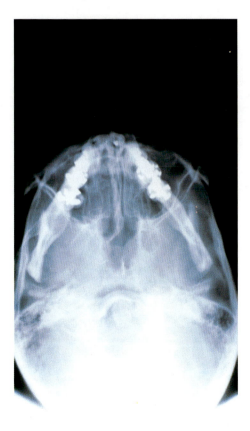

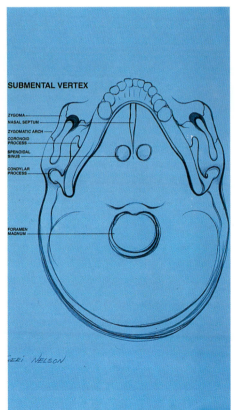

(C)   (D)

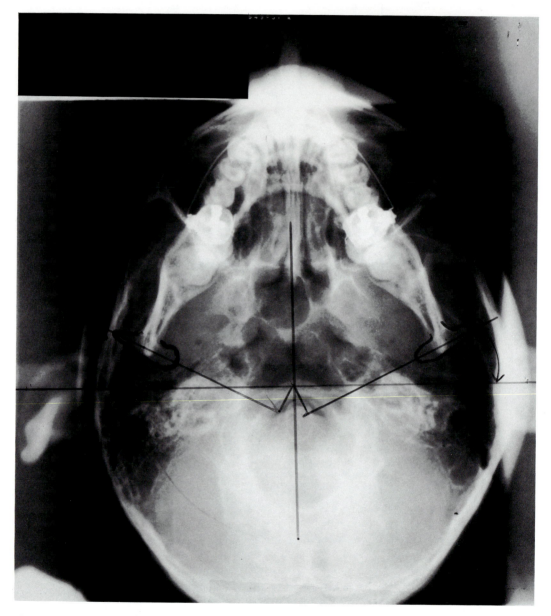

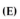

(E)

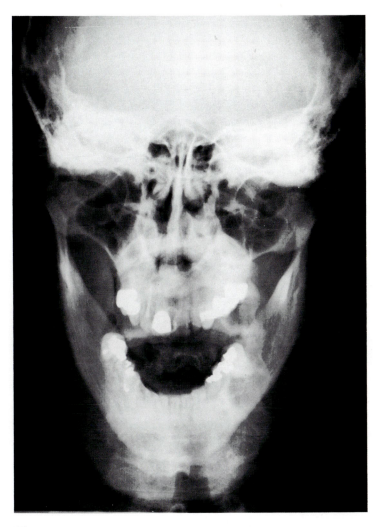

(F)

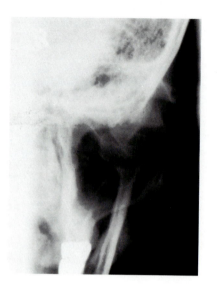

(G)

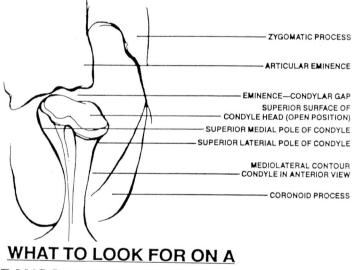

ZYGOMATIC PROCESS

ARTICULAR EMINENCE

EMINENCE—CONDYLAR GAP
SUPERIOR SURFACE OF
CONDYLE HEAD (OPEN POSITION)
SUPERIOR MEDIAL POLE OF CONDYLE
SUPERIOR LATERIAL POLE OF CONDYLE

MEDIOLATERAL CONTOUR
CONDYLE IN ANTERIOR VIEW

CORONOID PROCESS

WHAT TO LOOK FOR ON A
TRANSORBITAL RADIOGRAPH

(H)

units will prove satisfactory. For those patients for whom they do not, the polar corrections may be made by using the pilot film submental vertex technique in conjunction with fully adjustable equipment. Thus the undistorted joint space relationships of the all-important posterior joint space may be accurately analyzed, and obtaining excellent films no longer requires exceptional radiographic skills. The equipment that produces these films is dependable, economic, and easy to operate and govern. This places the availability of an excellent TMJ imaging method within easy reach of every practicing clinician, which is as it should be.

Since the transcranial film is obtained by means of the central beam passing through the cranial base, familiarity with not only the osseous anatomy of the target area but also the extraneous bony images that may be superimposed over the area helps make for a clearer interpretation of the film in the mind of the clinician. The three traditional views taken with the transcranial technique are the fully clenched or closed position, the rest position, and the fully opened position.[86] By the rest position is meant the position to which the patient allows his mandible to drop after holding it in the fully clenched position of habitual occlusion and being told to "just relax and let your jaw fall naturally to where it wants to or where it is most comfortable." The current mechanisms for holding cassettes allow for all three views to be produced along the bottom half of a 5 × 7-in. film for one joint. When the cassette holder is switched to the other side of the head to image the other joint, the cassette is turned upside down, and the process of fully closed, relaxed, and fully opened positions are shot in the same sequence so that they show up in the same locations on the film. Thus all six views appear on one film. The relaxed position is always the middle view, and it is obvious which is the closed and which is the fully opened position. Of all three views, the most important by far is the fully closed position, for it is in that position that the maximum invasion of the condylar head into the posterior and superior joint spaces may be evaluated. In the event the patient may have had a number of radiographs taken recently due to medical conditions, an auto accident, etc., or if concern is expressed over the number of incidents of exposure to radiation he may have had, restricting the transcranial film to the fully closed views will be more than adequate to tell the diagnostician all that is needed for confirmation of a diagnosis of functionally induced TMJ arthrosis.

In corrected views of the joint, the condylar head, the outline of the fossa, and the intervening joint space will be clearly seen. It is important to note here that the outline of the condylar head seen on a transcranial film represents the *lateral pole* of the condyle. Also, it must be remembered that what appears as the dome of the fossa and anterior slope of the articular eminence is actually the lateral inferior transitional border of the supra-articular crest. The actual osseous surface of the slope of the articular facet of the eminence is slightly medially and superior to this white

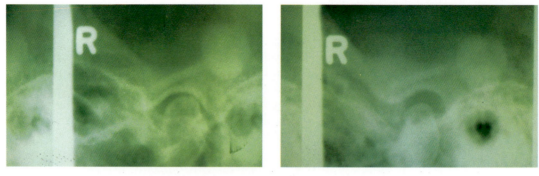

(A)

(B)

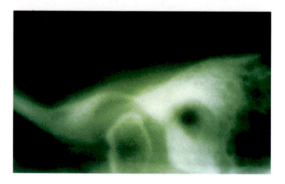

(C)

Figure 4–12 **(A)** Transcranial radiograph, noncorrected. **(B)** Transcranial radiograph of the same joint, corrected. This view was produced after using corrections made on an adjustable transcranial unit that were produced from measurements of condylar polar axis angulations on the submental vertex view. **(C)** Tomogram of the same joint through the middle portion of the condyle. Note flattening of the anterior condylar surface that does not show up on the transcranial lateral pole view. (Courtesy of Dr. James Colt, Denver.)
Figure 4–13 **(A)** Transcranial oblique projection landmarks; **(B)** variations in projection. Note the alignment of structures and how they change with variations in angulation of the central ray. Also note the superimposition of structures. (Courtesy of Dr. Ronald Levandoski, Erie, Penn.)

Figure 4-13(A)

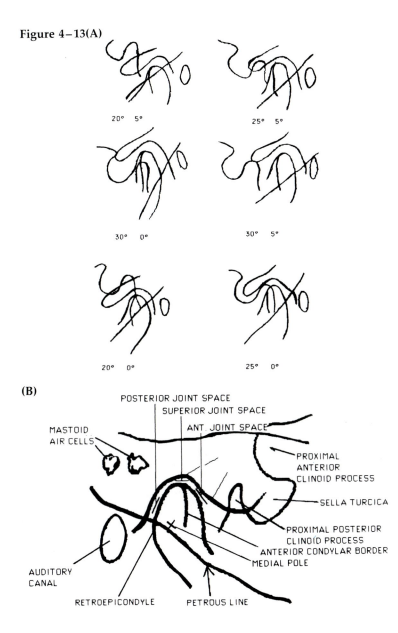

20° 5°

25° 5°

30° 0°

30° 5°

20° 0°

25° 0°

(B)

POSTERIOR JOINT SPACE

SUPERIOR JOINT SPACE

ANT. JOINT SPACE

MASTOID
AIR CELLS

PROXIMAL
ANTERIOR
CLINOID PROCESS

SELLA TURCICA

PROXIMAL POSTERIOR
CLINOID PROCESS

ANTERIOR CONDYLAR BORDER

MEDIAL POLE

AUDITORY
CANAL

RETROEPICONDYLE

PETROUS LINE

demarcation line of the outline of the superior and anterior portions of the fossa. Therefore, the anterior and a portion of the superior joint spaces are actually a bit wider than they appear on the film. But the discrepancy is not great. The superior border of the supra-articular crest provides a handy reference point for two things. First, it is nearly always parallel to the patient's Frankfort plane and therefore serves as a quick reference as to how level the patient's head was when the radiograph was taken. It should be parallel to the upper and lower borders of the film. Second, the angulation of the articular eminence may be evaluated relative to the line of the supra-articular crest. The average inclination ranges from 30 degrees (considered a "flatter" joint) to 60 degrees (a "steep" joint). Flatter joints are often associated with Class II, Division 1 malocclusions, and steeper joints are often associated with Class II, Division 2 malocclusions. Steeper joints are also more prone to subluxation of the mandible.

Other osseous landmarks that appear are the external auditory meatus and the petrotympanic fissure, which often appears as a sharp little invagination on the outline of the posterior wall of the fossa at the level of the middle of the anterior border of the external auditory meatus. Another thin demarcation line that appears is the petrous line of the petrous portion of the temporal bone. It runs at about a 45-degree angle across the target area, starting superiorly from the external auditory meatus area and running down and forward toward the base of the condylar neck. It may be so faint an image at times as not to be seen. When it is visible, the petrous line should not cross the condyle below the upper third. The outline of the sella turcica with its anterior and posterior clinoid processes may also be seen on some films. Mastoid air cells may also appear in the area above the auditory meatus and posterior to the posterior dome of the fossa.

Variation of the central beam away from the ideal horizontal angulation particular for that patient will cause the superimposed images of structures within the depth of field of the target area to shift in a manner similar to the way buccal and lingual images shift when the angulation of *bitewing* radiographs are changed. A deviation of the central beam away from the ideal individualized projection angulations will, as previously alluded to, produce a narrowing of the joint space. Also, as the vertical

---

Figure 4–14 (A) The supra-articular crest is often very nearly parallel to the Frankfort horizontal plane, a handy relationship for orienting and standardizing transcranial projections. (B) The transcranial radiograph on the left shows that the patient's head was tilted forward. A black line is drawn along the supra-articular crest. On the right is a radiograph of same joint without the black line for a better view of crest demarcation (black arrows).

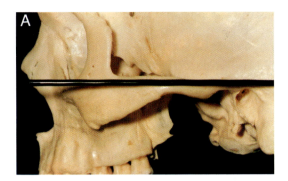

Figure 4–14(A)

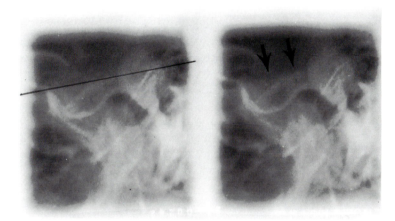

(B)

tube angulation is increased, as might be expected, the petrous line and the posterior clinoid process move inferiorly. At 0 degrees horizontal angulation, the clinoid process is superimposed over the fossa and condyle. As the horizontal angulation changes to 4 to 6 degrees posteriorly, the clinoid process will be over the eminence area. At 8 to 12 degrees posterior, the clinoid process will be anterior to the eminence and within 1.0 cm of the condyle.

The condylar outline of a properly angulated transcranial film reveals many things. We have learned that the old concepts of the TMJ being immutable and anatomically stable with respect to its hard tissues (except for arthritic changes) is fallacious. Adaptive and degenerative changes do take place in both soft and hard tissues as a result of punishment dished out to the joint by the occlusion or, in this case, malocclusion. Increased functional loading of the condyle can cause proliferative changes in subarticular layers of bone and thickened cartilagenous layers. Bony remodeling, usually most prominent on the condylar head, (although it can occur in the fossa), can take place as the result of excessive loading and other noxious stimuli. It may take place either as an internal change that is associated with no outward changes in shape (but that can be detected with magnetic resonance imaging [MRI]), or it can take place as an outright external change with clearly discernable changes in external morphology. If the increased loading of the condyle is gradual and within certain physiological limits of the body's ability to deal with it, adaptation will occur without any untoward symptoms or signs of trouble. But if occlusal changes are rapid or if the abuse the system sustains is beyond these physiological limits, beyond the body's ability to adapt, rapid remodeling or outright degeneration can occur. Thus if changes in the condylar outline are obvious, it is a sign of excessive functional abuse of the joint (barring of course the aforementioned exceptions such as rheumatoid arthritis, etc.). It is a general consensus among authorities on the subject that up to 30% loss of bone mineralization can occur before the first signs of radiographic changes become observable.

The outline of the condylar head can be examined for such osteoarthritic changes. It should be smooth, continuous, and gently rounded. Any surface irregularities or interruptions of the condylar outline or the outline of the fossa (which are more difficult to detect) are indicative that advanced changes in both the articular tissues and subarticular osseous tissues are already present. It must be remembered that we are viewing the lateral pole of the condyle on the transcranial film, but that is the first area usually to undergo osseous breakdown. Erosions appear as irregular, jagged, or pitted areas and are usually a sign of highly localized osteochondritis dissecans or more generalized avascular necrosis. Flattening the condylar head or bending over of the head are usually signs of remodeling that is getting "physiologically desperate." Flattened condyles are also commonly associated with lipping and other forms of osteophytic formations.

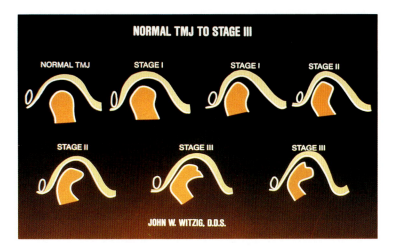

Figure 4–15 Stages of TMJ degeneration.

Although these hard-tissue findings are important and add valuable information to the total diagnostic picture of the patient's TMJ condition, the chief area of concern for modern TMJ clinicians is not so much the white images of the transcranial radiograph but rather the dark images, i.e., joint spaces. All sorts of opinions have been generated as to what constitutes proper joint space or how important it is. The controversy over this issue could almost be expected since it is such an integral part of an already very controversial subject. One of the hottest arguments is that even if satisfactory images free of distortion could be produced of the joint, one could not make linear or angular measurements from them act as a therapeutic guideline. It was claimed by certain dissenters that there was too much variance from one patient's joints to another. The condyle was a highly movable entity anyway. Agreement couldn't even be reached as to where it belonged or where it should reside if one were to try to measure things around it. Or so it seemed.

The new wave of thought concerning the interpretation of joint spaces feels that under the right conditions these spaces can be very revealing, they can be measured, these measurements can have a great deal of clinical significance, and they can be used as guides for treatment goals. Needless to say, this is also steeped in controversy, but only among those who have no experience in employing the methods of treatment predicated on their use.

The first and most important premise concerning analysis of the joint spaces, other than that it be done with an adequate transcranial film (i.e., polar corrected if need be), is that these spaces must be analyzed when the condyle is fully seated in the fully closed, fully interdigitated, fully clenched position of habitual occlusion. Analysis of the joint spaces at the rest position has only the most limited usefulness. The spaces could vary greatly from film to film because the patient's so-called rest position is highly subjective and arbitrary and may change slightly from day to day anyway. The same holds for the fully opened position. This view has only limited significance. The main view we should be interested in is the fully closed position.

The second consideration is that although modern TMJ clinicians do in fact use actual linear average measurements as guidelines and treatment goals, they are not so concerned with the actual linear value as they are with the relative proportions of these spaces, especially the proportions of the posterior joint space to the anterior joint space. Quite simply, the posterior joint space should be decidedly larger than the anterior joint space. The disc is biconcave, being thinnest at its middle. Healthy discs vary in thickness at their center from individual to individual to be sure. But the range of variance is not great. An inordinate number will be found to be in the 1.5- to 1.8-mm range through their narrowest central portion. The same holds true for the width of the posterior joint space. Other than the fact that it should be decidedly larger than the anterior joint space (especially for the types of patients we see), a great many people will do well if their posterior joint space is larger than 3.0 mm. It should be perferably 4 to 5 mm! When patients have less than a 3.0-mm posterior joint space, they usually have some sort of TMJ trouble. It has been the clinical experience of your authors as well as many other expert clinicians in the field that after analyzing hundreds upon hundreds of films and treating these types of patients to remission of symptoms and joint health over the last decade, the 3.0-mm guideline appears to be the consensus boundary line between a healthy joint and a compressed, compromised joint. Now this is meant to be a guideline, of course, and is subject to the intelligent interpretation of the clinician, like any other therapeutic and diagnostic guideline. In a small, 90-lb ballerina, a 2.5-mm posterior joint space might in fact be adequate. Conversely, in a 6-ft, 4-in, 260-lb defensive tackle on a professional football team, a 4- to 5-mm posterior joint space may be needed as a bare minimum. But for the vast majority of patients of normal stature, it has been our overwhelming clinical observation that when the patient's posterior joint space starts dropping below 3.0 mm, the bilaminar zone starts suffering condylar compression, the muscles of mastication start overworking and becoming sore and cramped, the supportive ligaments of the joint start distorting, the headaches and myofascial pains start to appear, and the patient is on his way on the gradual path of TMJ degenerative arthritic problems.

Another thing to consider in this regard is that as the condyle is displaced progressively superiorly and posteriorly, the anterior joint space in turn is progressively enlarged at the full occlusion position. This should not be. As previously stated, in a healthy joint, the posterior joint space should be decidedly bigger than the anterior counterpart. There are those who propose that a concentric condyle at full occlusion, i.e., an equal anterior superior and posterior joint space all around, is the ideal in Nature. To this, the more forward-thinking TMJ clinicians reply first, "even if it is a natural position (which it isn't), the patient is 'sitting on the fence' *physiologically* with respect to tolerance of condylar position," and second, "regardless if it were a naturally occurring relationship or not, the TMJ patient is suffering from a joint that exhibits distorted and elongated ligaments." This means that little other than the newly developed posttreatment therapeutic occlusion and the newly retrained neuromuscular sling will hold the condyle down and forward out of the battered bilaminar zone. Therefore, it is important to see to it that these entities hold the condyle down and forward in the fossa far enough to absolutely ensure that the bilaminar zone will not be violated again in the future. This in conjunction with extensive clinical observation is what is responsible for the formulation of the now classic "Gelb 4/7 position" as a treatment goal.

Therefore, in light of the above, it has long been accepted by various authorities that the anterior joint space of a normal uncompromised joint in the full-occlusion position should range from 1.5 to 1.8 mm and the all-important posterior joint space should be at least 3.0 mm and is more likely to be 4 to 5 mm. Another way of describing the posterior joint space is that an average distance from the center of the external auditory meatus to the back edge of the outline of the image of the condyle should range from 7 to 9 mm.

In light of the above, if the posterior joint space and/or superior joint space reflect smaller-than-average measurements in the fully occluded position, it may be a sign that the bilaminar zone is being impinged upon. If clicking and classic TMJ-type headache, neck ache, and myofascial pains are present, and these joint spaces are less than average; it would be difficult for the experienced TMJ clinician not to conclude that condylar impingement of the bilaminar zone is taking place at full occlusion. If the above scenario of signs and symptoms exists with superior and posterior joint space narrowing and the anterior joint space is correspondingly *larger* than average, it would be nearly impossible not to conclude that the condyle is posteriorly displaced and the disc is anteromedially displaced.

Another assumption that would be reasonably safe to make is that if crepitus is present and if the articular surface of the condylar head (capitulum) is flush against the articular facet (tuberculum) of the eminence such that it appears to obliterate a portion of the anterior or most likely superior joint space altogether, the chances of a perforation existing in the posterior attachment are extremely high. Perforations of the discal posterior attachments by the condylar capitulum with concomitant arthritic-type remodeling of subarticular bone and consequent joint space compression are much more common at the lateral pole of the condylar head than at the central or medial portions. This is the advantage of the transcranial film in this regard, for it is the lateral pole that forms the image of the superiormost border of the condylar outline.

As previously noted, the purpose of the transcranial film is to confirm the diagnosis made from the history, anamnesis, and clinical examination of the patient. If the joint spaces are compressed superiorly and posteriorly by the condylar head and the anterior joint space is correspondingly larger than normal, treatments must entail some form of mandibular advancement/posterior joint space decompression techniques. Once completed, the patient's symptomatic picture will reveal whether enough mandibular advancement and joint decompression has taken place. But once again the transcranial radiograph may be called upon to confirm that the posttreatment joint spaces have been returned to their normal average widths or preferably even slightly overcorrected by a millimeter or two for the critical 3-mm posterior joint space.

With the importance of proper medicolegal documentation being what it is today and with our current understanding of the importance of proper disc-condyle-fossa relationships with adequate superior and posterior joint spacing being what it is today, it would be difficult to justify treating TMJ problems without first obtaining an image of the joint. And as an initial screening procedure, the transcranial film, if properly angulated or used in conjunction with pilot films if need be, is the initial technique of choice. So much is revealed by the transcranial film that more sophisticated (and expensive) studies may be called for on demand for special reasons. A transcranial film should also be a part of the preliminary diagnostic procedure for any major orthodontic case or any major prosthetic or rehabilitative case. The corrected transcranial film compares favorably with other techniques for producing a joint image and yet is the hands-down winner when it comes to practicality and economics. Although originally viewed by some as an unworthy radiological stepchild, the transcranial projection of the joint has been proved capable of a high percentage of concordance between the image produced and the actual condition and is deserving of its new found respect as an important diagnostic and treatment-planning modality.

Tomography

The tomogram is a radiographic image that is the result of the x-ray source and the film being moved in a precise mechanical way such that the x-ray beam is only focused at a given depth through the target area.[87] Structures on either side of the focused "slice" are subsequently blurred and leave no superimposed images to obscure the target area. Thus a relatively clear and accurate image of the TMJ may be produced at any depth through the entire mediolateral thickness of the structure. The machines that move the x-ray source and the film may operate via two types of motion. It may be circular-type motion (polytome) or a figure-eight type of motion (polycycloidal). The tomogram represents the most accurate image of the joint available by a conventional x-ray source. Although tomography may provide an accurate view of the central and medial portions of the condyle, views much less frequently required, it offers little advantage over the conventional transcranial projection as far as the lateral portion of the joint is concerned. And as many authorities have already noted, this is the area of the condyle most subject to arthritic-type bony changes since it is the area of the condyle that suffers the most compressive abuse in posterior displacement situations. There is the problem of added expense, however, because equipment of the tomographic type radiograph is usually available only to institutions or the most affluent of private practitioners. There is also a problem of significant radiation exposure. Hence the tomogram is usually relegated to the role of a supplemental film to be used when initial transcranial films uncover defects that may need further clarification by including views of the central and medial portions of the condyle.

Arthrography

The arthrogram is another technique devised to make some sort of visualization of the disc possible. The process consists of injecting a radiopaque contrast medium into the synovial sac of the joint prior to taking the radiograph. Arthrography has been used in large joints such as the knee. Synovial fluid was withdrawn, and the exact same amount of contrast media could then be reinjected so as to reproduce original intrasynovial hydraulic pressures. However, early investigators who tried to apply the technique to the TMJ faced several problems. The arthrographic injection method was first applied to human TMJs during the period of World War II.[88] Its use as a joint imaging technique quickly faded only to be reintroduced again a generation later in the late 1970s.[89] Its use as a method for divulging the status and location of the disc made it popular with those concerned with treating disc-interference disorders that would be handled surgically. Refinements in technique had to be made to make the method safe and practical. When properly performed, the technique is excellent for imaging torn or anteriorly displaced discs.[90-94]

The basic objective of arthrography is the opacification of the synovial spaces of the joint with injected contrast media so that radiographic imaging of that joint in various stages of the function throughout the opening and closing cycle will divulge silhouette images of the disc and its relative location during the various phases of that cycle. The problem with applying the technique to a small joint like the TMJ is that it is difficult to aspirate fluid from the relatively small synovial sacs of the upper and/or lower compartments. Therefore, when contrast medium is injected into the synovial space, the hydraulic pressure within the joint is increased, a condition referred to as a hyperbaric joint. This can increase the size of the superior and/or inferior joint spaces slightly as the increased hydraulic pressure pushes the articular surface of the condyle and disc away from each other. This of course can interfere with normal joint function. The pressure in effect is increased in the posterior portions of the synovial space, which results in a hydraulic pressure being exerted in an anterior direction on the disc. In a noninvolved joint with a normal disc, the contours of the widened posterior heel of the disc allows this pressure to displace it only as far forward over the capitulum of the condyle as the extra little increase in joint space due to the pressure and the contours of the heel of the disc itself will permit. It is not much. It consists of a slight forward rotation of the disc over the condyle until it is secure between the capitulum of the condyle and the tuberculum or articular facet of the eminence when the jaws are fully closed. However, if there is extensive disc and posterior attachment damage or if the heel of the disc has suffered distortion and "disc ironing" from the chronic abuse of the overloading of a posteriorly displaced condyle, the increased synovial pressure can exaggerate the amount of forward displacement of the disc slightly due to the small increase in anterior joint space as a result of the hyperbaric condition brought on by the injected contrast medium.

Once the joint has been injected, the conventional transcranial-type angulation of the central beam proves unsatisfactory due to the angulation-induced overlap of the upper and lower synovial joint spaces. Therefore, the tomographic method (arthrotomography) must be used to produce the image. However, it must be remembered that this only produces an image slice through the central two thirds of the joint.

Although some investigators advocate injections of contrast media into both upper and lower compartments, it has been found that arthrography of the upper joint space involves more difficult techniques and is less dependable.[95] Hence injection of the lower compartment is the more popular method. The disc itself of course is totally radiolucent. However, its position is evaluated by observing the extent of distribution of contrast medium at the limits of the joint space, i.e., the point of attachment of the retrodiscal inferior lamina posteriorly and the inferior anterior capsular wall at the anterior end of the disc. The inferior border of the disc limits the distribution superiorly, as does the condylar head inferiorly. Since the retrodiscal tissues of the bilaminar zone and the superior head and anterior wall of the capsule are also equally radiolucent, the points at which the disc ends and they begin can only be estimated. It must be remembered that the image of the contrast medium against the inferior disc contours cannot be relied upon to determine where the disc itself actually ends and retrodiscal tissues begin because disc distortion and loss of contour (ironing) is a product of functional abusive overloading and is necessary for most forms of discal displacement anyway.

Interpretation of the arthrogram consists of analysis of the image of the contrast media with the particular phase of the translatory cycle represented by the film. In the fully closed position of habitual occlusion in the normal joint, the distribution of contrast media in the synovial spaces should be fairly even between the anterior synovial joint recess and the posterior synovial recess. The posterior recess (or reservoir) may be slightly larger. As the condyle starts to move down and forward in the beginning stages of the translation cycle, the disc starts to rotate backward over the capitular surface of the condylar head (the reciprocal movement of the condyle rotating forward in the rotation phase of the beginning of the opening movement). As the forward condylar motion steadily proceeds, the anterior capsular recess and synovial spaces become progressively more tensed as the disc reciprocally rotates backward over the top of the condyle as it in turn moves forward and rotates more and more open. This action relaxes the posterior inferior lamina between the heel of the disc and posterior condylar neck and allows the posterior reservoir of the inferior synovial compartment to distend, which it does because at the same time the synovial fluid–contrast medium mixture is being steadily displaced posteriorly by the tensing action of the disc and condylar head on the anterior capsular recess and synovial reservoir areas. In the fully opened position, most all of the synovial fluid–contrast medium mixture in the lower compartment will be displaced posteriorly in the posterior inferior synovial reservoir. The arthrotomographic image will readily display this characteristic distended posterior inferior synovial space, with little or no contrast media seen anterior to the condylar head.

However, arthrography was not designed to image normal joints. In the abnormal joint, something a bit different happens to the synovial fluid–contrast medium mixture during translation when anterior displaced discs are present. When the disc is anteriorly displaced in conjunction with a posteriorly displaced condyle in the full-occlusion position, the anterior displacement stretches the inferior laminar attachment running between the posterior condylar neck and heel of the disc and keeps it somewhat tensed. This increased tension of the lamina, which forms the posterior wall of the posterior reservoir of the inferior compartment, restricts the amount of joint fluid that may be expressed into it. Thus in the fully closed position, the anterior synovial reservoir of the inferior compartment may appear more distended and filled. At the fully opened position, two scenarios may occur. First, if the anteriorly displaced disc is reduced, i.e., if the condyle renegotiates the disc at some time during the opening motion and "hops back onto it again," the fluid distribution will be seen to be displaced to the posterior, similar to the normal joint configuration, with possibly some small amount retained in the anterior recess area. This area it must be remembered has been forced to stretch somewhat due to the chronic anterior displacement of the entire disc at the fully closed position, hence a slightly larger than normal reservoir area forms that retains some of the fluid at the fully opened position. In the second possible scenario, the condyle does not renegotiate the disc but merely pushes it ahead of itself during the entire opening motion. This of course results in a reduced range of opening due to anterior disc jamming. In this case the posterior attachments to the disc remain tensed and taut and restrict fluid flow into the posterior reservoir area when the condyle is as far down and forward as the anteriorly displaced and jammed disc will allow. Fluid is retained in the anterior reservoir and assumes a characteristic shape on the film, not unlike a small fat crescent shape with the convex part of the crescent outlining the anterior wall of the synovial recess while the concave portion of the image reflects the bulge into that space of the crumpled, "balled-up," anteriorly displaced disc. Thus in spite of being radiolucent, the position of the disc may be deciphered by analysis of the shapes produced on the film by the contrast medium in the synovial compartments. Although the position of the disc may be confirmed, how far it actually extends, i.e., where the unions are with the anterior portion of the joint capsule and the posterior bilaminar attachments, must be estimated.

Another advantage of the single-injection method is that it is ideal for the detection of perforations in the disc or posterior bilaminar attachments. If the contrast media is injected into the lower compartment but the film reveals that there is fluid in both upper and lower compartments, the presence of a perforation is confirmed. As might be expected, such a radiographic finding is most often accompanied by the clinical observation of crepitus.

In recent times the discipline of arthrotomography has evolved to even one higher level of sophistication. It is known as double-contrast arthrotomography.[96-98] It merely consists of a clever little technique whereby both the upper and lower synovial compartments are injected with contrast medium, which is then in turn aspirated back out again, followed by injection of air (pneumatization of the joint). This leaves a thin film of contrast medium spread out all over the lining of the upper and lower synovial compartments. Thus by default the entire disc, even though it is radiolucent, is outlined on both its superior and inferior surfaces, as is the condylar surface and articular surface of the eminence.

Arthrography provides the most accurate information regarding the presence of anteriorly displaced discs or discal or posterior attachment perforations. But the technique is not without its problems. They consist of significant radiation exposure, considerable discomfort at the injection site, and the presence of an altered occlusion or acute malocclusion due to the temporarily distended synovial compartments of the transient hyperbaric joint. Other factors to consider are possible needle damage to joint structures, allergic reaction to contrast medium, or iatrogenic joint infection.[99] It is also the kind of technique that requires high levels of training

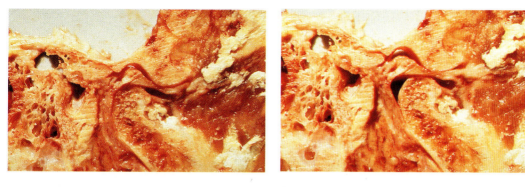

(A)   (B)

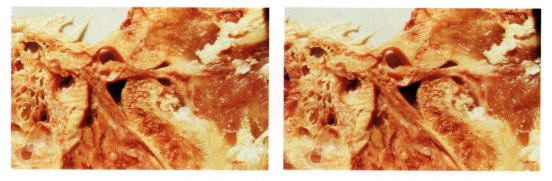

(C)   (D)

Figure 4–16   Anatomical sagittal sections through the right TMJ. Note how the upper and lower synovial compartments change as the condyle is moved from a fully closed position **(A)** to the beginning of the opening movement **(B)**, through the intermediate opening movement **(C)**, to the fully opened position **(D)**. (Courtesy of Dr. James Colt, Denver.)

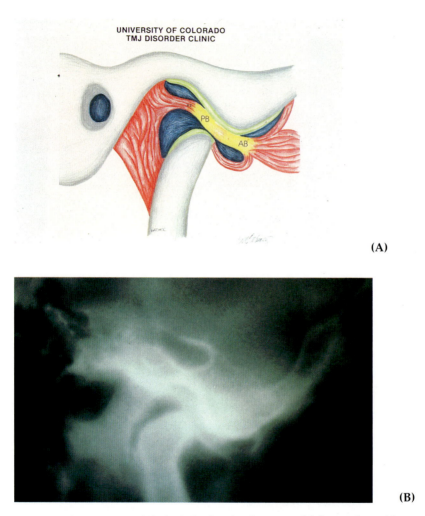

(A)

(B)

Figure 4–17 **(A)** Artist's sketch of a normal joint at the mid opening position. **(B)** Double-contrast arthrotomography of the joint from which the sketch was made. In these and the following illustrations in this series note how the outline of this upper and lower compartments change. (Courtesy of Dr. James Colt and the University of Denver.)

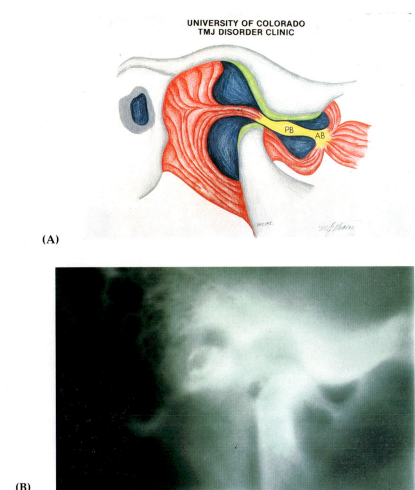

(A)

(B)

Figure 4–18 **(A)** Artist's version of anterior displacement of the disc. **(B)** Double-contrast arthrogram of an anteriorly displaced disc. (Courtesy of Dr. James Colt and the University of Denver.)

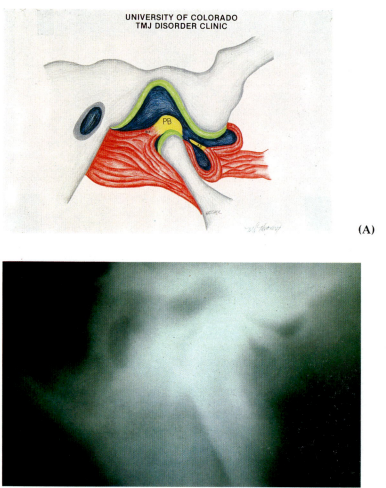

(A)

(B)

Figure 4–19 **(A)** Artist's sketch of a perforation in the articular disc (most perforations occur in the posterior attachment). **(B)** Double-contrast arthrogram of a discal perforation (rare). (Courtesy of Dr. James Colt and the University of Denver.)

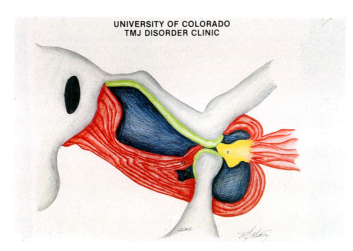

UNIVERSITY OF COLORADO
TMJ DISORDER CLINIC

Figure 4–20   Artist's sketch of a "normal" perforation, i.e., the most frequent type through the posterior attachment. (Courtesy of Dr. James Colt, Denver.)

and skills and is therefore not a mere casual office procedure. Also, it must be remembered that the contrast medium is injected only after the joint is anesthetized, which may have some effect on how the muscles operate it.

Although arthrotomography exhibits high levels of accuracy in depicting the actual condition of the joint, anterior disc displacements may be easily diagnosed by proper clinical examination in conjunction with conventional transcranial radiographic projections. Therefore, although it was more popular in times when surgery was considered the answer to anterior displacement and/or perforation problems, the use of arthrotomography in these modern times of FJO and that technique's ability to once again place a condyle back in its proper location make the use of the arthrotomographic technique a redundancy. Its use may now be confined to cases of inexplicable pain, chronic subluxation, the detection of perforations, or unexplained limitations of jaw movement. Most authorities familiar with both the capabilities of arthrotomographic technique as well as proper transcranial technique who are fortified by the additional knowledge of the capabilities of FJO technique feel that arthograms may be only indicated less than 1% of the time for truly exceptional cases.

Magnetic Resonance Imaging

MRI represents a sophisticated and exotic application of the modern advanced technology of nuclear magnetism and wave mechanics to the business of producing diagnostic images of specific anatomical areas of concern.[100–110] The main difference between the process of MRI and that of conventional radiographic methods is that the more complicated nuclear magnetic method does not rely on ionizing radiation for the production of an image. Rather it is a result of computer-reassembled signals received from the atomic nuclei of the molecules of the patient's own tissues that have been first magnetized and then "energized" by radio waves. Once excited to a higher energy state in such fashion, as the energizing radio frequency is shut off, the nuclei emit back radio wave signals that may be discretely collected by finely tuned radio receivers placed over the target area. These signals may be then used to produce the image of the area. Therefore, the first advantage noted with image production of this type is that there is no health risk involved due to ionizing radiation (x-rays). Another feature that makes MRI different from standard radiographic images is that calcified tissues emit little or no signal during the magnetization and excitation process and therefore appear dark. Conversely, soft tissues such as muscle and fat emit more of a signal and therefore appear brighter. The stronger and longer the signal received from the tissue, the brighter the resultant image. Even things such as increased levels of synovial fluid in joints may be detected. And what turns out to be one of the most incredible features of all, the entire process may be so finely tuned as to often even be able to display a contrast in image between diseased and normal soft tissues!

Although production of MRI requires skilled expertise, extremely sophisticated equipment, and a good deal of interpretation by experienced radiologists, their use as an adjunct to the diagnostic process is becoming steadily more popular with a percentage of TMJ investigators. Therefore, it would be handy for the TMJ clinician who may be considering employing such modalities to be familiar with some of the most basic MRI parameters such as spin density, T1 relaxation time, T2 relaxation time, repetition time (TR), echo time (TE), and the spin-echo pulse sequence. This in turn requires a modest review of basic physics.

One of the physical factors intrinsic to tissue that affects the strength

---

Figure 4–21 **(A)** Arthrogram correlated with condylar path measurement. In these sketches of arthrograms (dye in the lower compartment only) note how the shape of the lower compartment changes from normal condylar function **(A)**, intermediate click **(B)**, to complete anterior jamming of the disc (C and D). **(B)** Various patterns of arthrograms: lower compartment injected only. A = normal joint; B = early opening click; C = intermediate opening click; D = late opening click; E = complete anterior dislocation of articular disc, disc jamming, or clinical closed lock. (From Solberg WK, Clark GT: *Temporomandibular Joint Problems, Biologic Diagnosis and Treatment*. Chicago, Quintessence Publishing Co, 1980, pp 157, 159. Used by permission.)

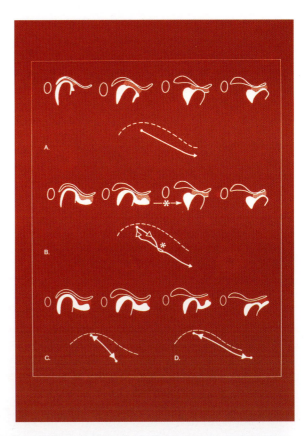

Figure 4−21(A)

(B)

of the signal it produces during the MRI process is the number of hydrogen nuclei present in the target area. Both the proton and the neutron of the atomic nucleus exhibit magnetic dipole moments, like a common north-south bar magnet. Therefore, they are capable of being torqued when placed in an external magnetic field. When an *even* number of protons and neutrons are present within a given atomic nucleus, their dipoles align such as to cancel each other out, resulting in a net magnetic dipole moment of these nuclei equal to zero. However, when an *odd* number of protons and/or neutrons exist in an atomic nucleus, a net magnetic dipole moment exists for that nucleus. This is what makes the MRI technique possible. Examples of naturally occurring atomic nuclei exhibiting this feature are carbon, 13 (protons, 6; neutrons, 7); sodium, 23 (protons, 11; neutrons, 12); and phosphorus, 31 (protons, 15; neutrons, 16). Yet by far the most commonly occurring nucleus of this type in tissue is, of course, hydrogen with 1 (proton, 1; neutron, 0). With few or no hydrogen atoms present in a target tissue, little or no signal will be produced (darkness of image). If a great deal of hydrogen nuclei are present in a target tissue, a strong signal will be produced (brightness of image). For example, cortical bone produces very little signal because it consists of little hydrogen. Therefore, a condylar outline would appear dark along the outer layer of cortical bone. Soft tissues, on the other hand, emit stronger signals because of the abundant hydrogen nuclei within the water of these tissues. Fats also emit strong signals because of the large concentration of hydrogen in lipids.

Although production of MRI is a complex process, several basic steps in that process should be understood. In the natural state, the magnetic dipole moments of the uneven atomic nuclei are totally out of phase and exist in completely random alignment. However, when placed in an external magnetic field, the nuclear magnetic dipoles want to align themselves as parallel as they can to that field, the direction of which we shall call B_0. But they don't necessarily all align themselves "heads to tails." That is, some nuclei (somewhat more than half) align in parallel fashion like a compass needle to the direction of the external static magnetic field B_0. But some nuclei (somewhat less than half) align their dipoles parallel, yet opposite to the field. This state is referred to as antiparallel alignment (compass needle parallel to the magnetic field but with the north end pointing south). This is also a higher energy state. Random interactions between these magnetic dipoles of the hydrogen nuclei and other dipole moments of adjacent macromolecules cause a constant "flipping back and forth" of the proton magnetic dipole moments between the parallel (low-energy) and antiparallel (high-energy) states. Eventually, an equilibrium of this process is reached, M_0. As long as the external static magnetic field is maintained, the magnetic dipole moments of susceptible nuclei will attempt to align in parallel or antiparallel fashion to that field. Well, almost.

It is as if the tissue itself becomes a very weak magnet. Yet this field

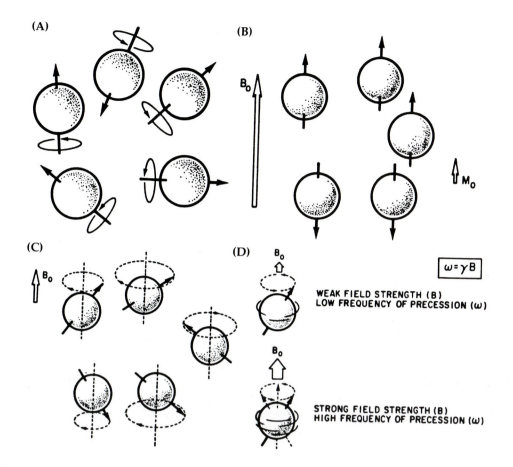

$$\omega = \gamma B$$

Figure 4–22 **(A)** In the absence of an external magnetic field, the spinning unpaired protons in hydrogen nuclei are randomly oriented; therefore the net sample magnetization is zero. **(B)** When placed in a strong external magnetic field (B_o), slightly more than half the magnetic dipoles align with the field, while slightly fewer than half assume an antiparallel orientation. This creates a net magnetization of the sample M_o. **(C)** The aligned dipoles "precess" around the axis of the external magnetic field B_o. Since the precessional frequency is determined solely by the magnetic field strength, all the dipoles have the same rate of precession. **(D)** The relationship between magnetic field strength and precessional frequency is described by the Larmor equation. Weaker magnetic fields result in slower rates of precession; stronger magnetic fields result in high precessional frequencies. (Courtesy of Anne G. Osborn, MD, Department of Radiology, University of Utah School of Medicine, Salt Lake City; and R. Edward Hendrick, PhD, Department of Radiology, University of Colorado Health Sciences Center, Denver.)

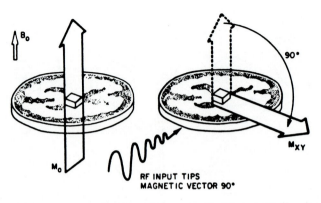

Figure 4–23   The net magnetization of the sample M_o is initially aligned with the main magnetic field B_o but is so small in comparison with B_o that it is undetectable. An RF field applied at the Larmor frequency tips tissue magnetization into the transverse plane, and this renders it measurable as transverse magnetization M_{xy}. (Courtesy of Anne G. Osborn, MD, Department of Radiology, University of Utah School of Medicine, Salt Lake City; and R. Edward Hendrick, PhD, Department of Radiology, University of Colorado Health Sciences Center, Denver.)

or magnetization vector (M_z) of the target tissue cannot be measured since the externally applied magnetic field (B_o) is millions of times stronger than the minuscule magnetic field it induces in the tissue. However, the net magnetization vector of the tissue (M_z) can be measured if it is tipped into the XY plane *perpendicular* to the direction of the external magnetic field (B_o) and its parallel net tissue magnetization (M_z). The Z plane is called the longitudinal plane (B_o, M_z), and the plane perpendicular to it (which is two dimensional) is, of course, the XY plane, or transverse plane. With a cue from the Larmor condition and the Larmor frequency (that frequency of precession of nuclear magnetic moments as a function of magnetic field strength), as might be guessed, the gimmick used to tip the net tissue magnetization vector 90 degrees (transversely) to the original B_o plane is a pulse of radio frequency, the RF pulse. Fight fire with fire, electromagnetic waves with electromagnetic waves. This is how we excite nuclei—now we're getting close to getting a picture. Well, almost again.

Immediately after the tuned RF pulse that is aimed 90 degrees to the longitudinal axis of the external magnetic field (B_o) and its resultant parallel net tissue magnetization vector (M_z) to tip it 90 degrees onto the transverse (XY) plane, the M_z is zero. The 90-degree RF pulse has caused the magnetic dipoles of hydrogen nuclei to now be precessing in phase in the XY plane (90 degrees to the original plane M_z), and the transverse net tissue magnetization vector M_{xy} is momentarily at its maximum. But with

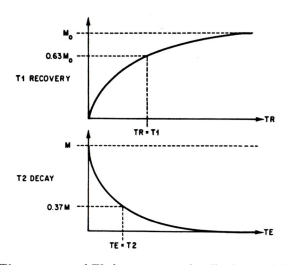

Figure 4–24 T1 recovery and T2 decay are graphically depicted. T1 is defined as the time delay required for 63% of the tissue magnetization to recover along the direction of B_o. T2 is defined as the time required for the transverse magnetization to decay to 37% of its original level. (Courtesy of Anne G. Osborn, MD, Department of Radiology, University of Utah School of Medicine, Salt Lake City; and R. Edward Hendrick, PhD, Department of Radiology, University of Colorado Health Sciences Center, Denver.)

the 90-degree transverse-tipping RF pulse shut off, all the precessing magnetic dipole moments in the transverse plane (XY) start losing their phase coherence. It's as if the magnetic dipole axes of the energized or excited nuclei that were all precessing parallel to the RF pulse in the XY plane start assuming random directions once again, some precessing faster, some precessing slower as the net tissue magnetization in the transverse plane M_{xy} starts to fade. Some start to precess around the original external static magnetic field again (B_o), and slowly a regrowth of magnetic dipole moments in the original Z plane, or longitudinal plane, starts to occur in which they are aligned (in precessing fashion) in parallel-antiparallel fashion along the B_o. Thus the M_z starts to reappear again in an exponential "regrowth rate" until the M_z (net tissue magnetization vector) in the longitudinal plane approaches an equilibrium state (parallel-antiparallel) once again (M_o). Now what must be remembered about the loss of the net tissue magnetic vector M_{xy} in the transverse plane once the RF pulse is shut off and about the regrowth of the longitudinal net tissue magnetization vector M_z along the longitudinal plane is that, although they occur almost simultaneously, they *do not* occur in direct inverse proportion on a one-for-one basis. When the 90-degree RF pulse is shut off, some of the dipole moments start to precess (regrow) along the B_o direction; others (the majority) merely lose phase coherence along the XY plane and assume a more random arrangement. The exponential regrowth of the M_z or longitudinal net tissue magnetization vector is described as the *spin-lattice* relaxation time, or T1. It is essentially an assembly process. T1 differs from tissue type to tissue type. It represents by definition the time required for just under two thirds (63%) of the longitudinal net tissue magnetization vector (M_z) to recover (realignment of magnetic dipoles) along the direction of the original external magnetic field (B_o) after the 90-degree RF pulse is shut off. This process gives off radio wave energy from the "RF pulse–excited" atomic nuclei, and this is what is used to produce an image. But additional radio wave energy is also being given off from the excited nuclei of the tissues by other things occurring at the same time.

To keep things clear in one's mind, it must be remembered that magnetic dipole (axis of rotation) alignment in a state of parallel-antiparallel equilibrium is not the same as coherence (phase coherence) of the precessional frequencies about that axis of rotation of magnetic dipole moments. When the "Larmor frequency–tuned," 90-degree RF pulse is applied to the tissue to tip the net tissue magnetization vector (M_z) from the longitudinal plane onto the transverse plane (to form the M_{xy}), not only does that radio pulse have the ability to align the magnetic dipole moments all in parallel alignment (in the new XY plane perpendicular to the original Z plane), but it also has the ability to force all the precessional rates of these dipole moments to precede at the same frequency (coherence). Thus magnetic dipole alignment (axis of rotation or spin of the proton) and frequency of precession about that axis are two different, albeit related things.

Actually, only a small part of the decay of the transverse net tissue magnetization vector (M_{xy}) is due to the realignment of some of the magnetic dipoles along the original B_o static magnetic field (T1 relaxation). A greater amount of loss of the M_{xy} is due to the loss of coherence of nearby

---

Figure 4–25 **(A)** Immediately after a 90-degree RF pulse, the magnetic dipoles of individual nuclei are precessing in phase, and the transverse magnetization vector M_{xy} is maximal. **(B)** As time progresses, magnetic dipoles lose phase coherence, some precessing faster, some slower, due to the local magnetic environment. This loss of phase coherence causes a decrease in transverse magnetization, with the new transverse magnetization M_{xy}' less than M_{xy}. (Courtesy of Anne G. Osborn, MD, Department of Radiology, University of Utah School of Medicine, Salt Lake City; and R. Edward Hendrick, PhD, Department of Radiology, University of Colorado Health Sciences Center, Denver.)

Figure 4–25(A)

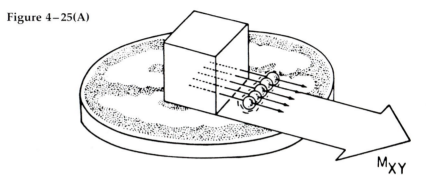

M_{XY}

(B)

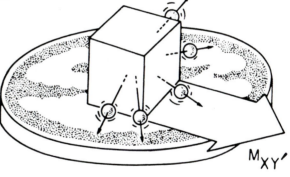

$M_{XY'}$

magnetic dipoles along the XY plane (dipoles going from all being in phase to a state of random-phase directions but not necessarily in the Z axis direction). Loss of coherence entails a change of precessional frequency among individual dipoles, some precessing faster, some precessing slower due to both the static magnetic field's influence and that of local fields of adjacent macromolecules (lattice). This difference in precessional frequencies of individual hydrogen nuclei magnetic dipole moments results in a loss of coherence. The decay rate of the coherence of the transverse net tissue magnetization vector M_{xy} after the 90-degree RF pulse is shut off is a second magnetic relaxation time referred to as the *spin-spin* relaxation time, or T2. It is essentially a disassembly process. It represents the time required for the transverse net magnetization vector (M_{xy}) to decay (largely due to a loss of phase coherence and less so due to magnetic dipole realignment to M_z) to 37% of its original M_{xy} signal value the instant the RF pulse is stopped. This process also gives off radio wave energy (again, as a result of the nuclei having been excited), which contributes to the signal used for image production. Thus it may be seen that to generate a signal from tissue, it has to be magnetized in one direction (the B_o in the Z axis); then the resultant net tissue magnetization vector (M_z) of that direction must be flipped out 90 degrees onto the transverse plane and excited so that the protons are in effect raised to a higher (more organized) energy state. This is done by specific tissue-dictated frequencies of radio waves (Larmor frequency) aimed 90 degrees to the longitudinal (B_o) original magnetic field. Once the RF pulse is shut off, the net tissue magnetization vector M_{xy} starts to decay and gives off its newly acquired "higher" energy in the form of radio waves as it does so. The loss of precession coherence of the magnetic dipoles (T2) is an energy loss, as is the realignment of the dipole moments back parallel to the original B_o external magnetic field (T1) in a state of parallel-antiparallel equilibrium M_z approaching M_o as the limit of that equilibrium (reassembly). This is compounded by background "noise" also. To get an actual image, all these sources of radio signals being given back to the receivers over the target area have to be "separated" by a complex series of gradients. This amounts to nothing more than a series of electromagnetic "filters and focusers." Since signal production depends on the amount of magnetic dipole alignment and precession phase coherence (precessional frequency) for the strength of its signal, tissue with a long T1 value (a long time required after the RF pulse to realign magnetic dipoles along the longitudinal Z axis and regenerate the M_z once again) will appear dark. They haven't been given the time they need to realign and regenerate the M_z before another 90-degree RF pulse is fired and flips them all 90 degrees out onto the XY plane (creating the M_{xy} net tissue magnetization [and excited] vector). If the tissue has a short T1 value, more of the magnetic dipoles align in the allotted time interval before the next RF pulse and therefore create a stronger M_z component, hence a stronger or "brighter" signal. However, to see the T1 component of the entire radio wave emission of T1, T2, and background emissions after excitement, the electronic "filters and focusers" (gradients) are used in a fashion similar to the way ultraviolet (UV) filters are used in color photography to get a truer blue color to pictures of the sky, etc. This process is called weighting the total emission after excitation to produce a "T1-weighted" image. A short T1 (stronger signal/brighter image) is due to a quicker regeneration of the M_z in the allotted time frame due to quicker realignment of the protons' magnetic dipole moments with the original B_o.

To see the T2 component of the total energy emission after RF excitation, a few extra steps must be carried out. T2 relaxation time describes a decay process, a loss of precession-phase coherence (going from a state where all precession frequencies are not only aligned in the same direction but also precessing at the same frequency) to a state where they precess at higher and lower or uneven frequencies and in different directions as the proton magnetic dipole axes bounce around to random directions. What we want to measure is the rate of the loss of phase coherence (evenness of precessional frequency). But with the dipole moments starting to randomly point all over the place once again after RF excitation (some of which start realigning along the original B_o longitudinal plane to regenerate an M_z once again), it is difficult to measure energy loss (radio wave emission) when such random disorganization exists. We would like the precessional frequencies to all be in phase coherence to measure the T2-governed component of energy emission. Therefore, physicists devised a sneaky little electromagnetic trick that can be played on the tissue during this sequence of events that allows this to happen. A 180-degree pulse is fired to reverse the polarity of the entire field or "flip" it back and forth between one direction and another. In doing so, there is one point during the "flipping" at which the precessing magnetic dipole moments all momentarily come into phase once again, at which time the true radio wave energy remaining (which originally came from the RF excitation) may be detected. This "flipping" process to obtain true readings of the decaying energy governed by the T2 relaxation time may be likened to opening an Oriental umbrella. When it is half open, all the bamboo spokes point toward your hand but angularly in all directions. Opening the umbrella all the way places the bamboo spokes all at a 90-degree angle to the central shaft of the umbrella (phase coherence); overextending the umbrella "flips" the bamboo spokes past this point to where they all point in different directions *away* from your hand. Imagine further that we want to measure the circumference of the umbrella at the exact 90-degree position of the spokes to the shaft. Also imagine that the total circumference of the umbrella gradually gets smaller (energy of emission loss or decay) each time it is flipped back and forth.

The 180-degree rephasing pulse is applied within milliseconds of the RF pulse that energizes the target area. It is applied in the transverse (XY)

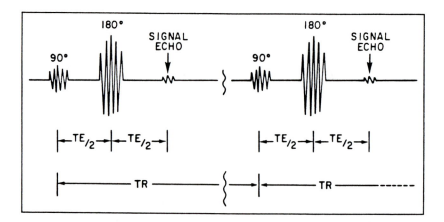

Figure 4–26 RF pulses and signal echoes in spin echo (SE) pulse sequence. (Courtesy of Anne G. Osborn, MD, Department of Radiology, University of Utah School of Medicine, Salt Lake City; and R. Edward Hendrick, PhD, Department of Radiology, University of Colorado Health Sciences Center, Denver.)

plane from the opposite direction of the RF excitation pulse that flips the M_z onto the XY plane to create the M_{xy}. The signal from the tissue, which is gradually decaying in a fashion similar to the way the chime of a struck crystal wine glass dies away, is measured in the XY plane during the rephasing of the transverse magnetization vector (umbrella spokes 90 degrees to the shaft). Between the 90-degree RF excitation pulses and the 180-degree rephasing pulses, dipoles within a pixel (a given area of target tissue) "dephase" due to (1) irreversible dipole-to-dipole interactions (what we are not interested in) and (2) reversible relaxation due to applied magnetic fields and magnetic field inhomogeneities across the area of the pixel. (This combination of irreversible with reversible relaxation of transverse [XY] magnetization is called most eloquently "T2* relaxation"!) The important thing desired for imaging purposes is that these can be separated and, at an equal point in time after the 180-degree rephasing pulse, the reversible (desired) effects are rephased so that a little signal output or "echo" may be detected, which is purely a product of only the reversible T2 relaxation (originally a function of the RF excitation pulse) and describes the signal decay (chiming wine glass effect) between the 90-degree pulse and the signal measurement. All other random "distortions" have in effect been eliminated. This entire process of obtaining a T2-weighted image out of the entire energy emission milieu is referred to as a "spin-echo pulse sequence." The more straightforward T1-weighted image, which is a product of the amount of regeneration of longitudinal magnetic dipole (M_z) in a given time frame, may be obtained without all this. But to obtain a T2-weighted image that shows different tissue characteristics on the final image and is a product of the degree of loss of phase coherence after RF pulse excitation, the spin-echo pulse sequence must be used. It allows a true T2-weighted image to be drawn out of all the surrounding and interferring "electromagnetic camouflage" in which it is hiding.

Thus since T2-weighted images are related to the speed of decay of phase coherence of a given target tissue's hydrogen nuclei (a disassembly process), tissues with short T2 times (time to reach only 37% of the original post-excitation value) appear dark (remember, this is in contrast to short T1 times, which give brighter images). Tissues with short T2 relaxation times quickly lose their phase coherence, hence strength of signal, hence darkness of image. Not much lasting "ring" to the wine glass when struck. Tissues with long T2 relaxation times, on the other hand, retain phase coherence longer and hence have more energy for signal production at the time intervals when measured (rephasing). Therefore, they have a brighter image (long T1 relaxation times in contrast only produce a weaker signal and darker image).

T1 and T2 relaxation times are determined for a certain type of tissue by that tissue's own specific localized macromolecular microenvironment. Hence different tissue types have different chemical makeups and therefore different T1 and T2 relaxation times. This in turn is responsible for the contrast between tissues seen on an image produced by MRI technique. As previously noted, there even exists an image contrast between normal and diseased tissues of the same type.

Finally, not only is the final production of the actual MRI image subject to inherent tissue parameters and their effect on received signal intensity, but also some control may be imparted to image production by means of "user-selectable" parameters. Some of the factors that are inherent to the target tissue itself are not under the control of the operator and affect MRI signal (radio wave) intensity and therefore the blackness or whiteness of the image are things like proton density (spin density), T1 relaxation time, and T2 relaxation time. Other factors of less importance also have an effect on signal strength. The factors that are under the control of the radiologist are things like the type of pulse sequence used (spin-echo pulse sequencing just described being one of them), interpulse delay times, section thickness of the target tissue being imaged, matrix size, field of view, gradients used (filters and focusers), and flip angles. Since spin density, T1 longitudinal relaxation time, and T2 transverse relaxation time all have a bearing on the total radio signal emission back from the excited hydrogen nuclei of the target tissue, it is impossible to control and set all the imaging parameters so as to obtain a pure spin-density (proton density), pure T1 spin-lattice, or pure T2 spin-spin–type image free of contributions of signal from the other two types of sources.

This is why gradients (filters and focusers) and electromagnetic tricks (transverse magnetization [of the M_{xy}] rephasing with 180-degree rephasing pulses as in spin-echo pulse sequencing) must be employed to maximize the contrast of one or more of the tissue parameters while minimizing the contrast loss from other contributing sources. The final image is weighted in favor of the accumulation of one type of image over another in a fashion distantly related to the manner in which contrast, color, and intensity may be adjusted on a common television set.

The TR of the 90-degree RF pulse that does the excitation and TE are user-controllable parameters in the spin-echo pulse sequencing process of obtaining T2-weighted images. TR is defined as the time interval between the 90-degree RF excitation pulses. It is often on the order of 2 seconds. The TE is the time interval between the 90-degree RF excitation pulse and the maximum signal output (echo) of the rephasing M_{xy} from the patient. Remember that this specific signal gradually dies away like the chime of a struck crystal wine glass (T2 relaxation time) and may only be clearly detected (pulled out from under the surrounding electromagnetic camouflage) during 180-degree rephasing (flipping) of the M_{xy} vector. The signal expression (strength) is a "simple" product of the inherent spin density, T1 and T2, in such a fashion that TR governs T1 weighting and TE governs T2 weighting.

One final factor that must be appreciated in MRI is the time necessary to produce an image. Simply, it is a factor of several basic things. One of the tricks radiologists use to obtain better images is to collect and store in the computer more than one "reading" of a planar acquisition (slice) of the target tissue. This improves the signal-to-noise ratio. But a price must be paid. The total imaging time (T total) increases with the number of planar acquisitions (N_{aqs}) taken at each "encoding step." Phase encoding steps allude to the "filters and focusers" (gradients) previously mentioned. There are 256 phase encoding steps (N_{pe}) commonly used. The number of phase encoding steps (N_{pe}) and the TR (time required for

---

Figure 4–27 **(A)** T1-weighted MRI of a normal joint. The large arrow delineates the posterior band (heel) of the disc; the small arrow delineates the anterior band (toe) of the disc (mandible in fully closed position). **(B)** By contrast, note the different appearance of the same joint in a T2-weighted image. Note the appearance of bone marrow in the T2-weighted image vs. the T1-weighted image. **(C)** Again the same joint as in **A** and **B** except in an open position. This is a T2-weighted image; note how the biconcave disc is positioned under the articular eminence and on top of the condyle. **(D)** A T1-weighted image of a different joint shows a disc in the closed, clenched position. Arrows delineate the anterior and posterior borders of the disc. **(E)** T2-weighted image of the same joint as **D**. Note the lack of signal from the condyle and the appearance of marrow. (Courtesy of Dr. James Colt, Denver.)

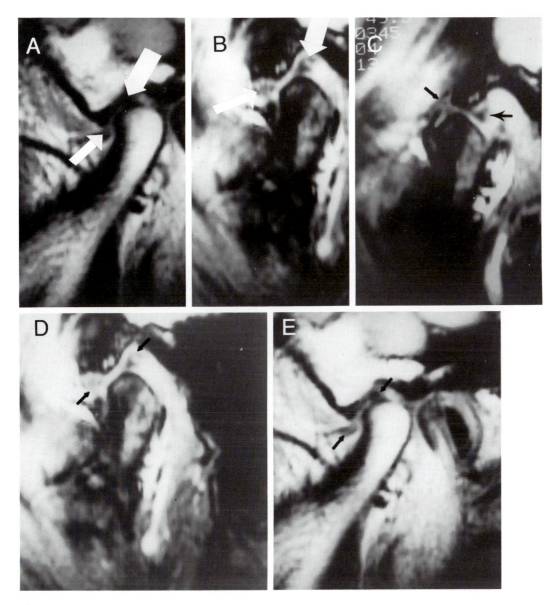

Figure 4-27

the repetition of a single 90-degree RF excitation pulse) each affect the total time required for production of the MRI according to the following formula:

$$T \text{ total} = (N_{aqs})(N_{pe})(TR)$$

If, for example, the number of planar acquisitions (done to sharpen the picture), or N_{aqs}, is 2, the phase encoding steps (N_{pe}) are set at 256 (which they commonly are), and the repetition time interval for 90-degree RF pulse excitations is 2 seconds, then

$$T \text{ total} = (2)(256)(2) = 1{,}024 \text{ seconds}$$

That represents the chink in the armor; 17.1 minutes is a long time for a patient to hold still in the tomblike confines of the noisy MRI machine. All of the world's really great gems seem to come with a curse!

T1-weighted images are achieved by selecting short TR settings (TR < 500 ms) and short TE settings (TE < 30 ms) in spin-echo pulse-sequencing procedures. T2-weighted imaging is achieved by choosing longer TR settings (TR > 2 seconds) and longer TE settings (TE > 60 ms) in spin-echo pulse sequencing.

The following protocol has been suggested as advisable by those knowledgeable with the discipline of MRI. MRIs of the TMJ may reveal not only condyles and articular fossa outlines but also changes in bone marrow status, cortical plate integrity, and joint effusion. They do in fact reveal articular discs but are inadequate to detect perforations.

1. T1-weighted images are indicated for most TMJs. Bilateral views in the open and closed positions (full occlusion) are taken to reveal disc displacement or reduction.

2. T2-weighted images are best to check for joint effusion and the intrinsic status of the articular disc itself. Excess fluid in the synovial spaces (indicative of joint inflammation and intracapsular edema) appears white. Such images are also good for the detection of the presence of any inflammatory process in the muscles.

3. Coronal views may at times be handy to identify mediolateral displacement of the disc.

4. T1-weighted images generally show the outline of the disc and bone clearly. They also image the marrow spaces quite well due to the T1 relaxation times inherent in these types of tissue.

5. T2-weighted images do reveal soft tissues better. However, they also require longer TR and TE times. This, of course, as per the dictates of the previously described formula for total time to obtain an image, greatly increases the time the patient must remain still in the machine. This, in turn, increases the chances for motion artifacts.

6. The thinnest possible planar acquisition (slice) should be taken, 3.0 mm or less.

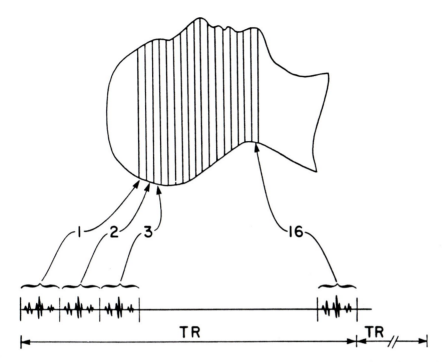

Figure 4–28 Multisection acquisitions are obtained without extending the total imaging time by exciting and measuring the signal from different sections in the patient during a single TR. (Modified from Sprawls P: Spatial characteristics of the MR image, in Stark DD, Bradley WG (eds): *Magnetic Resonance Imaging.* St Louis, CV Mosby Co, 1988, pp 24–34.)

7. To improve image quality, the field of view should be as small as possible, and the smallest surface coil (radio wave receiver over the target area) should be used.

8. Ideally, it would of course be best to obtain simultaneous bilateral acquisitions. However, this can lead to complicated gradient problems and requires very sophisticated (and expensive) software.

9. A high-resolution matrix of the 256 × 256 variety should be employed.

Although all this may at first seem intimidating to the referring TMJ clinician who may be considering employing MRI as part of a total TMJ diagnostic procedure, the radiologists who perform these procedures will read the images and send a report to the referring clinician that outlines their interpretation of what the MRI reveals. What is there may not be as important as what is done about what is there!

Cephalometrics

Along with the transcranial view of the joint, a thorough radiographic survey of the patient with TMJ problems should also include a cephalometric view of the rest of the entire maxillofacial complex. The purpose of the conventional cephalogram is not further analysis of joint relationships but rather analysis of the apical base and dental relationships that contribute to the overall retrusive mandibular arc of closure and its resultant superior posterior displaced condyles. The cephalogram

Figure 4–29 **(A)** T1-weighted MRI of a TMJ with an anteriorly displaced disc when the mandible is in the fully closed position (the large arrow delineates the condyle; small arrows delineate the disc). **(B)** T1-weighted image of the same joint during partial opening. The large arrow delineates a perforation through retrodiscal (bilaminar) tissue. The small arrow indicates folding of the disc upon opening. **(C)** T2-weighted image of the same joint again, also during a state of partial opening. The arrow delineates a perforation in retrodiscal tissues. **(D)** Same joint again, this time viewed from a coronal aspect. A T1-weighted image shows medial displacement of the disc. Arrows indicate borders of the disc. Note the inferior portion of the temporal lobe of the brain above the joint area. (Courtesy of Dr. James Colt, Denver.)

Figure 4–30 **(A)** T1-weighted MRI of an anteriorly displaced disc. Note the loss of cortical plate signal. **(B)** Anatomical cryosection of the same joint. (Courtesy of Dr. James Colt, Denver.)

Figure 4–31 **(A)** T1-weighted MRI of a coronal view of a medially displaced disc. **(B)** Artist's sketch of the same view. C = condyle; arrows denote the disc beginning to be displaced medially. (Courtesy of Dr. James Colt, Denver.)

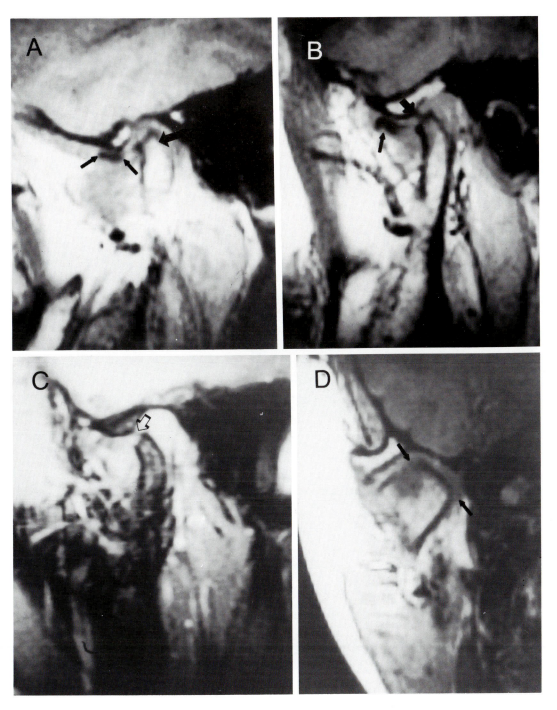

Figure 4–29

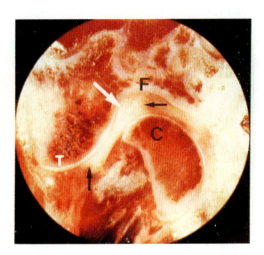

Figure 4–30(A)

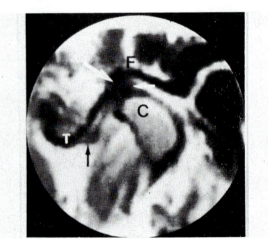

(B)

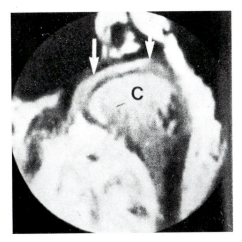

Figure 4–31(A)

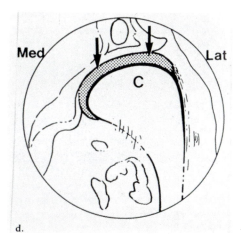

(B)

may be analyzed by anyone or a number of different cephalometric analysis systems, optimally including members of the more orthopedically oriented group such as the McNamara (Functional Orthopedic), Bimler, Sassouni, or Bowbeer.

The key to interpretation of the cephalometric film is the search for that combination of orthopedic and/or orthodontic imbalances that might be responsible for the retruded "big MAC," mandibular arc of closure. The most obvious example of this is the classic Class II, Division 2, deep-overbite case. Here the causes of the retruded mandible and displaced condyle and disc are obvious. But at other times the agents responsible for the posterior deflection are less obvious. They can be at times subtle and more hidden. This can be deceiving when the mere molar alignment is traditional Angle Class I.

The first thing that should be evaluated is the location of the maxillary apical base and the extent, if any, of any retrusion present. For all things being equal, a retruded maxilla is sufficient to cause a functionally induced TMJ arthrosis due to the fact that the mandibular arch, which is housed under it, may be forced so far distally in the mandibular arc of closure to full dental interdigitation that the condyles are forced up and back off the disc even if the molar relationship is traditional Angle Class I and upper anterior incisors appear angled far enough forward. The study casts of such a case would harmlessly appear at normal dental Angle Class I. But the combination of the reduced superior and posterior joint spaces and increased anterior joint space as revealed by the transcranial film analyzed in combination with the retruded maxillary apical base (i.e., a full-scale maxillary retrusion of the apical base and upper dental arch) as revealed by the cephalometric film soon divulges the source of the problem.

The dental components of the upper of the "two jaw bones of the skull, the craniomaxillary bone," i.e., the maxillary teeth, should also be analyzed as a possible source of posterior mandibular deflection. Again, the retroclined Division 2 upper anterior incisors are obvious culprits. But sometimes the Division 2 angulation is not great. Yet when combined with a retruded maxillary apical base (which would place the upper anterior teeth relatively more posterior regardless of their individual degree of angulation) and/or forward-tilted lower anteriors or an extra long mandible, the combination can result in what is referred to as a "Division 2 ef-

---

Figure 4–32 **(A)** T1-weighted MRI of an anteriorly displaced and "hammered" disc (arrow) and a posteriorly displaced condyle (C). Note again the loss of cortical plate signal, bending over of the condyle, and the superficial temporal artery in the lower posterior joint space area. **(B)** Anatomical cryosection of the same joint. (Courtesy of Dr. James Colt, Denver.)

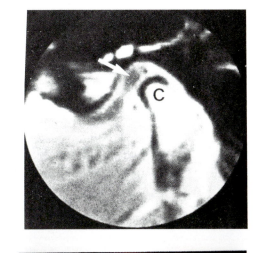

Figure 4–32(A)

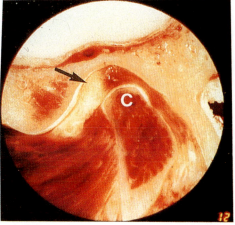

(B)

fect." Its net result is still retrusion of the mandibular arc of final closure, superior posterior displacement of the condyle, anteromedial displacement of the disc, and all the other trappings (no pun intended) of the classic NRDM/SPDC phenomenon.

Likewise, the mandibular apical base, its overall size (as expressed by cephalometric measurements such as the Bimler DLM, the McNamara effective mandibular length, or the archial relationships of the Sassouni), and the degree of forward angulation of the lower anterior incisors may be evaluated for their contributions to the posterior displacement of the mandible at full occlusion. The maxilla may in fact be far enough forward and the maxillary anteriors may in fact exhibit adequate proclination, yet with a crowded forward lower anterior incisor coupled with a mandible that may be just a bit on the long side, the net result is still the same. The mandibular arc of closure with its lower dental arch ends up being housed under the upper dental arch in full occlusion in such a way that the entire mandible is forced too far posteriorly for the joints to be able to stand it.

Evaluation of the vertical dimension of occlusion also contributes to this entire scenario and is an indirect reflection of the status of something totally unseen on any type of diagnostic radiograph, muscles. It may be safely assumed that gross deficiencies in the anterior vertical dimension of occlusion imply a muscular problem in a fashion similar to the way in which excessive deficiencies in the posterior vertical dimension of occlusion imply a condyle that is being forced too far superiorly and posteriorly at full occlusion. When the anterior vertical dimension is grossly lack-

Figure 4–33 **(A)** T1-weighted MRI of a TMJ with severe damage and a severely anteriorly displaced disc (white arrow). The superior head of the lateral pterygoid appears white. Also note extreme superior posterior displacement of the condyle (C) and condylar lipping. Also note the loss of condylar and eminential cortical plate signal. **(B)** Anatomical cryosection of the same joint corroborates the MRI findings. (Courtesy of Dr. James Colt, Denver.)

Figure 4–34 Deceptive MRIs **(A)** T1-weighted MRI of advanced TMJ arthrosis: F = fossa; T = articular eminence of temporal bone; C = condyle. Note the erroneous identification of the disc (white arrows), which is actually the superior head of the lateral pterygoid muscle. The actual disc is thinned (ironed) and very well hydrated, i.e., full of proteoglycans that are imaged brightly, just as soft tissue would. **(B)** Anatomical cryosection of the same joint. (Courtesy of Dr. James Colt, Denver.)

Figure 4–35 **(A)** T1-weighted MRI of a TMJ with an anteriorly displaced disc and loss of cortical plate signal on the posterior edge of the displaced condyle **(C).** The large arrow points to the anterior band of the disc. **(B)** Anatomical cryosection of the same joint. E = external auditory meatus. (Courtesy of Dr. James Colt, Denver.)

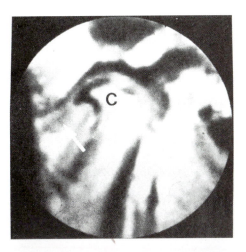

Figure 4–33(A)

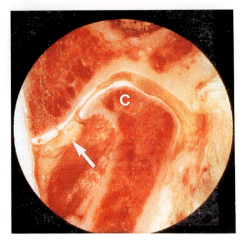

(B)

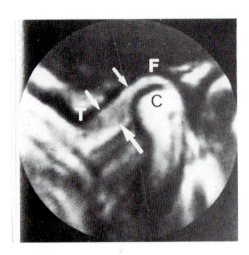

Figure 4–34(A)

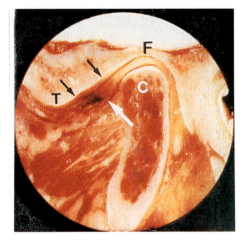

(B)

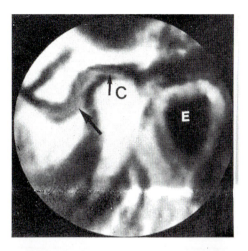

Figure 4-35(A)

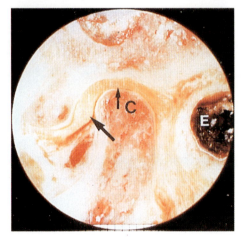

(B)

ing, the elevator muscles of mastication must often overconstrict past their ideal working length, which can result in myostatic contracture, loss of resting vertical, and the usual myogenic problems associated with chronic muscle abuse.

Thus we look at the entire maxillofacial complex cephalometrically to see whether the upper jaw and/or its teeth are in too far or the lower jaw and/or its teeth are out too far. Any combination of all four of these entities may conspire to result in a more retruded mandibular arc of closure than the entire system—joint, muscles, ligaments, and all—can tolerate. This is the essence of discovering the true nature of the patient's functionally oriented TMJ problems.

Not only is cephalometrics important in deciphering where the source of the patient's TMJ problems arise, but it also helps the clinician make important decisions with respect to just which orthodontic/orthopedic techniques will be the treatments of choice in the effort to untie the stubborn knot of the malocclusion and in turn relieve the distressed joint. By analyzing which components of the maxillofacial complex are deficient or excessive, the clinician can determine whether the upper front teeth need to be moved forward so that the mandible may in turn be brought forward or whether the lower anteriors should be condensed back in order to clear the way for unobstructed mandibular advancement procedures. The purpose of cephalometrics in treatment planning is not to present a goal of normative standards that force the clinician to "treat to the numbers." The fallacy of that premise has been adequately exposed in a previous volume. One must not treat to norms, but to the patient's needs. And the patient's needs are first and foremost dictated by the needs of the joint, regardless of what the pretreatment cephalometric measurements say about the other components of the maxillofacial complex. *The joint comes first.* When the history, anamnesis, and clinical examination, staunchly fortified by the findings of the transcranial radiograph, indicate a dire need for mandibular advancement procedures to decompress a compromised joint, cephalometrics provides information that allows the clinician to determine the quickest, easiest, most logical, and most stable way of meeting those needs. The former tells the doctor what must be done, and the latter tells the doctor how it will be done. The net result of this will in turn be a posttreatment upper jaw and teeth that combine at full occlusion with the lower jaw and teeth in such a way as to lock the mandibular condyle in its proper position down and forward in the joint as per its original design intent while also allowing the muscles to work at their proper increased vertical as per their design intent. Radiologically, the transcranial radiograph is what determines the goal, cephalometrics is what determines the method.

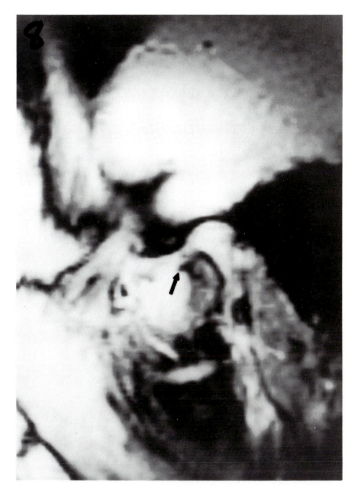

Figure 4–36   A T1-weighted MRI of a TMJ shows gross deformity of the condyle and lipping (black arrow) at the anterior rim of the condylar head in a 14-year-old girl. (Courtesy of Dr. James Colt, Denver.)

OCCLUSAL ANALYSIS

The term *occlusal analysis* often brings a shudder to both dental students and experienced practitioners alike, for it has long been associated with face bow transfer devices, mounted study casts in complicated articulators, red and blue articulating paper marks in endless profusion across the occlusal table of the teeth, pristine theories of cusp-fossa relationships, working occlusion, balancing occlusion, centric relation, centric occlusion, etc., and an endless variety of theories as to what constitutes proper occlusion. Fortunately for the TMJ clinician, occlusal analysis is straightforward, simple, logical, and easily understood. It consists of examining the occlusion of the TMJ patient both clinically and with the aid of study models to determine just what it is in the occlusion that might be contributing to or wholly responsible for the retruded mandibular arc of closure that results in the patient's functionally induced TMJ arthrosis.

Again, the obvious example of a Class II, Division 2 malocclusion may be cited as an occlusal relationship, observable clinically, that has an untoward effect on the functional integrity of the TMJ. However, there are other occlusal relationships that are also capable of seriously contributing to the NRDM/SPDC phenomenon. After all, it must be remembered that this phenomenon is mitigated at the first point of occlusal contact of the teeth in the arc of closure, and as a result of the dental relationship, if you will forgive a play on words, these teeth in turn are prime movers in the retrusive mandibular problems of the TMJ patient. (Actually, as previously noted, the muscles do the moving of the mandible rearward. The teeth merely send the initial-contact, warning proprioceptive signal that mandibular retrusion is needed.)

One of the chief offenders in the NRDM/SPDC league, besides the retroclined upper anteriors, is the proclined lower anterior that usually manifests itself in the form of a labially crowded-out incisor. Sometimes the combination of the retroclined uppers and a single excessively proclined lower add up to a net effect that is devastating to the joint. The discrepancy may be as subtle as the interference represented by the accumulative effect of mere rotations. Any portion of a tooth may act as the source of interference, even the interproximal mesial or distal marginal line angle areas that become exposed due to the rotation.

Another easily detectable occlusal relationship that can drive the mandible back on full occlusion is the loss of the proper maxillary arch form. Ideally, the maxillary dental arch should resemble a gracefully rounded Roman arch, an outline not unlike the rounded end of a common chicken egg. However, when the arch form becomes compromised such that the outline resembles a Gothic arch due to progressive lateral collapse in just the bicuspid and cuspid area with resultant forward protrusion of the anteriors in a manner resembling the outline of the pointed end of an egg, the mandible is forced back. The lower arch usually retains

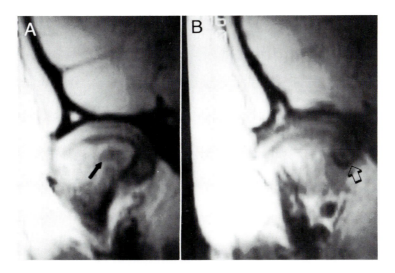

Figure 4–37 **(A)** A T1-weighted coronal MRI view of a TMJ shows avascular necrosis (arrow) deep in the condylar head. **(B)** T1-weighted coronal MRI view of a TMJ. The arrow depicts medial displacement of the disc as well as "balling up" of the disc. (Courtesy of Dr. James Colt, Denver.)

a more correct rounded arch form. As a result, the transarch distance across a given point on the lower arch must progressively seek an equivalent width farther back on the Gothic-shaped upper arch so that the teeth will interdigitate. This, of course, results in a retruded arc of closure, which if severe enough can trigger a TMJ problem.

Occlusal analysis can also divulge another dental interference relationship that is universally hard on both the orthopedic components of the TMJ and the musculature: balancing side interferences. Observable only by direct intraoral clinical examination during lateral excursive movements, the balancing side interference, between the lingual cusps of the uppers and the buccal cusps of the lowers, is an occlusal relationship that accentuates functional TMJ problems before treatment and may linger to haunt the patient somewhat after treatment. Fortunately, postorthodontic treatment of these particular types of interferences is an easy matter of changing the cusp slope angulations (and maybe even the cusp tip heights if need be) just enough so as to eliminate the interference on the balancing side when the patient executes a lateral excursive movement to the working side. Patients notice the relief of the increased freedom of lateral excursive movement almost instantly. Elimination of such interferences represents quick and easy "touch-up," finishing-type work in a considerable number of treatment plans.

To enhance the examiner's clinical impression of the occlusion, study models become a necessary part of any comprehensive clinical examination of a patient with TMJ-type signs and symptoms. Not only do they serve to clarify the nature of the problem in the mind of the clinician, when compared with ideal models of the human dentition, they serve as excellent patient education material during case presentations. But their true meaning only becomes clear when interpreted in the light of the revelations of the clinical examination, the cephalogram, and the all-important transcranial radiograph. Without these, they are merely grinning hunks of plaster.

"But they asked one another the reason,
No sooner knew the reason but
They sought the remedy."

William Shakespeare
As You Like It *Act V, scene ii*

References

1. Gelb H (ed): *The Clinical Management of Head, Neck and TMJ Pain and Dysfunction.* Philadelphia, WB Saunders Co, 1977, pp 92–110.
2. Bell WE: *Temporomandibular Disorders: Classification/Diagnosis/Management,* ed 2. Chicago, Year Book Medical Publishers, Inc, 1986, pp 117–118.
3. Gross A, Gale EN: A prevalence of the clinical signs associated with mandibular dysfunction. *J Am Dent Assoc* 1983; 107:932–936.
4. Bush FM, Butler JH, Abbott DM: The relationship of clicking to palpable facial pain. *J Craniomandib Pract* 1983; 1:43.
5. Farrar WB, McCarty WL: The TMJ dilemma. *J Ala Dent Assoc* 1979; 63:9.
6. Westesson P: Double contrast arthrography and internal derangement of the temporomandibular joint (abstract 1218). *Swed Dent J Suppl* 1983; 13:1–57.
7. Marciani RD, Haley JV, Roth GI: Facial pain complaints in the elderly. *J Oral Maxillofac Surg* 1985; 43:173–176.
8. Solberk WK, Woo M, Houston J: Prevalence of signs and symptoms of mandibular dysfunction (abstract 432). *J Dent Res* 1975; 54.
9. Solberg WK: Epidemiology, incidence and prevalence of temporomandibular disorders, a review, in *The President's Conference on the Examination, Diagnosis and Management of Temporomandibular Disorders,* Chicago, American Dental Association, 1983, pp 30–39.
10. Jones P: Personal communication, Indianapolis, March, 1983.
11. Laskin DM: Etiology of the pain-dysfunction syndrome. *J Am Dent Assoc* 1969; 79:147–153.
12. Bell WE: Recent concepts in the management of temporomandibular joint dysfunctions. *J Oral Surg* 1970; 28:596–599.
13. Bell WE: Management of masticatory pain, in Alling CC, Mahan PE (eds): *Facial Pain,* ed 2. Philadelphia, Lea & Febiger, 1977, p 185.
14. Gelb H (ed): *The Clinical Management of Head, Neck and TMJ Pain and Dysfunction.* Philadelphia, WB Saunders Co, 1977, p 75.

15. Kraft GH, Johnson EW, LaBan MM: The fibrositis syndrome, *Arch Phys Med Rehabil* 1968; 49:155–162.

16. Simons DG, Travell J: Letter to the editor. *Pain* 1980; 10:106.

17. Travell J, Simons D: *Myofascial Pain and Dysfunction: The Trigger Point Manual.* Baltimore, Williams & Wilkins, 1983, p 17.

18. Travell J, Berry C, Bigelow N: Effects of referred somatic pain on structures in the reference zone (abstract). *Fed Proc* 1944; 3:49.

19. Sharav Y, Tzukert A, Refaeli B: Muscle pain index in relation to pain, dysfunction, and dizziness associated with myofascial pain-dysfunction syndrome. *Oral Surg* 1978; 46:742–747.

20. Moran JH, Kaye LB, Fritz ME: Statistical analysis of an urban population of 236 patients with head and neck pain: Part III, treatment modalities. *J Periodontol* 1979; 50:66–74.

21. Meyerowitz M, Rosen H: Myofascial pain in the edentulous patient. *J Dent Assoc S Afr* 1975; 30:75–77.

22. Goharian RK, Neff PA: Effect of occlusal retainers on temporomandibular joint and facial pain. *J Prosthet Dent* 1980; 44:206–208.

23. Isberg A, Isacsson G, Williams WN: Lingual numbness and speech articulation deviation associated with temporomandibular joint disc displacement. *Oral Surg Oral Med Oral Pathol* 1987; 64:9–14.

24. McNamara JA Jr: The independent functions of the two heads of the lateral pterygoid muscle. *Am J Anat* 1976; 138:197–206.

25. Lipke DP, Gay T, Gross RD, et al: An electromyographic study of the human lateral pterygoid muscle (abstract 713). *J Dent Res* 1977; 56:230.

26. Wilkinson TM: The relationship between the disk and the lateral pterygoid muscle in the human temporomandibular joint, *J Prosthet Dent* 1988; 60:715–724.

26a. Johnstone DR, Templeton M: The feasibility of palpating the lateral pterygoid muscle. *J Prosthet Dent* 1980; 44:318–333.

27. Burch JG: Occlusion related to craniofacial pain, in Alling CC, Mahan PE, (eds): *Facial Pain,* ed 2. Philadelphia, Lea & Febiger, 1977, p 77.

28. Shore NA: Temporomandibular joint dysfunction: Medical-dental cooperation. *Int Coll Dent Sci Educ J* 1974; 7:15–16.

29. Mahan PE: Differential diagnosis of craniofacial pain and dysfunction. *Alpha Omegan* 1976; 69:42–49.

30. Franks AST: Masticatory muscle hyperactivity and temporomandibular joint dysfunctions. *J Prosthet Dent* 1965; 15:1122–1131.

31. Butler JF, Folke LEA, Bandt CL: A description of signs and symptoms associated with the myofascial pain-dysfunction syndrome. *J Am Dent Assoc* 1975; 90:635–639.

32. Green CS, Lerman MD, Sutcher HD, et al: The TMJ pain-dysfunction syndrome: Heterogenicity of the patient population. *J Am Dent Assoc* 1969; 79:1168–1172.

33. Kaye LB, Moran JH, Fritz ME: Statistical analysis of an urban population of 236 patients with head and neck pain. Part II, patient symptomatology. *J Periodontol* 1979; 50:59–65.

34. Reynolds MD: Myofascial trigger point syndromes in the practice of rheumatology. *Arch Phys Med Rehabil* 1981; 62:111–114.

35. Travell J: Mechanical headache. *Headache* 1967; 7:23–29.

36. Travell J: Temporomandibular joint pain referred from muscles of the head and neck. *J Prosthet Dent* 1960; 10:745–763.

37. Williams HL: The syndrome of physical or intrinsic allergy of the head: Myalgia of the head (sinus headache). *Proc Staff Meet Mayo Clin* 1945; 20:177–183.

38. Rubin D: An approach to the management of myofascial trigger point syndromes. *Arch Phys Med Rehabil* 1981; 62:107–110.

39. Rocabado M, Johnston BE Jr, Blakney MG: Physical therapy and dentistry: An overview. *J Craniomandib Pract* 1982; 1:47.

40. Greene CS, Olson RE, Laskin DM: Psychological factors in the etiology, progression and treatment of MPD syndrome. *J Am Dent Assoc* 1982; 105:443.

41. Fearon CG, Serwatka WJ: Stress: A common denominator for inorganic TMJ pain-dysfunction. *J Prosthet Dent* 1983; 49:805–808.

42. Rugh JD: Psychological factors in orofacial neuromuscular problems. *Int Dent J* 1981; 31:202–205.

43. Greene CS: Myofascial pain-dysfunction syndrome: The evolution of concepts, in Sarnet BG, Laskin DM (eds): *The Temporomandibular Joint.* Springfield, Ill, Charles C Thomas Publishers, 1979, pp 277–288.

44. Ingle JI, Beveridge EE: *Endodontics,* ed 2. Philadelphia, Lea & Febiger, 1976, pp 514–531.

45. Rugh JD, Solberg WK: Electromyographic studies of bruxist behavior before and during treatment. *Calif Dent Assoc J* 1958; 3:56–59.

46. Mercuri LG, Olson RE, Laskin DM: The specificity of response to experimental stress in patients with myofascial pain-dysfunction syndrome. *J Dent Res* 1979; 58:1866–1871.

47. Olson RE: Myofascial pain-dysfunction syndrome: Psychological aspects, in Sarnat BG, Laskin DM (eds): *The Temporomandibular Joint.* Springfield, Ill, Charles C Thomas Publishers, 1980.

48. Lupton DE: Psychological aspects of temporomandibular joint dysfunction. *J Am Dent Assoc* 1969; 79:131–136.

49. Grieder A, Cinotti WR, Springob HK: *Psychological Aspects of Temporomandibular Joint Dysfunction and Neuromuscular Dysfunction in Applied Psychology in Dentistry.* St Louis, CV Mosby Co, 1972.

50. Dawson P: *Evaluation, Diagnosis, and Treatment of Occlusal Problems.* St Louis, CV Mosby Co, 1974, pp 18, 48–107.

51. Shore NA: *Temporomandibular Joint Dysfunction and Occlusal Equilibration,* ed 2. Philadelphia, JB Lippincott, 1976, pp 193–205, 237–249.

52. Faulkner KDB, Atkinson HF: An analysis of tooth position on initial tooth contact. *J Oral Rehabil* 1983; 10:257–267.

53. Jemt T: Positions of the mandible during chewing and swallowing recorded by light emitting diodes. *J Prosthet Dent* 1982; 48:206–209.

54. Suit SR, Gibbs CH, Benz ST: Study of gliding tooth contacts during mastication. *J Periodontol* 1976; 47:331–334.

55. Nevakari K: An analysis of mandibular movement from rest to occlusal position Acta. *Odont Scand* 1956; 14(suppl 19):1–129.

56. Clark GT, Beemsterboer PL, Solberg WK, et al: Nocturnal electromyographic evaluation of myofascial pain-dysfunction in patients undergoing occlusal splint therapy. *J Am Dent Assoc* 1979; 99:607–611.

57. Staz J: The treatment of disturbances of the temporomandibular articulation. *Off J Dent Assoc S Afr* 1951; 6:314–335.

58. Walsh JP: Temporomandibular arthritis, mandibular displacement and facial pain. *Off J Dent Assoc S Afr* 1950; 5:430–436.

59. Lindblom G: Disorders of the temporomandibular joint. *Acta Odont Scand* 1953; 11:61–85.

60. Hankey GT: Discussion: Affections of the temporomandibular joint. *Proc R Soc Med* 1956; 49:983–994.

61. Posselt U: *Physiology of Occlusion and Rehabilitation.* Philadelphia, FA Davis Co Publishers, 1962, p 88.

62. Soderberg F: Malocclusion-arthroses-otalgie. *Acta Otolaryngol Suppl (Stockh)* 1950; 95:85–98.

63. Weinberg LA: Practical evaluation of the lateral temporomandibular joint radiograph. *J Prosthet Dent* 1984; 51:676–685.

64. Rieder CE, Martinoff JT: Comparison of the multiphasic dysfunction profile with lateral transcranial radiographs. *J Prosthet Dent* 1984; 52:572–580.

65. Updegrave WJ: Temporomandibular articulation x-ray examination. *Dent Radiogr Photogr* 1953; 26:41–52.

66. Richards AG, Alling CC: Extraoral radiography, mandible and temporomandibular articulation. *Dent Radiogr Photogr* 1955; 28:1–7.

67. Updegrave WJ: Roentgenographic observations of functioning temporomandibular joints. *J Am Dent Assoc* 1957; 54:488–505.

68. Bell WE: Standards of normal for temporomandibular diagnosis. *Proc Inst Med Chic* 1960; 23:168.

69. Updegrave WJ: Practical evaluation of the techniques and interpretation in the roentgenographic examination of temporomandibular joints. *Dent Clin North Am* 1961; 421.

70. Schier MBA: Temporomandibular joint roentgenography: Controlled erect technics. *J Am Dent Assoc* 1962; 65:456–472.

71. Mongini F: The importance of radiography in the diagnosis of TMJ dysfunctions: A comparative evaluation of transcranial radiographs and serial tomography. *J Prosthet Dent* 1981; 45:186–198.

72. Eckerdal O, Lundberg M: The structural situation in temporomandibular joints: A comparison between conventional oblique transcranial radiographs, tomograms, and histologic sections. *Dentomaxillofac Radiol* 1979; 8:42.

73. Yale SH: Radiographic evaluation of the temporomandibular joint. *J Am Dent Assoc* 1969; 79:102–107.

74. Farrar WB, McCarty WL: *A Clinical Outline of Temporomandibular Joint Diagnosis and Treatment,* ed 7. Montgomery, Ala, Normandie Publications, 1982.

75. Preti G, Arduino A, Pera P: Consistency of performance of a new craniostat for oblique lateral transcranial radiographs of the temporomandibular joint. *J Prosthet Dent* 1984; 52:270–274.

76. Robinson M, Lytle J: Simplified method for office roentgenograms of the temporomandibular joint. *J Oral Surg* 1962; 20:217–219.

77. Updegrave WJ: Interpretation of temporomandibular joint radiographs. *Dent Clin North Am* 1966; 567.

78. Pharoah M: Radiology: A commentary on its use for TMJ examinations. *Oral Health* 1986; 76:7–8.

79. Eckerdal O, Lundberg M: The structural situation in temporomandibular joints. *Dentomaxillofac Radiol* 1979; 8:42–49.

80. Eckerdal O, Lundberg M: Temporomandibular joint relations as revealed by conventional radiographic techniques. *Dentomaxillofac Radiol* 1979; 8:65–70.

81. Lundberg M, Welander U: The articular cavity of the temporomandibular joint. *Medicamundi* 1970; 15:27–29.

82. Omnell K, Petersson A: Radiography of the temporomandibular joint utilizing oblique lateral transcranial projections. *Odont Rev* 1976; 27:77–92.

83. Levandoski R: Personal communication, Erie, Penn, Feb 1989.

84. Dixon DC, Graham GS, Mayhow RB, et al: The validity of transcranial radiography in diagnosing TMJ anterior disc displacement. *J Am Dent Assoc* 1984; 108:615–618.

85. Donovan RW: Method of temporomandibular joint roentgenography for serial or multiple records. *J Am Dent Assoc* 1954; 49:401–409.

86. Ricketts RM: Laminography in the diagnosis of temporomandibular joint disorders. *J Am Dent Assoc* 1953; 46:620–648.

87. Norgaard F: Arthrography of the mandibular joint. *Acta Radiol* 1944; 25:679–685.

88. Wilkes CH: Structural and functional situations of the temporomandibular joint. *Northwest Dent* 1978; 57:287–294.

89. Blaschke DD, Solberg WK, Sanders B: Arthrography of the temporomandibular joint: Review of current status. *J Am Dent Assoc* 1980; 100:388–395.

90. Oberg T: Radiology of the temporomandibular joint, in Solberg WK, Clark GT (eds): *Temporomandibular Joint Problems*. Chicago, Quintessence Publishing Co, 1980, pp 49–68.

91. Graham GS, Ferraro NF, Simms DA: Perforations of the temporomandibular joint meniscus: Arthrographic, surgical, and clinical findings. *J Oral Maxillofac Surg* 1984; 42:35–38.

92. Wilkes CH: Arthrography of the temporomandibular joint. *Minn Med* 1978; 61:645–652.

93. Farrar WB, McCarty WL: Inferior joint space arthrography and characteristics of condylar paths in internal derangements of the TMJ. *J Prosthet Dent* 1979; 41:548–555.

94. Dolwick MF, Lipton JS, Warner MR, et al: Sagittal anatomy of the human temporomandibular joint spaces. *J Oral Maxillofac Surg* 1983; 41:86–88.

95. Westesson P, Omnell K, Rohlin M: Double-contrast tomography of the temporomandibular joint: A new technique based on autopsy specimen examinations. *Acta Radiol (Diagn) (Stockh)* 1980; 21:777–785.

96. Westesson P: Double-contrast arthrotomography of the temporomandibular joint: Introduction of an arthrographic technique for visualization of the disc and articular surfaces. *J Oral Maxillofac Surg* 1983; 41:163–172.

97. Westesson P: Diagnostic accuracy of double-contrast arthrotomography confirmed by dissection, in Moffett BC (ed): *Diagnosis of Internal Derangements of the Temporomandibular Joint*, vol 1. Seattle, University of Washington, 1984, pp 31–34.

98. Salon JM, Ross RJ: Computerized tomography with multiplanar reconstruction for examining the TMJ. *J Craniomandib Prac* 1983; 1:27.

99. Kean DM, Smith MA: *Magnetic Resonance Imaging: Principles and Applications.* Baltimore, Williams & Wilkins, 1986.

100. Partain CL, James AE, Rollo FD, et al: *Nuclear Magnetic Resonance Imaging.* Philadelphia, WB Saunders Co, 1983.
101. Higgins CB, Hricak H: *Magnetic Resonance Imaging of the Body.* New York, Raven Press, 1987.
102. Bushong SC: *Magnetic Resonance Imaging: Physical and Biological Principles.* St Louis, CV Mosby Co, 1988.
103. Margulis AR, Higgins CB, Kaufman L, et al: *Clinical Magnetic Resonance Imaging.* San Francisco, Radiology Research and Education Foundation, 1983.
104. Curry TS, Dowdey JE, Murry RC: *Christensen's Introduction to the Physics of Diagnostic Radiology,* ed 3. Philadelphia, Lea & Febiger, 1984.
105. Johns HE, Cunningham JR: *The Physics of Radiology,* ed 4. Springfield, Ill, Charles C Thomas Publishers, 1983.
106. Young SW: *Nuclear Magnetic Resonance Imaging: Basic Principles.* New York, Raven Press, 1984.
107. Partain CL (ed): *Nuclear Magnetic Resonance and Correlative Imaging Modalities.* New York, Society of Nuclear Medicine, Inc, 1983.
108. Morgan CJ, Hendee WR: *Introduction to Magnetic Resonance Imaging.* Denver, Multi-Media Publishing, Inc, 1984.
109. Morris PG: *Nuclear Magnetic Resonance Imaging in Medicine and Biology.* Oxford, Clarendon Press, 1986.
110. Witzig J, Spahl TJ: *The Clinical Management of Basic Maxillofacial Orthopedic Appliances:* vol II. *Diagnostics.* Littleton, Mass, PSG Publishing Co, 1989.

*"It would not be enough even if the stars
came down to earth to bring witness
about themselves."*

Galileo Galilei, 1564–1642

*(Reply to a letter from one of his
students, Fr. Benedetto Castelli, concerning
the rejection of certain of Galileo's
astronomical discoveries by the hierarchy
of the Church.)*

CHAPTER 5
Eliminating the NRDM/SPDC Phenomenon: Physiology Put Right Again

TREATMENT: THE COMPLETE DENTITION

In no other discipline of dentistry is the spectrum of employable treatment modalities as broad as those available for the treatment of temporomandibular joint (TMJ) pain-dysfunction conditions. Likewise, with the possible exception of the field of endodontics, no other discipline is as replete with controversial and hotly debated issues ranging from the broadest of philosophical concepts of approach to the most specific entities of technique. Yet the ultimate purpose in all this is the same: the deliverance of the patient suffering from functionally induced TMJ arthrosis to a posttreatment pain-free state of normalcy of jaw function from a former pretreatment painful state of *ab*normalcy of jaw *dys*function. The development of a wide variety of legitimate treatment modalities capable of making temporary contributions to the alleviation of some of the patient's symptoms is a result of the varied nature of symptomatic manifestations that might be exhibited in the overall TMJ pain-dysfunction condition. As previously alluded to, the therapeutic regimens used to treat TMJ problems might be thought of in the past as having been roughly divided into the two large subdivisions of those concerned with *stress* and those concerned with *structure*. Each of these two therapeutic subdivisions may of themselves consist of a variety of techniques for a given patient. And as also previously noted, although stress is of itself extremely important, the single most mitigating factor in the long-term course of the patient with TMJ problems is ultimately related to the status of the patient's own gnathologic structure. For if the patient undergoes a great deal of physical, physiological, emotional, or mental stress, given an excellent condyle-disc-fossa relationship in an excellent overall maxillofacial structure, the chances are that the individual will most likely do fairly well. Yet on the other hand, if a given individual is under minimal stress (an extremely unlikely circumstance in this day and age) but possesses an extremely unbalanced gnathologic structural status, i.e., anteriorly displaced discs and posteriorly displaced condyles, that particular patient will no doubt do poorly because an improperly coordinated and dysfunctioning structure is of itself a major physiological stressor. Stress merely exhausts the body's physiological adaptation mechanisms prematurely and in turn allows by default the problems of the abuses taking place within the TMJs to more readily rise unchecked to the surface. In the area of TMJ arthrosis, stress is not a true etiological agent. The phenomenon of neuromuscular reflexive displacement of the mandible causing superior posterior displacement of the condyle (NRDM/SPDC) is the true etiological agent. Condyles riding on the posterior attachments, overclosed musculature due to a lack of posterior vertical dimension, and excessive mandibular retrusion cause the patient to brux. Stress merely leaves the patient with less of a capacity to recover from the damages caused by such gnathologic dysfunction. When muscles do not receive proper attention physiologically from the body due to exhaustion and dissipation of healing and adaptive mechanisms because of increased periods of stress, they react in the usual way. They send initial warning signals of pain, hypertonicity, muscle splinting, or even myospasm effects and other myogenic problems as a call to the body that more intense recuperative attention be paid them in their plight. Unfortunately, this needed attention is sometimes not available because it has been spent elsewhere by the body in its efforts to deal with (or adapt to) increased periods of stress in whatever variety of forms it may present itself. Structure is the key. Sound structure is the answer when unsound structure is the problem. You simply cannot let the patient's condyles ride hard off the disc and get away with it. Sooner or later pain ensues. Stress or no stress, the problem is in how the occlusion affects the anatomical integrity of the disc-condyle-fossa assembly.

The key to selection of specific and proper treatments, from the many available for a given case, lies in first determining what physical attributes the patient is actually presenting and then differentiating between those signs and symptoms that are pertinent to the dental practitioner from those that pertain to the field of general medicine. This represents the differential diagnosis. If it has been determined that the signs and symptoms the patient presents are in fact within the realm of dentistry, a specific diagnosis has been made. Once it has been determined that maxillofacial functional jaw orthopedics (FJO)-type techniques are indicated, the purpose then becomes a deduction in turn of a differential form of treatment specifically designed for the peculiarities of the specific type of malocclusion exhibited by the individual patient. This is the first and most important step in treatment modality selection because the determination of a specific diagnosis reflects, by its very nature, the needs of that specific individual. And as already established, the needs of a given individual are intimately related to the treatments selected to correct and fulfill those needs. Accepting that structure is the most important factor that treating clinicians might directly address; a therapeutic system that is based on determining the needs of patients according to the status of that structure is an obvious aid in clearing the way through the maze of extraneous and ancillary TMJ therapeutic possibilities.

THE MAXILLOFACIAL TRIANGLE
AND STRUCTURAL IMBALANCE

All malocclusions, including those that affect the TMJ, may be thought of as being composed of three main areas of concern: teeth, bone, and muscle. They may be thought of as three legs of a triangle, the maxillofacial triangle. In a healthy maxillofacial complex with no attendant joint problems, the triangle of teeth, bone, and muscle may be thought of as being in structural balance. However, when malocclusion exists, when functionally oriented TMJ problems are present, the triangle may be thought of as being distorted, each member to its own degree. The structure of the maxillofacial complex, the structure represented by the teeth, bone, and muscle, has gone from a state of balance to a state of imbalance. Structural imbalance is the etiological source of the patient's problems. Structure is what should receive the lion's share of the clinician's therapeutic attention. This is where FJO principles fit in.

With respect to TMJ pain-dysfunction therapeutics, the chief area of employment of the FJO series of techniques and methods is for that patient who might be categorized as being in a state of *structural imbalance.* It must always be remembered that for most instances in this series of texts the word "structural" equates with "skeletal." This category of structural imbalance implies the presence of one or several of a set of very important physical characteristics pertinent to the status of both the patient's TMJs as well as the maxillomandibular, or jaw-to-jaw, relationship. This category comprises by far the vast majority of TMJ pain-dysfunction patients.

With respect to the joint, structural imbalance implies some form of disc-condyle-fossa malalignment during function and rest that is defined as internal derangement of the articular disc. Since the disc is situated such that it cannot be displaced an excessive amount either superiorly or laterally by the very essence of the biomechanical and osseous architecture of the joint itself, the only displacement or derangement that will be possible in a true structural imbalance is for the disc to be displaced *forward* more anteriorly and medially down the anterior slope of the tuberculum and articular eminence. The rest of the glenoid fossa and the osseous contours of the petrous portion of the temporal bone form a sort of anatomical bony cul-de-sac that, in conjunction with the tough fibrous ligamentous tissue of the capsule, forms an anatomical dead end as far as disc displacement either superiorly or posteriorly is concerned. With the addition in this fossa area of the head of the condyle, the disc's posterior ligaments, both superior and inferior, and the soft tissues, nerves, and blood vessels of the bilaminar zone, there is very little room left in the area of the bowl of the glenoid fossa—not much room for a soft cartilagenous disc to work its way superiorly and posteriorly, especially since it would have to compete for that space with the condylar head. But there is plenty of room for the disc to move (or maybe more correctly "to be squeezed") anteriorly and inferiorly down the slope of the tuberculum by a condyle that is being simultaneously forced superiorly and posteriorly. When the disc may be displaced anteriorly and inferiorly slightly, it naturally facilitates in turn the displacement of the condylar head superiorly and posteriorly past the bulbous heel of the disc.

The basic source of all functional TMJ problems is intracapsular. *The condyle is riding off the disc,* and as it hops back on again by sliding over the bulbous posterior heel to the discal concavity as it begins its translatory movement, the telltale click or "pop" is made clinically audible. If no sound is heard during such a circumstance and full-range opening to 45 mm or better still exists, it would be because the posterior heel has been worn or "ironed" flat from chronic abuse by the condylar head riding on and off. Where the disc resides at full occlusion is important, but such information can't hold a candle to the importance of where the condyle is at full occlusion. There's where the action is!

As for the head of the condyle, unlike the soft cartilagenous disc, the hard bony surface of the capitulum has no trouble stretching the ligaments of its surrounding capsule while forcing its way up into the soft posterior attachment area past the heel of the disc and invading the bilaminar zone, an area of meek resistance. Given time and enough force behind the closing actions of the mandible, it's a wonder the superiorly,

---

Figure 5–1 (A–C) The maxillofacial triangle. Conceptually all malocclusions that induce functional TMJ problems may be thought of as imbalances in the three main components of the maxillofacial complex; teeth, bone, and muscle.

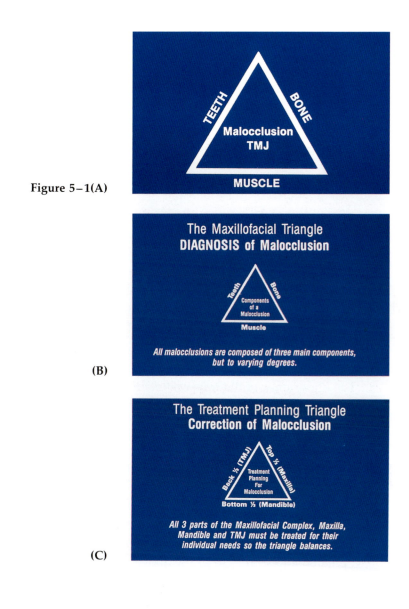

Figure 5–1(A)

(B)

(C)

posteriorly invading capitulum doesn't pulverize the tissues of the retro-discal area. Even Nature's naturally made shock absorber, the articular disc itself, has been shown to perforate through its central isthmus due to the improper application of the tremendous and unrelenting forces of oc-clusion. How much more so would the fragile tissues of the posterior at-tachment and/or bilaminar zone be expected to suffer when they are sub-jected to such forces. No wonder patients complain of pain! You just can-not take an anatomical area that is designed to absorb the enormous amount of physical stresses that a TMJ is designed to accept and discon-nect its component parts, as the appropriate kind of dental malocclusion can easily do, and still expect it to work right! Although willing to comply and make an honest attempt to adapt to untoward situations, Nature will tolerate a certain level of deviation from Her grand plan of design for only so long before She answers back in the common language of such abuse: disarticulation, dysfunction, degeneration, and pain. As long as there is life, Nature will always make an honest effort to heal, but only when given what She determines as a fair chance. For the structurally imbal-anced patient, the FJO series of techniques represent not only a fair chance but also a loving and protective helping hand.

Though a purely dental Class I malocclusion of a specific variety is capable of forcing a full-sized mandible back entirely on its own, another way in which the structural status of a given case may become compro-mised is due to a deviation during the years of growth and development from the normal maxillomandibular relationship, specifically in the form of a *skeletal* Class II mandibular deficiency or retrusion and/or insufficient vertical dimension of occlusion, although the latter nearly always follows on the heels of the former. Maxillary size and position also play an impor-tant role here.

The importance of the full-scale mandibular deficiency and its result-ant skeletal mandibular retrusion in some form or other, along with the usual attending and culpable lack of vertical, is so intimately related to the superior posterior displacement of the condyle (SPDC) that it would be difficult to think of one without the other. The mandible may actually be deficient in size due to underdevelopment and be in a true Class II skeletal deep-bite situation with its attending "Class II musculature," or it may be only slightly underdeveloped and of near-normal size, as per the standards represented by the Bimler DLM or McNamara effective man-dibular length, the Sassouni arcs, or other cephalometric standards, only to be forced posteriorly by the anterior incisal interferences of the NRDM-SPDC phenomenon. In light of the above it may now easily be seen how a severe Class II, Division 2–type malocclusion could be responsible for both types of the aforementioned forms of structural imbalance, both dental and skeletal, occurring simultaneously in the same case. This also makes it clear as to why that particular type of malocclusion, the Class II, Division 2, deep-bite case, on the whole is the most physiologically destructive with respect to the proper function of the TMJ! The NRDM/ SPDC aspects of the incisal interference represented by the deep-bite Division II dental malocclusion compounded by what may also be an already retropositioned maxillary apical base can trap a mandible in a skeletal (and dental) Class II situation, retard its overall down and forward growth to full size, and/or force condyles back up and off the discs at full occlusion. Throw in plenty of bruxism and a high-stress/poor-nutrition American life-style for good measure, and it is easy to see why these types of patients (and their bilaminar zones) are walking "TMJ time bombs."

Occlusal imbalances anteriorly may be such as to also cause a sideways deviation of the mandible upon full closure. This, if great enough, can cause the disarticulation of the joint unilaterally on the side of the direction of the shift and result in clicking upon opening and closing on that particular side. Both joints may also be disarticulated, with the worse of the two being on the side of the direction of the mandibular lateral midline shift. This is perfectly logical since the side to which the mandible shifts from midline on closing would be the side with the more posteriorly displaced condylar head at the completion of the arc of closure to full-contact habitual occlusion. Conversely, both joints might click equally in the presence of no midline shift. Yet regardless of how it comes about, joint clicking or "popping" upon opening and closing is probably the single most important telltale sign of a joint that is structurally imbalanced.[1] Symptoms, on the other hand, tell their story in their own way.

As previously described, a simple and easy confirmation of the presence of this NRDM/SPDC-type of structural imbalance in a given case may be demonstrated by having the patients assume the now famous "as if" position, i.e., have them slide their mandible forward to a dental end-to-end position of the incisors that would be near the same orthopedically as if they had their mandibles advanced with a Bionator. Once the patients bite together with their anterior teeth somewhere around an incisal end-to-end position (sometimes past), they then open and close to that same approximate advanced mandibular position without allowing the mandible to regress back to more habitual retruded arc of closure. If the clicking of the joint disappears, as it often will, it is because the condyle has been relocated, albeit temporarily, to a new, more structurally balanced and correct position *on the disc,* a position more anterior and inferior than its usual uncorrected, retruded starting place. In so doing, it moves from its former position of riding off the disc back down onto the disc again and "recaptures" it. Then in beginning its transition movements from that position *on* the disc, no click of the passage of the capitulum over the bulbous heel into the discal concavity during opening is possible because it is already there. If the patients are instructed to return to their "normal" (actually retruded) bite or habitual occlusion, one will observe that the clicking returns upon opening and closing to that retruded habitual position again. This clearly confirms that the habitual occlusion is such that it forces the entire mandible posteriorly upon full interdigitation of the teeth, hence effecting the superior posterior movement of the condyle in the glenoid fossa to a point where it has skipped (or has actually become jammed) past the discal heel and is riding off the disc on the "retrodistal" tissues of the posterior ligament and/or bilaminar zone, a place Nature never intended mandibular condyles to be! Such is the most clear-cut example of classic structural imbalance, disarticulation, derangement, and dysfunction within the joint. As a clinical procedure, it is incredibly simple. As a diagnostic procedure, it is incredibly profound.

Again, as previously noted, radiologically the patient who is suffering from a full-fledged structural imbalance will have a reduced posterior and even superior joint space.[2] As the disc is displaced forward, the capitulum of the condyle may be driven superiorly and/or posteriorly in the posterior joint space of the glenoid fossa. This also in turn results in a reduction of the joint space superiorly and posteriorly. If clicking exists in only one joint due to a severe mandibular shift upon full occlusal interdigitation to that same side, the corresponding transcranial film may logically be expected to divulge a more reduced joint space on that side than in the unaffected side, which it almost always will. If full bilateral Class II retrusion of the mandible exists, the radiographs may be expected to support the clinical signs and symptoms by revealing a reduced joint space as small as 2+ or even 1 mm bilaterally. However, it must be remembered that a 1- to 2-mm posterior joint space is only a rough clinical guide for intrusion of the condylar head into the posterior joint space. For some patients whose normal posterior-superior joint space might be 4 to 5 mm, a 3-mm space may actually reflect condylar intrusion. This is why the measurement of such spaces should only be judged *relative to the clinically observed signs and symptoms,* which are what actually determine the diagnosis. Radiographics are supportive; clinical observation is definite, not vice versa. Yet the experienced clinician will be amazed at the large number of cases that hover around a 3.0-mm posterior joint space as a safe minimum. Less than that, and the patient and his joints are often in trouble.

At this point it would serve well to briefly discuss a concept that may prove at first a bit vague and nondescript when compared with the review above of structural imbalance of the hard tissues of the stomatognathic system. It involves an imbalance of a true physical nature that is a major contributor to the total picture of overall structural imbalance in the TMJ pain-dysfunction patient. However, its presence is nearly impossible to physically measure but rather must be inferred, and even then its presence may be inductively inferred only after having observed a considerable number of clinical situations. It is the notion of "Class II musculature," or the Class II "neuromuscular sling." At the risk of being oversimplistic and for the sake of discussion, if we discount some genetic, hormonal, and nutritional influences, it might be stated that the bones

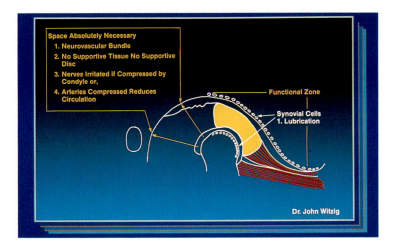

Figure 5–2   The TMJ is designed to transmit forces of occlusion up and *forward*, not up and back. No stress-absorbing tissues are present there, only sensitive nerves and blood vessels. (Courtesy of Dr. John Witzig.)

essentially follow the dictates of the muscles during growth and development in the maxillofacial complex. Empirical observations soon lead one to conclude that muscles or, more correctly, the improper functions of muscles are the chief etiological culprits in the development of most malocclusions (barring genetic aberrations, true birth or growth defects, trauma, etc.). It must also be remembered that muscles are "creatures of habit." Their persistent function in a skeletal Class II, deep-overbite situation causes them to adapt physically to the mechanics of the skeletally retrusive mandibular situation the best they can. Relieving the problems of uncoordinated, traumatic, overclosed movements (overworking at a less than physiologically ideal length) is an important consideration of treatment for muscles that are engaged in function. Yet an equal consideration must also be given to these same muscles when they are at "rest." Where do they rest; in what position and how much do they actually rest or relax in that position? How much myostatic contracture or muscle splinting is present? In the case of Class II musculature, the "rest" position may not be sufficient to allow the mandible to "relapse" far enough down and forward from its Class II retruded position to allow sufficient decompression of the joint. In the more severe cases of chronic mandibular retrusion and deep overbite with its attending TMJ pain-dysfunction problems, such observations may actually be made clinically. But in the less severe, less obvious cases, its presence must be inferred, and it should be assumed to be present so that it may be taken into account and directly addressed therapeutically in the treatment plan. Merely altering the occlusal table by one means or another in order to rearticulate the condyle in proper relationship to the disc during function *may not always be enough* to provide complete full-time decompression of the joint if the residual effects of Class II musculature remain uncorrected and formidable. Occlusal correction confined exclusively to the dental apparatus only would allow the mandible to be positioned forward due to the guiding surfaces of the inclined planes of the occlusal table during function. But without the benefits of retraining the muscles of mastication, this may very well also result in the mandible being carried at rest more rearward than it should be in the "sling" of the unretrained musculature while the mandible is not in function, which is its status most of the time. The elongated damaged capsular ligaments of the entire joint complex allow for this. When major structural TMJ imbalances exist, treatment plans must be constructed that directly address not only the occlusal table and its relationships and the structural status of the internal joint components and their relationships but also the guiding force that brings these two factors into play, the perpetually functioning masticatory musculature. All three components of the maxillofacial triangle, teeth, bones, and muscles, must be considered in every treatment plan. Sometimes treatment will merely take the form of the muscles learning new habits of motion as per the guiding influences of the newly reconstructed or altered occlusal table. Other times actual muscular retraining by means of functionally altering their lengths down to a cellular level must be effected to properly complete the case. And that means functional appliances like the Bionator or the Orthopedic Corrector, for one way or another, musculature must always be a major consideration in the formulation of therapeutics for Class II mandibular retrusion-type TMJ problems. They are often one of the most neglected of the three sides of the famous bone/teeth/muscle triangle of malocclusion. They simply cannot be ignored.

The patient who might be categorized as having structurally irreparable anatomical relationships by the traditional standards of what is considered normal has a twofold problem. First, the condyle is riding off the disc, and it is suffering from the problems of chronic capitular intrusion into the posterior joint space and has been in this state for a long period of time. Second, due to such severity of intracapsular damage as separation of the posterior attachment from the heel of the disc, discal perforation, full-scale condylar resorption, or irrecoverability of the disc, complete reconstruction of the internal joint structures to their normal status becomes impossible by means of traditional noninvasive conservative procedures. One of the most common problems in the category of structural irreparability is that state whereby the disc is displaced so far forward and its posterior attachments are so compromised (either due to separation or overelongation) as to render the disc irrecoverable or what is termed "nonreducible." Another frequent occurrence in this category is where the disc is so chronically displaced forward as to be compressed or distorted past the point where it is usable again even if recovered. In such instances, not only will the transcranial film divulge the commonly seen reduced superior and posterior joint space, but should the patient be subjected to the process of arthrography, the arthograms would also reveal a confluence between the superior and inferior cavities of the posterior attachment area or patentcy through the center of the joint space in the case of discal perforations. However, arthrography not yet being that common a procedure, the procurement of such radiographs as these may not be practical, especially in less densely populated areas. Therefore, under such circumstances, a greater weight is placed on the clinical diagnosis of such advanced states of joint degeneration. Since the condyle at no time rides on the disc, which is perpetually down and forward ahead of it, there is no clicking upon jaw movement. There also is almost always some relative degree of limited opening. Sometimes referred to as "the silent stage" of the TMJ degenerative process, the disc will not remain far enough up on the slope of the tuberculum to allow the capitulum to hop back into it again regardless of how the mandible is either voluntarily moved by the natural efforts of the patient or manually manipulated by the therapeutic efforts of the clinician. This inability to recapture the disc may also be due to the aforementioned chronic forced distortion of the disc making articulation with the condylar head a totally unstable situation even if the capitulum could be repositioned back onto the disc's misshapened surface. A history of past TMJ problems such as pain, dysfunction, unilateral or bilateral limited opening or locking, and clicking will usually be revealed by the patient, all of which might paradoxically at present seem to be in remission except for the telltale myofascial and/or headache-type pain that remains. Forcible retrusion of the mandible manually by the clinician will sometimes elicit a painful response in most patients with this level of degeneration because there is nothing to stop the forces of the manually induced retrusion from being transmitted directly to the chronically traumatized posterior joint areas. Chronic low-grade (and sometimes not so low grade) inflammation of the soft tissues of the intracapsular area will eventually produce the same effects on surrounding bone that chronic soft-tissue inflammation would produce on bone anywhere else in the body. Bony dissolution, avascular necrosis, remodeling or "lipping" of the condyle or other osseous components of the joint may be evident. Extremely tight joint spaces of the 1 to 1.5-mm variety will commonly be seen on the transcranial film. Muscle splinting or trismus may frequently occur to limit movement of the joint as a reflexive protective mechanism while the body rallies its components in an effort to reduce trauma to the area. However, this usually only occurs during acute exacerbations of the problem. Yet even though torn discs might not be recoverable, severed posterior ligaments can be conservatively repaired. Autopsy studies[3] of patients with known histories of tears in the posterior attachment and subsequent treatments that advance the mandible and bring the condyle back down and forward once again in the fossa (but in these cases not back onto the nonreducible discs) showed that a form of fibrotic scar-type tissue forms over the tear. And with the condyles thus repositioned, they function on this surrogate articular scar tissue in a state of pain-free functional compatibility. Although it is not the original discal tissue, it serves the purpose nonetheless. The basic objectives of treatment have still been achieved, i.e., a restored state of improved function and elimination of pain. Although a full or totally complete structural repair of damaged joint structures back to their original nondamaged state might not be achievable with conventional conservative treatment, the ability of such methods to accomplish in essence the same treatment objectives of restored function and alleviation of pain keeps these techniques on the forefront of treatments of choice. It must be remembered that altering internal joint relationships is only one of the three main areas of concern in treating the total TMJ problem. Favorable alteration of internal joint relationships is also only one of the three main capabilities of the FJO technique. In addition, the other two major aspects of the functional TMJ degenerative arthritis process may and should be directly addressed by such traditional and conservative methods, i.e., alteration of the distal-driving occlusal table to a less damaging relationship and correction of the harnessing "sling" of Class II musculature. This "triple-header" approach will achieve the one very important goal in TMJ treatment as far as the patient is concerned, and that is the *relief of pain through decompression of the joint!* Invasive procedures may always be resorted to if needed once more basic biological issues have been addressed by the above-mentioned conservative means. However, clinically, this proves almost never to be the case when the initial source of the problem is functional in nature.

THE HERITAGE OF THE OCCLUSAL SPLINT

For over a generation the intraoral acrylic occlusal splint in any one of an endless variety of designs has been associated in one way or another with TMJ therapeutics.[4-10] Splint usage represented state-of-the-art methodology for the treatment of TMJ problems of a functional nature until recent times when its position of supremacy in the TMJ world has been overthrown by the discipline of FJO. However, some of the most fundamental principles of splint therapy have been carried over and form part of the overall picture of the treatment regimens of the newer methods. There are a number of times when splints of various types may still be used, either as part of an investigative or diagnostic procedure or as supplements to larger, more comprehensive treatment plans due to their palliative effect. They also form a conceptual basis for much of what modern clinicians do with the newer appliance techniques, i.e., utilizing the "splinting effect" in the design of the treatment appliance itself. This allows these appliances to provide the palliative relief of the patient's symptoms while the active components of the appliances are engaged in actual mechanical correction of the initial problem. Therefore, a proper knowledge of just how they work and what they are intended to do serves as a foundation point from which a deeper understanding of their role in overall TMJ therapeutics may be gained. Although their day in the sun has now been overshadowed by more advanced methods, there is no reason to discard the technique altogether. Even in spite of their now limited use, they still have an important auxiliary role to play at times in modern-day TMJ treatment planning. They have made great contributions to our present-day knowledge of how to address the functionally oriented TMJ problem. To gain a comprehensive understanding of the total picture in TMJ therapeutics, we cannot divorce ourselves from becoming familiar with their basic effects. They have been with us for a long time. We must build on what they have laid down for us from out of the past.

The Proprioceptive Occlusal Neuromuscular Circuit

Understanding the basic principles of the occlusofunctional proprioceptive neuromuscular circuit is fundamental to understanding not only how intraoral removable acrylic splints of various types work but also as to why and when they will work. The occlusion, the muscles, and the joint are all intimately related in the function of the stomatognathic system. When the three are in proper anatomical balance and functional harmony, the phenomenon of functionally induced TMJ-type pain and dysfunction will not appear. However, if the occlusion becomes imbalanced due to some form of prematurity, interference, or cuspal slide, the muscles are the first to take note. By a somewhat neurologically complicated mechanism, the biochemical and neuroanatomical details of which may be dispensed with for the sake of brevity, as the teeth first come into contact with one another, the exquisitely sensitive proprioceptive fibers in their respective periodontal ligaments send *efferent* electrical impulses to the central nervous system (CNS), which in turn sends *afferent* motor signals to the muscles of mastication so as to best direct the movement of the mandible to the most balanced and biomechanically stable position of dental interdigitation that the existing occlusion will permit. Like all striated muscular functions in the body, this muscular process has an optimal range of motion at an *optimal* muscular length that the muscles tolerate well. Conversely, this process also has a *suboptimal* range of motion in which the muscles and, consequently, their balancing antagonists can only work in a less harmonious fashion and at less than optimal length. Now muscles, especially the muscles of mastication (as well as the whole masticatory system itself) are relatively adaptable to the circumstances under which they must operate. But there are limits to this adaptability. Thus the notion of "functional frequency" becomes an important factor. Not only is the level of suboptimal operation of a muscular system a factor in its performance, but also the frequency at which suboptimal operation occurs. A major, albeit infrequent suboptimal circumstance may bring about a rapid muscular dysfunction (spasm) and attending pain (as in the simple act of attempting to reach the middle of one's back with one's hand), but an only slightly suboptimal functional circumstance that occurs with a great deal of frequency might also bring on the same unfavorable responses from the participating muscles, especially muscles as small and *well innervated* as those muscles concerned with mastication. It is easily understood how an occlusal imbalance can bring about muscle soreness during heavy mastication. Yet less dramatic functional stimuli may also accumulate to exhaust muscles. The most common is deglutition. Swallowing occurs 1,500 to 2,000 times per day, and each time the individual swallows, the mandible is usually lightly braced against the maxilla by means of full occlusal contact *(in the most biomechanically stable cusp/fossa position available)* through the reflexive contraction of the muscles of mastication. Even though the primary muscles involved are the three major pairs of closing muscles, the masseter, medial pterygoid, and temporalis, their antagonists must also be called into play to modify the arc of closure just enough to guide the mandible and the searching cusps of its occlusal table past the raft of possible occlusal interferences onto the most stable point of "habitual occlusion" available. The more imbalanced the occlusion, especially if that imbalance is in an overall net posterior direction, the more work will be involved for the muscles (both protagonists and antagonists) at both suboptimal lengths and/or positions in order to unobtrusively guide the mandible home. Muscles are creatures of habit. They learn from repetition. For an occurrence with the high level of frequency as that of deglutition, the muscles quickly learn how to modify the arc of closure to just the right pathway to bring the jaws together with minimal "occlusal collision," but in a severe malocclusion with a major distal-driving interference of some sort, they are "overworking" in order to do it. Then there is the compounding problem of bruxism. To this might be added the mechanical "shock" of the type of noxious stimuli transmitted to the muscles during lateral excursive movements by that "devil of occlusal harmony," the notorious *balancing side interferences,* and it's a wonder such occlusally imbalanced patients do as well as they do! The human body possesses an incredible biological forgiveness for abuse! But only to a point.

This process of all but reflexively seeking the best arc of closure to the most stable jaw-to-jaw intercuspation is a product of the perpetual round trip represented by the initial and continuous neurological responses of the proprioceptive fibers of the periodontal ligaments that upon initial and continuous occlusal contact travel to the central nervous system where they are received, interpreted, transformed, and discharged in turn in the form of afferent motor neural responses to the muscles controlling the mandible. Upon receipt of these neurologically electrical commands, these muscles then modify their function to the degree necessary as represented by the information received via this circuit so as to effect the best available and most "cusp-collision–free" arc of closure. This final position of closure, in itself due to occlusal irregularities of this type of imbalanced case, is still neuromuscularly and biomechanically disadvantaged. The above type of action is repeated with such a level of frequency that it becomes secondarily reflexive. The individual can do it without even thinking about it. Yet voluntary overriding conscious motor control still exists. The result is a dual means of control, one voluntary, one reflexive, and it is all due to the acute sensitivity of the neurological proprioceptive fibers of the periodontal ligaments! With enough repetition, the proprioceptive fibers within the muscles themselves even begin to contribute. When the net result is excessive mandibular retrusion, this is the essence of the generation of the NRDM/SPDC phenomenon. Taken to such an extreme, what started out as a normal functional process of muscular modification of the arc of closure becomes petulant enough to cause an actual full-scale structural imbalance (disarticulation) of the condyle-disc assembly within the joint itself.

However, there are other factors that contribute to the plight of the muscles in their daily workings other than the mechanical problems represented by an imbalanced occlusion. It is known quite well that TMJ pain-dysfunction problems have always been thought of as stress-related conditions, or at least are believed to be exacerbated by excessive stress to the individual. We have just seen how the occlusion can act as a source of mechanical or, more correctly, structural stress. But emotional factors also have a direct bearing in exacerbating TMJ symptoms in their proclivity for permitting myogenic problems, which should be normally kept reasonably at bay, to rise more quickly to the surface and expose the true level of increased work load placed on the muscles of mastication through the phenomenon of bruxism, bracing, or clenching of the teeth. Yet in addition to this commonly observed process, an even more subtle and less well understood phenomenon may also possibly be taking place that belongs in the same "family" of factors that make things hard on the masticatory muscles: the admittedly highly theoretical process of "dysponesis" as defined by Whatmore.[11] Although difficult to prove via conventional procedures of the scientific method, it nevertheless seems to represent an evocative and interesting theory that bears its attractiveness in its ability to account for what may easily be observed in the anamnesis of the patients to which its principles are applied. In essence, this process is theoretically one of "inappropriate or unnecessary neurological signaling" and is thought by many to exacerbate the unnecessary chronic low-grade tensing or hypertonicity of the striated musculature. The larger muscles are powerful enough to tolerate this well, but for the smaller muscles it is another matter, especially those as well innervated as the muscles of the head and neck. Dysponesis is defined as a physiological response to the less than optimum (i.e., stressful) environment provided for the muscles by not only the aforementioned occlusal stressors but also the biochemical stresses placed on the system by an unbalanced, incomplete, or improper diet! It would not be possible in the space provided here to discuss all the implications of proper nutrition relative to the TMJ pain-dysfunction patient, but it is generally accepted by a large number of practitioners in this field that improper diets with an excess of refined sugars, caffeine, alcohol, tobacco, and processed foods seem to increase the patient's proclivity for headaches or head and neck muscle soreness and fatigue. This would theoretically lower the stamina and resistance of the muscles of mastication to the noxious stimuli provided to them by the abusive functioning of an occlusally imbalanced dentition. Not only are the muscles forced to overwork at a foreshortened (overcontracted) suboptimal level at an increased frequency, but they are expected to do so in a less than optimal chemical environment bereft of their normal ration of "biological ammunition." Extensive clinical observance appears to support these theories, and it has been observed that proper nutritional counseling alone without the benefit of any other forms of active treatment has been shown in certain instances to reduce the intensity and frequency of headache-type discomfort in certain patients. Inadequate or imbalanced nutrition is simply one more type of stress, this time a chemical one, that should be reduced for the patients to better enable them to do well. Yet oddly, some patients seem only little affected by nutritional deficiencies (or excesses), and for them the dietary form of stressor does not turn out to be a major factor in their condition. This must be evaluated on a case-by-case basis, and extreme caution should be used in evaluating the true role of nutrition in treatment of patients with TMJ problems. The main object of attention for the patient with a functionally compromised TMJ is still the joint. Yet the importance of dietary control for some must *not be underestimated,* for when such dietary sensitivities are present in a given individual, the effects on not only the musculature in specific but the general health as well may be profound.

In the light of the previous review, it may now clearly be seen how initial splint treatment for the patient with TMJ problems sometimes follows a twofold course of action. The first step is to attempt to reduce the stress load on the muscles of mastication by providing them with a more favorable *biological environment* through biochemical "stress-relieving" dietary adjustments if necessary and then, second, to reduce the physical stress load on these same muscles as well as the retrodiscal tissues of the

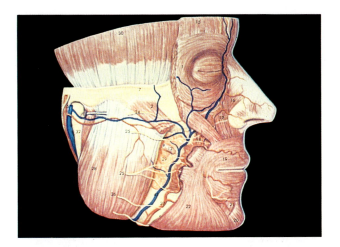

Figure 5–3 Muscles are creatures of habit. The musculature of the maxillofacial complex transmits all its power through the articular isthmus of the TMJ during mastication. Their physiological imbalance must be considered and many times directly addressed in every TMJ treatment plan.

bilaminar zone by providing them with a more favorable *mechanical environment* through "stress-eliminating" occlusal augmentation. These two categories of treatment essentially attempt to change things that dental professionals are most capable of changing and may easily directly control, i.e., occlusion and nutrition. Other forms of stress relief such as counseling of life-styles or mental or emotional conditions are beyond the dental practitioner's level of training and control. But if the patient's stomatognathic system is merely taken from a state of overfunctioning on a *suboptimal level* back to a state of functioning at a more acceptable degree of frequency (bruxism free) and at an *optimal level* once again, a great stride will have been taken in giving the patient relief from the headache, facial pain, and discomforts caused by occlusal imbalances. However, there is one problem. Often what ironically *prevents* a proper readjustment and prosthetic rehabilitation of the dental component of the problem (the occlusion) to a more proper biomechanically acceptable anteroposteriorly (AP) and vertically balanced form is that particular factor that this type of treatment is designed to help most, i.e., the muscles themselves! After the punishment that has been meted out to them over such long periods of time, the muscles of mastication can become dulled and somewhat desensitized. In their never-ending efforts to adapt, they have become so accustomed to positioning the mandible at the patient's habitual occlusion, albeit a position not optimal to the muscles own physiological demands and especially not optimal to the intracapsular demands of the joint, that they become temporarily resistant to other positions that might be biologically better for them. This is reflected in the untoward reaction of the muscles to impingement of an altered (raised) occlusal table into the habitual interocclusal freeway space. With respect to the mandibular arc of closure, the neuromuscular reflexive "memory" can become so ingrained due to the frequency of repetition of the act that the patient will close easily to this habitual occlusion every time. The demands of the proprioceptive occlusal neuromuscular circuit demand it. The myostatic contracture that foreshortens the muscles reinforces it. The cycle should be broken first not only to allow the muscles a chance to be relieved of the motor impulses of the CNS that direct them to these suboptimal, unfavorable retrusive working situations but also secondly to allow for better acceptance of the new impulses of information to be programmed into the CNS once the occlusion is changed. What is needed is a process whereby patients may close their jaws together in a manner that sends an entirely different, and if not favorable, then at least neutral proprioceptive set of signals to the controlling centers of the CNS—a set of signals that are kind and palliative to the muscles and allow them to work under more favorable or optimal conditions of physiological length, balance, and harmony. These neutral or more forgiving signals then allow the muscles to cease functioning at their former suboptimal levels. This is the concept behind the removable intraoral acrylic occlusal splint. It is a CNS deprogrammer; a biological circuit breaker!

"They sway'd about on a rocking horse
And thought it Pegasus."

"Sleep and Poetry"
John Keats, 1795–1821
English poet

Splint Usage and Design: The Mechanical Environment

The purpose of the intraoral, removable acrylic occlusal splint is to provide a surface of acrylic against which one or the other of the upper or lower dental arches may occlude so as to provide a new, more biomechanically balanced position of closure that is more compatible to the physiological demands of the joints and musculature. There are many different types and designs of splints for both upper and lower arches, yet they all serve the same purpose of providing what many refer to as a "vacation" for the overworked and distraught muscles by preventing their need to bring the mandible to its full point of occlusally imbalanced retrusive overclosure. Although splint types vary widely, they are of two basic types. The first is the articulated surface or, "occlusion-capturing," type of splints such as the Gelb splint or the Levandoski splint, which provides a new interdigitating occlusal surface of acrylic for the teeth to occlude against that *forces* the mandible to what is thought will be a new and more biocompatible position for the musculature (and disc-condyle-fossa assembly of the joint) upon closure. The second type is the flat-plane, or "occlusion-eliminating," type. Examples of this type would be the Witzig splint for the upper arch or the Sears pivotal splint for the lower arch. The purpose of these splint types is to provide a totally flat surface free of any inclined planes or cuspal guidances whatsoever against which an opposing dental arch might occlude. This allows the muscles the option of closing in a more two-dimensionally, physiologically acceptable AP and/or lateral arc of closure to a neutral and more forgiving surface of contact (the acrylic of the splint) that is more compatible with their demands, provided of course that the splint is properly balanced. The third dimension, vertical, can be controlled by the thickness of the occlusal acrylic of these types of splints.

The primary functions of splints over the years have turned out to be both palliative and diagnostic. If splint wear by the patient reduces symptoms, the clinician is more confident in permanently altering the occlusion in some way in an effort to obtain permanent symptomatic relief. If no symptomatic relief is obtained, especially with properly constructed splints like the Levandoski splint, the pathway of permanent corrective treatment may lie elsewhere.

In the light of our previous discussions of the proprioceptive occlusal neuromuscular circuit for muscular control of the arc of closure, it is now seen how the flat surface occlusion-eliminating splints effect such dramatic relief for patients of myofascial pains and/or headache discomfort. By providing a totally neutral surface for the teeth to occlude against, which means flat and generally bilaterally balanced in all excursive directions, the neuromuscular proprioceptive reflexive stimuli that the teeth normally transmit to the brain and hence to the muscles via the reflex circuits of the CNS are eliminated. Hopefully, if the splint is of proper thickness, another thing that will be eliminated is condylar impingement on the bilaminar zone. (Yet surprisingly, this does not always happen!) When the teeth occlude on the flat, smooth surface of the splint, the brain receives a totally new set of proprioceptive stimuli. The new proprioceptive occlusal stimuli tell the brain that no matter where the muscles close the mandible, no matter what position they bring it to, the effect is universally the same. Upon repeated deciphering of this incoming information, along with consideration of all the negative "complaints" the muscles and joint structures have been feeding the brain due to their displeasure at working in a manner in which they do not like, the controlling centers in the CNS soon make a logical value judgment and, if the vertical is acceptable, in effect issue new orders to the muscles to go ahead and close any AP or lateral excursive the way they please, for the CNS knows this may be done with impunity. There are no interfering guiding planes of opposing teeth to crash into and no requirements for sudden alterations of the mandibular arc of closure rearward at the last minute to avoid untoward cuspal or incisal-edge collisions. There is, quite simply, no occlusal feedback as to what particular arc of closure is required at all. Only the vertical remains fixed. Given their freedom, what are the muscles going to do? Continue in their old ways of overworking in order to produce a disharmonious, uncoordinated, canted, or twisted arc of closure? Hardly. Surely they may persist in their old ways out of habit for a while (we all do)—but sooner or later (and most likely sooner), for the patient in this first type of category, the muscles will begin to work more easily in a more optimal, coordinated fashion, and the patient will notice a gradual (and sometimes not so gradual) diminution of discomfort or myofascial and headache-type pain. When the splint is taken out for eating, the muscles and joints have had so much time to recover during the extended periods of splint wear between meals that the extra stresses associated with chewing on an imbalanced occlusal table pose less of a problem because these noxious stimuli are of such a short duration. Yet if splint wear is ceased altogether, the old symptomatic picture quickly returns in full force.

Another action of the removable intraoral splint is that of artificially opening the vertical dimension of occlusion. If structural imbalance exists with respect to this dimension (i.e., overclosure), increasing the vertical by means of splint wear automatically decompresses the joint slightly and gives some degree of relief to the battered bilaminar zone. If the disc is not displaced too far forward, the extra 2 to 4 mm of vertical opening represented by the thickness of the intraocclusal acrylic of the splint's biting surface may be just enough to allow the head of the condyle to come down and forward enough in borderline patients to recapture the disc, thus eliminating the clicking upon opening and closing during splint wear.

Of the varied types of flat surface or occlusion-eliminating splints available, one considered by many to be the "sweetheart" of them all is undoubtedly the Sears pivotal splint. It is the sheer essence of simplicity of design, yet its palliative and diagnostic capabilities are far-reaching. It has only three major component parts: a lingual metal bar hand shaped to the linguogingival portion of a model of the patient's lower arch and an acrylic saddle covering the occlusal lingual surfaces of each posterior quadrant and extending from the occlusal surface of the first bicuspid back to the last posterior tooth in the quadrant. There is some slight controversy as to the thickness this type splint should be. One method of determining occlusal thickness advocated by Dr. W. Scheer of Las Vegas is as follows.[12] Have the splint processed with about 2-mm thickness or less

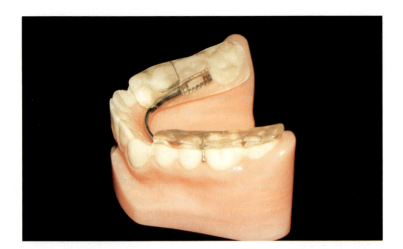

Figure 5–4 Sears pivotal flat-plane splint for the mandibular arch. (Courtesy of the Ohlendorf Co, St Louis.)

over the occlusal saddles, and have the lab grind it reasonably flat and unpolished at about this level. First, check the fit of the splint in the mouth by inserting it and pressing it with the fingers from side to side bilaterally and from front to back diagonally across the arch to check for rocking. It is important that the splint fit accurately in as stable a fit as possible. Should it rock either from side to side on firm finger pressure or front to back or diagonally, place a small amount of "wet" cold-cure acrylic on the underside of the particular saddle at fault and replace it in the mouth while holding it stable with finger pressure until the acrylic hardens. Should a "rock" be so slight as to escape initial detection, it usually will cause the tooth right underneath the void area responsible for the rocking to become slightly sore. The patient will usually detect this in a few days of splint wear, and if such occurs, the patient should be instructed to return for an adjustment. Correcting this problem is a simple matter of placing a drop of wet cold-cure acrylic onto the acrylic area of the underside of the splint immediately above the sensitive tooth and placing it in the mouth to cure under firm, yet gentle biting pressure.

To obtain the desired occlusal thickness of the splint, which in "deep-bite" cases routinely seems to hover around 2- and 3-mm thickness interocclusally, the clinician theoretically would like to have the body's own musculature aid in the selection of the best vertical dimension of occlusion. This is why the splint's occlusal biting topmost surface is left essentially "unfinished" and in the rough, flattened state. Cold-cure acrylic will then be added to these flattened occlusal saddles of acrylic at chairside by the clinician. To do this, first, make sure the acrylic surface of the splint is roughened by means of acrylic burs, etc., to facilitate bonding of the cold-cure acrylic to the splint. Next, place a few drops of monomer on the splint's roughened occlusal surfaces. This also facilitates bonding of the cold-cure acrylic to the splint. Now coat the thumb and forefinger of the left hand with common petroleum jelly and grasp the saddle of one side of the splint between the finger and thumb. The lubricated fleshy parts now act as a dam to prevent the cold-cure acrylic, which is mixed to a somewhat "runny" consistency, from flowing down over the edges of the saddle. After adding the cold-cure acrylic, which is mixed in a common dapping dish, allow it to reach a soft, doughy consistency so that it is soft enough to be shaped but not quite thin enough to run. This is done to each side of the splint in relatively short working time at chairside. The patients are instructed that the splint is going to be placed in their mouths and they should *not* bite into it, nor should they be alarmed by the volatile smell of the monomer or its unpleasant taste. Grasp the splint by its metal lingual bar. Place the splint in the mouth, and instruct the patient to remember not to bite into the doughy acrylic, but to merely give a "floating swallow", that is, to swallow as lightly as possible only by letting the lips seal, yet *without* clamping the teeth together. Distracting patients as they swallow by placing one's hand on their arm or shoulder with a word of encouragement also seems to help keep them from "clamping down" during swallowing. The splint is then removed and allowed to cure in warm water, and the depressions of the upper teeth are noted. It is felt that this method establishes the vertical dimension of occlusion on the splint at the nearest to physiological or ideal "rest" muscle length position for the closing musculature. After the splint is allowed to harden in hot water or a pressure pot to speed setting, it is retrieved, the indentations of the mesiolingual cusps of the upper first molars are marked with a lead pencil, and all other ridges and depressions of the newly added acrylic are ground flat and buffed smooth to that point. This allows the splint to be replaced, with the mesiolingual cusps of the upper first molars being the only teeth to contact. To balance each side of the splint—forward, right, and left—excursive movements are carried out while the patient occludes on thin articulating paper. All articulating paper markings on each side of the splint except those caused by the mesiolingual cusps of the upper first molars are removed. The splint is polished and replaced. As the patient closes and "slides around" on the splint while contacting only the mesiolingual cusps of the upper first molars in all protrusive and excursive movements, he will note that a "skating rink" effect is felt as all working, balancing, and protrusive interferences of the new acrylic occlusal table are eliminated.

Other dentists simply send upper and lower models of the dental arches to the lab, which in turn are mounted on a simple hinge articulator and opened to allow an approximate 2- to 3-mm covering of occlusal acrylic to be processed on the splint. Once returned, the clinician "articulates" and adjusts it in the mouth at its preexisting 2- to 3-mm vertical as in the "add-on" technique described above so that the same sliding "skating rink" effect is obtained. It is surprising how close both these methods come to each other in producing splints of similar occlusal thickness. Only in rare cases is the thickness of this type of splint critical. In such cases the 2- to 3-mm average thickness still does fairly well, and even then it is to serve a short diagnostic purpose of only several months anyway. Some patients are sensitive to variances in splint thickness of only fractions of a millimeter. However, these types of individuals are rare.

One type of sensitivity to splint thickness that is not rare, however, is muscle spasm that results from impingement on what has been referred to as "freeway space." The freeway space is the interocclusal distance between the occlusal surfaces of the back teeth when the patient's mandible is at rest. Hence it is also sometimes seen interchanged with that term and referred to as "resting" occlusion. It is commonly known that the insult represented by sudden changes in occlusion can cause muscle splinting and even myospasm. A splint that is thicker than the patient's own natural freeway space, which varies from individual to individual, is just such an acute insult. Some patients will complain of a "stiff mouth" or being unable to get their mouth open all the way, or maybe even hardly at all, due to sore and spastic muscles after wearing a new splint several days. This protective reaction is merely the body's effort to protect the elevator muscles of mastication from the equivalent of being physiologically "wrenched" during their working movements. The shock of too great an increase in the vertical dimension of occlusion effected too quickly by the insertion of the overly thick splint is more than the muscles can stand. They rebel. And when they do so, they do it in the way common to all forms of abuse-effected muscle rebellion, common muscle splinting or out-and-out myospasm. When this happens, splints are, of course, withdrawn. Temporary symptomatic relief is rendered, i.e., analgesics, muscle relaxants, vapocoolants, etc., and when things are under control once again, a splint of reduced thickness is used and usually "phased in" gradually over a week or so, being worn for progressively longer periods of time each day.

This brings us to another very important point concerning the longevity of splints. A splint such as the Sears pivotal type or others like it that do not provide full arch coverage should *not* be worn for longer than 6 months, for if worn longer than that, although it might not cause a depression of the posterior teeth as was formerly thought, it will definitely result in a supraeruption of the anterior teeth, thus deepening a bite anteriorly. This will only worsen the condition of the patient who is already suffering from a deficient mandible and inadequate vertical dimension because it increases the chances for occurrence of the NRDM-SPDC phenomenon.

Patients wearing such a splint as the Sears pivotal are checked every

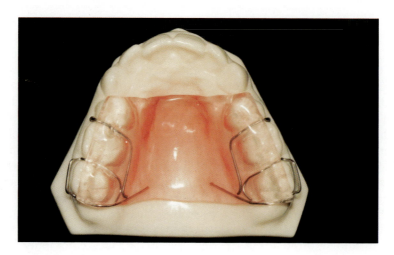

Figure 5-5   Witzig splint for the maxillary arch. (Courtesy of the Ohlendorf Co, St Louis.)

2 to 4 weeks, at which time the splint is rebalanced if need be and progress noted. If the vertical dimension is sufficient and myostatic contracture of the Class II neuromuscular sling is not too great so as to hold the mandible (and condyle) too far back in rest position, symptoms usually quickly subside.

Similar concepts are used for the fabrication of full-arch coverage, flat-plane occlusal splints for the maxillary arch. The advantage of the maxillary splint is that due to its coverage of the entire maxillary denture, the problem of the shifting of teeth, such as the bite deepening seen with long-term wear of a lower splint that covers only the lower posterior quadrants, is eliminated. The effects of palliative relief of myofascial discomforts (and even joint imbalances if the splint is constructed properly) are equally as dramatic with the use of upper splints as those seen with lower splints. Regardless of the direction, as long as the teeth hit on balanced, flat-plane acrylic, the circuit is broken, and relief is usually near at hand.

The Witzig Splint

Another splint that is easy to use and construct is the Witzig splint. It is nothing more than a transverse appliance without the midline expansion screws. The splint is similar to a full palatal Hawley-type retainer with Adams clasps on the molars, ball clasps between the bicuspids, and, of course, the important thing, 2 to 3 mm of acrylic covering the occlusal surfaces of all the posterior teeth. The acrylic occlusal "pads" of this device are made flat and smooth and are reasonably balanced over the posteriors in a manner similar to all upper splints. However, there is one important difference in the design and use of this splint, and it is a difference that reflects the complete opposite philosophy that governs other types of full upper splints. In the case of the Witzig splint, the acrylic is kept out of contact in the incisor area. The lower incisors never contact the acrylic of the anterior part of the appliance in either centric or excursive-type movements. Depending on the type of overbite and overjet present, the anterior teeth may contact one another at the outer ranges of border movements of straight protrusion and lateral excursion. This lack of lower incisor contact with the splint allows the appliance to be very thin in the anterior portion over the rugal area and as a result greatly facilitates speech and increases wearing comfort for the patient. One may easily see how this splinting approach is different from that of other types. In other types of upper splints that are products of a different philosophical approach, the acrylic in the anterior area serves as a ramp against which lower incisors occlude. In excursive movements of the mandible, this ramp of acrylic serves to disclude the lower posteriors from contact with the splint as the lower anteriors glide over the acrylic up front. In the process the joint is supposedly protected from occlusal shocks of an untoward variety. In the case of the Witzig splint, the anteriors are discluded by the acrylic over the posterior teeth in most all centric and excursive movements of the mandible. This definitely protects the joint because it prohibits initiation of the NRDM/SPDC phenomenon since the posterior acrylic of the splint prevents the anterior teeth from coming into contact. Being that the occlusal pads of the acrylic of the splint have an essentially flat plane, the mandible is free to "spring forward" if it wants to in a natural effort to seek its own AP level. This also allows for joint decompression and much-sought-after relief of TMJ-type headache pain. Obviously, an extreme case of a Class II, Division 2, very deep bite malocclusion precludes the effectiveness of this or any type of splint the posterior acrylic pads cannot open the vertical enough to allow the lower incisors to clear the upper anterior teeth.

The splint is used in the conventional manner similar to most temporary acrylic splints, i.e., only for a period of 3 to 4 months, but unlike the Transverse and Sagittal series of appliances, it is removed for eating. It is easily constructed from a set of models and a simple construction bite of 2-mm thickness.

The seeming "therapeutic nirvana" represented by the flat plane occlusal splint is not without its fair share of serious problems, however. Although these types of splints provide great relief for a goodly number of patients suffering from functionally induced TMJ problems, there are still a certain percentage of patients for whom they provide no relief at all. This may be due to a phenomenon that has been referred to as "horizontal posterior attachment pinching." Basically what happens under just the right (or actually wrong) set of circumstances is that a flat plane splint unlocks the occlusion, so that the mandible can slide forward. In certain relatively less frequently occurring combinations of splint thickness and a given patient's own joint anatomy, and level of degeneration, the splint could in effect not only offer no relief of symptoms, but paradoxically on rare occasion even seem to worsen them. Forgetting momentarily about minor muscle splinting problems (which are only temporary due to a sudden excessive change in the vertical dimension of occlusion effected by the splint), in patients with chronic anteromedial displacement of the disc, the disc is permanently deranged in a manner down and forward over the front of the condylar head. This can stretch the posterior attachments over part of the front of the condylar head. With the occlusion unlocked by a flat plane splint, some patients can execute a slight protrusive movement (as in bruxism) that allows the originally posteriorly displaced condyle to move straight forward (albeit only a short distance as per the size and shape of the fossa) in purely a horizontal direction before the condyle "unloads" in the joint by sliding down the eminence. In doing so, this brief period of horizontal forward motion pinches the posterior attachments, which are stretched forward over the face of the condyle due in turn to the forward and medial displacement of the disc to which they are attached. This traumatizes these tissues between the condylar head and the eminence. Under such circumstances, the splint simply is not unloading the condyle properly. This is a product of the degree (or lack thereof) of the posterior vertical dimension of occlusion on the splint. Of course the reciprocal of this process is also known to be a problem.

Once the occlusion is unlocked by the flat surfaces of a splint, certain patients will not only "grit" their lower teeth horizontally forward, but they also are able to clench them horizontally backwards even farther than before. This rearward movement is facilitated ironically by the flat "occlusion-eliminating" surfaces of the splint that was itself originally intended to prevent rearward condylar compression. This needless to say further traumatizes sensitive posterior joint space tissue making a bad situation even worse.

What this means to the patient is a failure to find relief of their classic TMJ type symptoms. What this phenomenon means to treating clinicians is that for all their often wonderful results, flat plane splints cannot always be relied upon to properly unload the condyle in certain of the more advanced functionally induced compressive derangement situations. The generic splint constructed from "bite" registrations produced by either patient volition or the "golden hands" of skilled operators and their noble attempts to manually "romance" the mandible to what is thought to be the correct physiologic location, simply cannot always be relied upon to do the job. "Almost always" is indeed very handy for clinicians but not for those patients suffering from functionally induced joint compression problems for whom conventional splint therapy will not work. What is truly needed for them is a consistently lenitive technique of splint construction that takes the guess work out of splint therapy and utilizes exact and scientifically verifiable methods that can place the operator in full control of final splint-determined condylar position. The clinician must be able to govern both horizontal and vertical condylar location within the confines of the glenoid fossa. What is needed is a superior splint construction technique. Fortunately, in the most timely and scientifically dramatic fashion, just such a technique has been evolved and has proven over time to be the long sought after solution to the splint construction debate, and it comes to us from the unobtrusive place of Erie, Pennsylvania.

> *"The reasonable man adapts himself
> to the world: the unreasonable one
> persists in trying to adapt the world
> to himself. Therefore, all progress
> depends on the unreasonable man."*
>
> *"Maxims for Revolutionists"*
> *George Bernard Shaw, 1856–1950*

Levandoski's Mandibular Stabilization Prosthesis: The Super Splint

The problem with all forms of splint technique is that although all varieties provide an interruption of the mandibular arc of final closure and most will prevent the condyle from going all the way back to the original starting point of full retrusion, thus effecting some modicum of relief, none is capable of positioning the condyle to an exact *predetermined* ideal location in the joint. Sometimes a certain type of splint could, in fact, reposition the condyle further down and forward in the fossa, but just *where* in that fossa the splint positioned it was still a guess. It has also been shown that many splints, although they may open the vertical, do not reposition the condyle AP within the joint at all.

All the elements were there, like pieces on a chessboard, but the right combination of moves had not yet been devised to result in a checkmate of the splint/condylar position problem. But then there transpired an event that seems to come along only once in a century. The technique of splint usage was showing the "TMJ discipline" that intraoral orthodontic mandibular repositioning devices could dramatically relieve TMJ-type pain symptoms. FJO was showing that in both children and adults mandibles could be developed down and forward to make better faces and better joints. Transcranial radiography was showing both disciplines just where the condyle was in the fossa and hinted at just where it should be. These elements were then gathered together by an individual who, with an injection of his own creative thought that may be described as nothing less than a stroke of pure genius, completely revolutionized not only the discipline of splint construction but also the equally expansive and time-honored methodology of mechanical articulator design and usage. The field of prosthodontics must now forever view its therapeutics from an entirely new TMJ-oriented frame of reference. The individual who is singularly responsible for the change in this view is the brilliant young prosthodontist Dr. Ronald Levandoski of Erie, Pennyslvania, and the appliance (for it cannot actually be considered just a splint) he developed that can position the condyle exactly as per the needs of that joint and the practitioner's clinical judgment he refers to as a "mandibular stabilization prosthesis." Others have nicknamed it the "super splint."

A graduate of the University of Pittsburgh, Levandoski served a 3-year residency in prosthodontics at the nearby Veterans Administration (VA) hospital. At the direction of his kindly and forward-looking superior, Dr. Paul Ruskin, who at that time was the chief of staff of the dental department of the hospital, Levandoski did a review of the literature on the subject of mechanical articulators. It was during this research that Levandoski came upon the works of the Swedish dentist Dr. Carl Christensen. A contemporary of men like G.B. Snow and W.G.A. Bonwill, Christensen published a critical yet almost totally forgotten paper in 1901.[13] It resulted in the definition of what has since been referred to as the "Christensen phenomenon." It was this phenomenon that served as the conceptual basis upon which Levandoski built his revolutionary ideas. The observations Christensen and others made at the turn of the century were of the most basic and elemental nature.[14-19] Yet their significance is far reaching in light of what we know about TMJ function and dysfunction.

The Christensen phenomenon may be explained in the following example. Let us construct the situation of an occlusion with a flat occlusal plane that happens to have a deep overbite and slightly retruded mandible at full occlusion. The angulation of the long axes of the anterior teeth would also be similar to that of a common Class II, Division 1–type malocclusion. Let us also assume just for the sake of our discussion here that at full occlusion our sample occlusal plane is perfectly horizontal. Now as the mandible is protruded while keeping the teeth in contact, the lower incisors start advancing down the lingual slopes of the upper anteriors. The condyle is also translating down the articular eminence of the temporal bone. What happens to the occlusion of the teeth, however, is where our interest lies. As the mandible advances, the posteriors are discluded, and an interocclusal space starts opening up between them. Yet the anterior teeth are still in contact. If the example is extended to protruding the mandible to an end-to-end anterior incisor relationship, even though the anteriors are still occluding, a posterior open bite of 3 to 4 mm has opened posteriorly between the occlusal surfaces of the molars. Thus when the mandible advances, the posterior vertical dimension *of occlusion* increases faster than the anterior vertical dimension of occlusion. This is due to the angle of the slope of the articular eminence with respect to the horizontal. The steeper the angle of the slope of the eminence, the greater this effect will be. To even intensify this effect, if the angle of the slope of the eminence with respect to the horizontal is steeper than the angulation of the path of the mandibular incisors across the lingual surfaces of the upper incisors, the occlusal plane of the mandibular arch will actually be canted downward slightly at the posterior, thus making it no longer parallel to the horizontal as in the full-occlusion starting point position of our example. Figuratively, this creates a wedge-shaped arrangement of interocclusal open space with the apex of the wedge at the anterior incisors.

However, Levandoski realized that the occurrence of this phenomenon in Nature's "human articulators" was the exact opposite of what was occurring in the basically hinge-type man-made articulators of the dental profession. In these artificial devices, the figurative wedge of interocclusal open space faced the opposite way, with its apex at the hinge. What makes this difference clear is our present knowledge that the opening movement of the mandible involves condylar translation from almost the very start.

Therefore, Levandoski endeavored to create an articulator that would be capable of allowing adjustments to be made that would match prescribed condylar changes and as a result correct for deficiencies in the *posterior* as well as anterior vertical dimension of occlusion. But in order to do this he would need a method of converting the pretreatment condylar position and the prescribed corrected condylar position into mechanical adjustments that such an appropriately designed articulator could accept. The articulator Levandoski designed to accomplish this is the first of its kind (now commercially available under the brand name of Logic Articulator), and the method he uses to transfer information from the pretreatment transcranial radiograph or tomogram to that articulator he refers to as the Levandoski "vector coordinate analysis." The beauty of this entire technique is that not only does it permit construction of intraoral devices that position the condyle exactly to a prescribed location but it is also a technique that can be easily incorporated into daily clinical practice with a minimum of investment of time and capital. It is a technique that finally gives the TMJ clinician the ability to completely control condylar positioning at will and is at the same time the essence of simplicity. Needless to say, it is a method that has caught both the prosthetic discipline and the TMJ discipline completely off guard.

Either transcranial radiographs or tomograms of the pretreatment joint may be used in this technique. The radiographs should be produced with the patient's Frankfort horizontal plane parallel to the floor. The transcranial head holder (cephalostat) should also be level. This is quickly verifiable by mounting a small bubble gauge (obtainable at any hardware store) on the top of the film cassette holder of the transcranial head holder. Properly standardized procedures as these allow for not only better image production but also the superimposition of serial radiographs of the same case.

Once the image is obtained, the radiograph is covered with tracing paper taped to the edge of the film similar to common cephalometric tracing technique. The outline of the fossa and condylar head and neck of the view of the fully closed position is traced onto the paper. Also a tracing is made of the top and side of that view to act as reference planes. A small reference hole is punctured by means of the sharp point of a compass or similar sharp object in the vicinity of the C-point (Bimler) in the center of the outline of the condyle. This first tracing is then set aside. Next, a second tracing is drawn of the condyle only. Care is taken to include the same C-point (Bimler) location on the second tracing of the condyle as the first. This is easily done by placing the mark right over the pinpoint hole in the actual film made during the production of the first tracing.

Now this second tracing, which is of the condyle only, is placed over the first tracing, which consists of both the condyle and the fossa. The C-point (Bimler) marks, and the condylar outlines of both tracings should coincide. The top tracing (condyle only) is then manually moved around over the bottom one until the condyle of the top tracing is properly positioned against the outline of the fossa of the bottom tracing. This will result in an image of the outline of the fossa (bottom tracing), and within the confines of that outline will appear the current pretreatment outline of the condyle (bottom tracing) and a second condylar tracing a bit inferiorly and anteriorly displaced from it (top tracing) that represents the proposed position of the condyle relative to that fossa at the end of treatment. That proposed position will be something very similar to the previously described Gelb 4/7 position. The two tracings are then secured by tape or staples before proceeding to the next step.

It will now be noted that two C-point (Bimler) reference dots also appear. One will be slightly inferior and anterior to the other. They may be connected by a small straight line. This line shows the direction of the relocation of the center of the condyle from pretreatment to proposed posttreatment locations. As with any line drawn on a two-dimensional, flat surface, its direction and magnitude may be described as the net result of the x and y components of the same plane. A reference line is

---

Figure 5–6 **(A)** Dr. Levandoski. **(B)** Levandoski Logic I articulator.

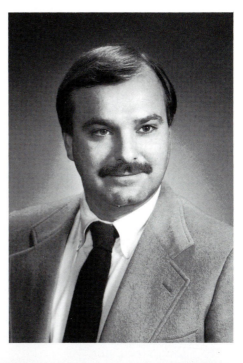

Figure 5–6(A)

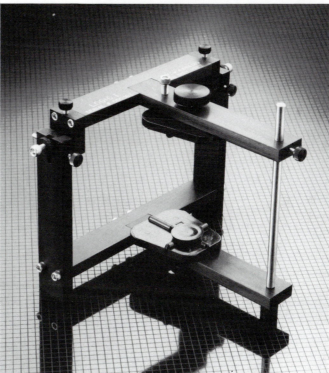

(B)

drawn vertically from the pretreatment or more superior and posterior of the two reference points. It is drawn parallel to the side edge of the film (which should be the same as the vertical reference line originally drawn at the edge of that view). The same is done for the horizontal component of the second reference point, or proposed position, and that line is made parallel to the top or bottom edge of the film (which should be the same as the horizontal reference line originally drawn across the top of that view). The vertical line then represents the y vector, and the horizontal line represents the x vector of the net movement of the condyle from actual to desired positions. These x and y vector components are, of course, perpendicular to each other and form the base and vertical side of a triangle. The hypotenuse of that vector triangle represents the actual net vector movement of the center of the condyle and is represented on the tracings as a direct line connecting the two C point (Bimler) reference points. It is the x and y vector components, however, that we are interested in. They represent the amount of vertical and horizontal components of the overall displacement of the two condylar reference points. This usually gives values of 1 to 3 mm each. The entire procedure is performed for both condyles. The linear measurements of these x and y vectors are what serve to transfer the information these tracings represent to the Levandoski articulator.

Before *every* usage the Levandoski's Logic I articulator must be "zeroed," i.e., adjusted to a static, neutral position. Adjustments are always

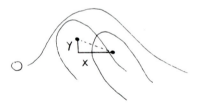

Verification with a Compound Bite Record.

Figure 5–7 Levandoski vector analysis. First, trace the transcranial projection of the condyle and fossa of a TMJ in the fully interdigitated position. Second, trace another transcranial projection (to be superimposed over the first) of the condyle only of same joint. Both tracings, with condyles exactly superimposed, are registered by arbitrarily placing the compass point through C point (Bimler) in the center of the condylar head. Then, the second, top tracing is moved to the ideal location (Gelb 4/7 position) against the background tracing of the fossa and articular eminence. The x and y components of the move from C to C' are then measured in millimeters.

Figure 5–8 **(A)** X, y, z hinge of the Levandoski articulator; **(B)** dial caliper; **(C)** mounting rings.

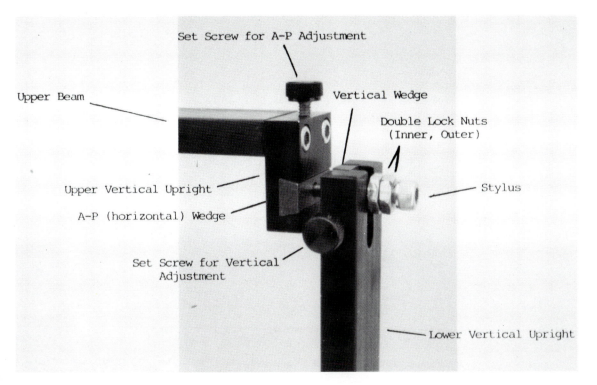

Set Screw for A-P Adjustment

Upper Beam

Vertical Wedge

Double Lock Nuts
(Inner, Outer)

Upper Vertical Upright

Stylus

A-P (horizontal) Wedge

Set Screw for Vertical
Adjustment

Lower Vertical Upright

Figure 5–8(A)

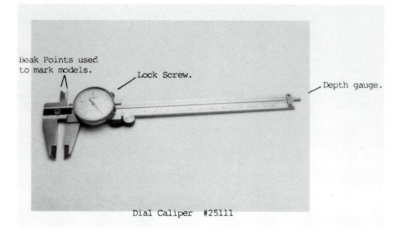

(B)

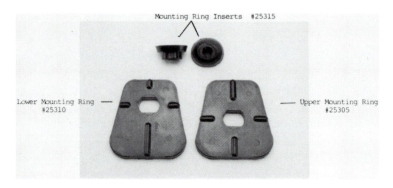

(C)

made from this neutral starting position. This not only places the hinges in a neutral starting position but also makes sure that the upper and lower beams of the articulator are parallel, as are the reference lines on the respective radiographic views at the joint.

To zero the Logic I articulator, the following steps are undertaken:

1. Check that the vertical uprights are 90 degrees to the lower beam and that the hex-head screws at the bottom of the lower vertical uprights are "squeaky" tight. Once this is done, it needs be rechecked only occasionally.

2. Slightly loosen the double-lock nuts on each stylus.

3. Zero each vertical wedge flush (by touch) across the *top* of each lower vertical upright.

4. Zero each AP wedge flush (by touch) with the *front* of each upper vertical upright.

5. Zero the z (transverse) axis by measuring with the depth gauge end of the dial caliper. Loosen the transverse stylus double-lock nuts on both sides to make any z-axis adjustments. Turn *both* stylus heads simultaneously (one clockwise, one counterclockwise) to adjust. Continue adjusting until the measurement is identical on both sides. Then tighten both *inner* lock nuts. Finally, tighten both *outer* lock nuts.

6. Set the upper and lower beams parallel. Use the dial caliper to measure the vertical distance between the upper and lower beams in the posterior part of the articulator. Lock that setting on the dial caliper. Then loosen the set screw for the incisal rod and adjust the distance between the upper and lower anterior portions of the beams to match the setting at which the dial caliper has been locked.

7. Scribe a line onto the incisal rod where it enters the upper anterior member. Thereafter, when zeroing the articulator, this scored mark is your reference.

Now the articulator is ready to receive the upper and lower models of the case and the all-important adjustments from the transcranial (or tomographic) vector analysis. The vector analysis provides vertical (y component) and horizontal (x component) adjustments for the three-way hinges of Levandoski's Logic I articulator. The transverse adjustments (z component) are obtained from analysis of the submental vertex radiographic view. However, unless gross asymmetries are present here, this component is usually not in need of correction. Measurements of the x and y vectors are made directly from the tracing with the dial gauge.

The Logic I articulator is adjusted for the x and y vectors as follows. The upper model should be mounted with a Levandoski custom-designed facebow. (For further details on use of this facebow see the next chapter.) The lower model is mounted in the same position in which the TMJ radiographs were taken, usually with teeth in full occlusion, without a wax record.

The incisal guide rod is opened temporarily to clear the anterior teeth since the relationship of the upper and lower models with respect to each other will change not only vertically but also *horizontally* as adjustments are made to the articulator as per the dictates of the vector analysis. Without clearing the occlusion temporarily by opening the guide pin, the anterior teeth might break off during horizontal movement of the models. Typically, 4 mm or so will do. Corrective adjustments are then made to the patient's right side. Adjustments are made for the y vector measurement on the articulator's right vertical wedge. Slightly loosen the double-lock nuts and setscrews so that the wedge will slide. Open the dial caliper the length of the y (vertical) vector on the Levandoski transcranial vector analysis of the TMJ film tracing. Lock in this setting on the dial caliper. Use the depth gauge end of the dial caliper (which automatically extends the equal measured distances) to adjust and set the vertical wedge. Gently tighten the double-lock nuts and setscrew. The y vector (vertical) correction has now been made for that one side (joint).

Next, follow the same steps for transferring the patient's right-side x axis (AP) measurements from the TMJ vector analysis to the articulator. (Consider the stylus to be the condyle.) After both the x vector and the y vector patient's right-side adjustments have been completed, *only then,* by using the same procedure as above, make appropriate adjustments to the patient's left side.

As mentioned previously, when necessary the z (transverse) vector can also be adjusted on this articulator. The measurements for this adjustment generally come from evaluating a submental vertex or posteroanterior (PA) cephalogram. The double-lock nuts must be loosened and both stylus heads turned simultaneously (one clockwise, one counterclockwise) to adjust.

Once the corrections for the x, y, and, if necessary, z axes or vectors have been made, return the incisal guide rod to the "zero" position. The correction for deficiencies in the *posterior* vertical dimension of occlusion has now been made.

And because the three-way hinges of the articulator move the upper base of the articulator in a compensating (opposite) fashion to the lower as per the dictates of the measurements of the vector analysis, the AP corrections have also now been made. The horizontal corrections are programmed into the hinges such that the upper base (and hence the model mounted to it) is moved backward (posteriorly), which is the mathematical equivalent of moving the lower base and model forward. Thus when

---

Figure 5–9 **(A)** Zero the z axis. **(B)** Measure the vertical distance between the posterior beams and lock that setting. **(C)** Match the anterior setting with the posterior.

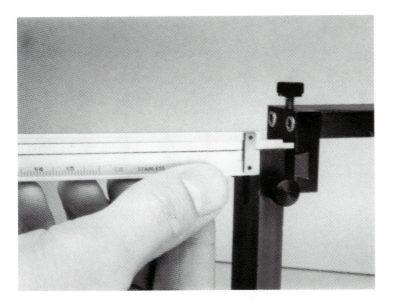

Figure 5–9(A)

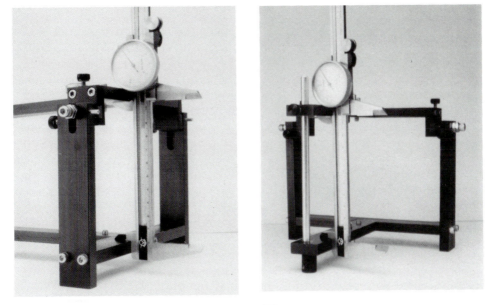

(B)   **(C)**

the x and y vector corrections are made and the anterior incisal guide rod is reset to the original starting position, the models of the upper and lower dental arches will now be juxtaposed in such a fashion as would be the real dental arches in the mouth if the patient's mandible were to be advanced in such a way that the condyles of the real mandible would move the corresponding amount represented by the x and y measurements of the vector analysis. The mounted models will now reveal a posterior open-bite equivalent to the actual posterior open bite exhibited in the mouth were the patient to advance his mandible to an ideal, near incisal, end-to-end or "as if" position. But further refinements may yet be made. The amount of anterior vertical opening desired (and some modicum is almost invariably needed, usually in the 2–4 mm range) can be determined by checking vertical face height cephalometric measurements. Assume for the sake of this example that a 3.0-mm increase is desired. To adjust for proper anterior vertical, open the dial caliper to 50 mm and lock in this setting. Place the beaks of the dial caliper against the bases of the upper and lower models and mark their points of contact on the plaster. Loosen the setscrew for the incisal rod. Open the dial caliper the desired amount (3.0 mm). With one beak point in the lower model reference mark, raise the upper anterior member of the articulator until the upper model reference mark reaches the other beak point at the new, more open setting. Finger tighten the incisal rod setscrew.

With the posterior vertical dimension of occlusion corrected and now the anterior vertical dimension of occlusion corrected, the articulator holds the dental arches in a position they would occupy if the mandible of the patient were in the orthopedically correct location at full occlusion as per the dictates of the disc-condyle-fossa relationships of the joint and the cephalometric requirements of cephalometrically balanced anterior and posterior vertical face heights. Of course, in such orthopedically balanced jaw-to-jaw alignment, it will be observed that the teeth now do not align. That is the purpose of treatment, i.e., to "fill in the gaps one way or another." The *"way"* we are concerned with here is with what will ultimately turn out to be Levandoski's mandibular stabilizaton prosthesis.

First we start with compound. Common brown denture compound is used to make a bite record *first on the mounted models* of the patient's jaws after all the articulator adjustments (corrections of jaw position) have been made. The compound is warmed in a water bath in the usual fashion, shaped into a horseshoe-shaped affair, and placed on the lower model. The patient's upper mounted model is then closed down into the soft compound. After cooling, this compound record is then transferred to the mouth, and a second transcranial or tomographic film is made to verify that the adjusted positions of the condyles produced by this bite record are in fact appropriate. If not, the articulator may be further adjusted in the appropriate manner, and the procedure for producing the compound bite record may be repeated until films verify that the record is putting the condyles in the desired place.

The mounted models with their mounting plates are sent to a full-service dental laboratory along with the compound bite record. An acrylic splint is then processed that duplicates the action of the compound bite record. The splint is constructed so as to snap into place on the mandibular dental arch, and it retains the detailed anatomical indentations of the upper teeth on its upper occlusal surface so as to lock the mandible upon closing into the desired position. The walls of acrylic adjacent to the buccal and lingual surfaces of the posterior teeth are left long enough to ensure that no lateral or excursive shifts of the mandible are possible when the patient bites into the splint because these types of movements are universally hard on joints that have been damaged due to functionally induced TMJ problems. Thus biting into the splint locks the occlusion vertically, horizontally, and laterally. It also locks both the mandible and the mandibular condyles in a calculated, predetermined correct position in the fossae.

The patient wears the splint 24 hours a day and especially when eating. This represents a great deal of difficulty for patients the first few days of splint wear until they become accustomed to it. They are also instructed to be careful not to close their mouths all the way shut when the splint is out for brushing. The purpose of this type of prosthesis is to allow the damaged joint structures to "heal" by virtue of never allowing the condyle to assume its fully retruded superior posterior displaced pretreatment position. Even lateral excursive movements are eliminated by this appliance. It is the closest thing to actually having the joint in a cast. This is why relief of symptoms is also so dramatic. Educated guesswork has finally been replaced by exact science, and the joints can tell!

Levandoski uses this mandibular stabilization prosthesis for a period of about 6 months prior to completing the case. Finishing may take the form of cast restorations of the fixed and/or removable type. If so, the construction bite will be taken in this corrected mandibular position, and the purpose of the prosthetics then is to merely "fill in the gaps." The 6-month period of splint wear acts to not only help the intracapsular tissues to repair but also importantly seems to retrain the musculature similar to Bionator wear so that the mandible has in effect been muscularly repositioned prior to finishing, thus making this corrected mandibular relationship all the easier to register in the construction-bite phase of treatment. Often it is best to construct a removable-cast, overlay-type prosthesis for these patients to use for several years prior to electing to go to the irreversible techniques of crown and bridge restorations. This ensures that the patient will be asymptomatic and that the patient's freeway space is not being unduly impinged upon.

Of course, if the patient is to receive orthodontic correction, the use of the mandibular stabilization prosthesis may be obviated in lieu of one of the active plate arch preparation appliances of the FJO-oriented treatment plan. But where a splint is needed, there can be no doubt that the Levandoski prosthesis represents a step up from generic splints and for the first time allows the clinician to truly treat the joint in a precisely prescribed manner that ensures correct orthopedic condylar corrective repositioning. And, of course, that repositioning will invariably be found to be down and forward.

The main thing in all this that should be remembered is that be they upper or lower, fancy or plain, occlusion capturing or flat plane, meticulously fabricated or "thrown in from across the room," *any splint will work* as long as it sufficiently unloads the condyles and interrupts the mandibular arc of final closure with a surface of acrylic that stops noxious stimuli from reaching the muscles and joints. This can always be accomplished by the indentations of the acrylic of a Levandoski appliance sharply "grabbing" the occlusal table and forcing the mandible and, as a result, its condyle to an exact and correct predetermined position, or if the case is still simple enough, it can be accomplished by a simple flat-plane surface providing an occlusal "skating rink" that allows the mandible to slide to a decompressed position of its choice, optimally at an acceptable splint-determined vertical. There is no "magic" in the acrylic. The results come from somehow properly positioning the condyle within the confines of the joint. Symptoms will often subside dramatically in the first month of wear. However, some patients will be seen to greatly improve in a matter of weeks or even days. This is a sure sign of how desperately the patient needs the help.

Figure 5–10 Super splint, Levandoski mandibular stabilization prosthesis. **(A)** Lateral view showing high buccal and lingual walls of acrylic and a built-in cuspid rise (black arrow). **(B)** Occlusal view. Note the deep occlusal indentations of the upper teeth. (Courtesy of Dr. T.J. Spahl, St. Paul, Minn.)

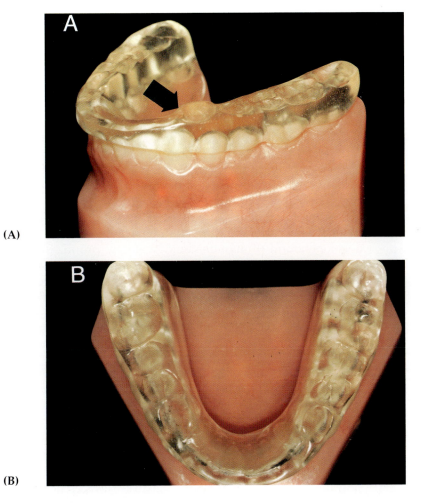

(A)

(B)

"All men are liable to error
and most men are, in many points,
by passion or interest,
under temptation of it."

Essay on Human Understanding xx, 17.
John Locke, 1632–1704

The Occlusal Splint as a Therapeutic Trap

As a result of the dramatic relief effected by the use of intraoral removable acrylic splints for patients with myofascial and TMJ pains and
dysfunction, these little devices have been the "darling" of the TMJ world
for several decades. Entire careers have been devoted to the perfection
and propagation of their use. Numerous varieties have evolved as a result, and the involved treatment modalities of their design and usage
have been brought to extremely high levels of sophistication. As far as the
palliative relief of intense and chronic TMJ pain-dysfunction problems
was concerned, splint usage was a tremendous boon to the awesome task
of treating the millions of patients who suffered so much from these conditions. Their arrival on the scene was an important event of which their
developers and promoters could be justly proud. But it was a dark victory. For although there were those patients who could benefit from a
program of preliminary splint therapy followed by occlusal balancing via
the rehabilitation route to a reasonably permanent level of myofascial harmony, stability, and comfort for their stomatognathic systems, there were
far too many who could not. There were always those who suffered from
more than just a simple occlusal imbalance. There were those who suffered from a greatly reduced vertical dimension of occlusion for which no
amount of equilibration could compensate. There were those whose
structural status placed their mandibles so far back in both rest and function that no amount of mere mechanical occlusal alteration could advance
the mandible/condyle unit enough to bring the condyle down forward
again out of the bilaminar zone and back onto the center of the disc.
There were those whose musculature was so overwrought from years of
holding the mandible too far posteriorly during fully interdigitated occlusion that a slight change in the occlusal surfaces of opposing teeth could
never retrain these muscles enough to allow the joint to permanently
rearticulate itself condyle to disc once again. There were those whose upper anterior incisors were either so retroclined or bodily placed so far posteriorly or whose lower anteriors were crowded so far anteriorly that the
mandible was permanently locked in its posterior position during full occlusion with a resultant NRDM-SPDC phenomenon in full force.

For these patients, equilibration in the long run worsened the situation. Splint therapy and other stress relieving procedures helped lessen

only somewhat the shock load and vectors of force that would have to be absorbed by a joint with a condylar head riding off the disc up in the bilaminar zone. For these patients and their frustrated clinicians, long-term permanent elimination of clicking, myofascial pain, and other joint symptoms remained elusive. For these types of patients often the only way to obtain full relief of such problems was to continue to wear their splint. The sure increase in vertical and the possible mandibular advancement that such properly designed splints provided helped decompress joints, relax muscles, and relieve discomfort but unfortunately did nothing to effect a permanent change in the factors responsible for the condition. For this particular type of patient, the splint represents a device that they become trapped into wearing as the only way to obtain palliative relief for their condition. For the particular clinician involved in treating this type of patient, splint usage per se represents a therapeutic dead end!

The reason lies in the nature of the patient's condition itself. These patients suffer from not only an altered occlusal relationship but also an altered muscular relationship and in addition, and surely most importantly, an altered skeletal relationship that displays its primary manifestation in the anatomical derangement of the articular structures internal to the joint. The occlusion and/or skeletal alignment forces the condyle partially or completely up and off the disc into the retrodiscal areas where it doesn't belong. This is a *major structural imbalance.* These are the patients who have "drifted over the line," who have crossed over that conceptual *"barrier of structural imbalance"* beyond which only treatments that effect major structural changes will succeed. We have now arrived at the domain of FJO. When condyles ride too far posteriorly, a TMJ problem always results, and to correct it, the condyle must be permanently brought down and forward again where it belongs. It's that simple.

The Tolerant Zone vs. the Intolerant Zone

To simplify the discussions of joint stability and correct anatomical intracapsular relationships, the following may prove useful. The condyle will ride and seat itself during function and full occlusal interdigitation in one of two basic areas. In a normal, healthy, structurally balanced joint, the condylar head rides at the center of the articular disc during the entire range of mandibular movements. At full occlusal interdigitation, the condyle is still cradled by the articular disc, albeit that stereoscopic position may not necessarily be at the most fully superior position on the bony dome above the tubercular eminence. It may be slightly forward or inferior on the tubercular slope. Nevertheless, the condyle-disc relationship is fully articulated and resides where it does as a result of the dictates of the occlusion. This broad area of anatomical acceptability might be referred to as the "tolerant zone" since the full shock absorber effect of the disc is in full effect and the posterior areas of the joint are not in the least way impinged upon.

However, in cases where the joint is structurally imbalanced, the condyle rides either partially or completely off the back end or heel of the disc during some or all of the functional movements of the mandible. Even if the condylar head rides only partially off the heel of the disc during full occlusion, it can cause irritation of the postcondylar tissues, and some degree of local inflammation can and often does occur. Whatever point in the stereoscopics of the condyle-disc-fossa relationship this process of impingement of the condylar head into the more posterior joint areas begins to take place might be referred to as the *"in*tolerant zone." This term intimates that forces of occlusion transmitted to the joint area by the condylar head are not totally absorbed by the disc but rather are partially or wholly absorbed by retrodiscal tissues that are not designed for this purpose. The localized traumatically induced posterior joint area inflammation caused by such a process can lead to increased synovial fluid in the superior and inferior joint spaces. Such inflammation can exert itself in the form of a biologically produced intracapsular hydraulic pressure, which resultantly increases pressure on the highly vascular and innervated retrodiscal tissues of the bilaminar zone. This is in addition to the mechanical trauma of direct condylar impingement.

Thus the main thrust of correction of the structurally imbalanced joint suffering from forced condylar intrusion past the heel of the disc may be seen to consist basically of permanently altering the structural circumstances such that the condylar head is taken out of the intolerant zone and brought back down into the tolerant zone once again where it will be made to permanently reside as per the dictates of what optimally would be the new occlusion and the readapted and/or retrained neuromuscular sling. Structurally imbalanced patients have their condyles riding, functioning, and sometimes even resting in the *in*tolerant zone, whatever and wherever within the confines of the joint space one may wish to consider it. Men may pompously argue over what they think is ideal in how the occlusion forcefully positions the condyle, but the only thing that is important is how Nature argues over how the occlusion positions the condyle.

Figure 5–11 The tolerant zone vs. the intolerant zone. **(A)** Right TMJ (lateral view) showing a double-sized fossa (atresia). Even though there is hardly any disc left, the patient functions well and has *no pain!* The reason is that the condyle does not seat on nerves and blood vessels of the bilaminar zone of the posterior joint space. It seats and operates forward. **(B)** Left TMJ in a similar condition in another patient. The joint functions without pain. (Courtesy of Dr. Arnold Berrett and Dr. Harold Gelb, New York City.)

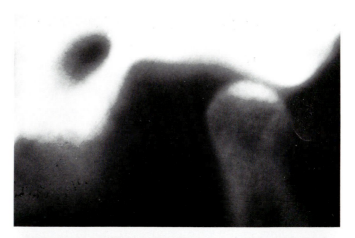

Figure 5–11(A)

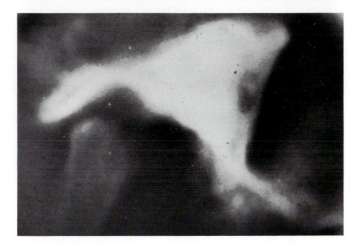

(B)

The one thing that these types of patients all have in common is that these structural imbalances must be corrected as a top priority before any other form of corrective therapy is undertaken. Ignoring these structural imbalances will only result in a compromised case or possibly even complete failure, regardless of how expertly other treatments ancillary to this basic concept are implemented. Patients must simply be taken out of this category of structural imbalance and therapeutically "moved back over the line" or "barrier" down into the category of structural balance once again. Once back out of the former, whatever additional measures that may be necessary to complete the case may be performed within the boundaries of the latter, with an extremely high percentage of success. When major structural imbalances exist, until they are directly addressed by techniques specifically designed to correct them, other techniques that were not originally designed to correct them can never be expected to result in total success. First things first. Get that condyle out of the bilaminar zone back onto the disc where it belongs! The orthodontics and/or prosthodontics in this approach is also then employed to make a newly created occlusion lock it there in function. It's a simple matter of first lining up the jaws right and then, if spaces exist between the teeth, merely filling in the gaps one way or another. But primarily, get the condyle out of the posterior part of the fossa.

The patients for whom FJO techniques are most effective are those who have lapsed fairly far over the conceptually defined barrier line from the category of structural balance into the category of obvious full-scale structural *im*balance. They may also have traditionally defined occlusal interferences and prematurities and may for a short time respond to preemptory attempts to eliminate them, but never permanently. This is simply due to the fact that the shock-absorbing effect of the joint has been either partially or completely lost due to the occlusion forcing the condyle up and back off the disc. Equilibrating away prematurities might help the muscles work more smoothly, but it cannot lessen the shock load that intense and ever-present function transmits to the posterior attachment area and bilaminar zone by a condylar head. For the classic functionally induced TMJ arthrosis patient, prematurities are not the real problem, but posterior condylar displacement is. These structurally compromised types of patients often routinely exhibit three major types of imbalances: severe loss of vertical, full Class II dental and skeletal mandibular retrusive relationships, and middle-to-late opening and closing clicks. Yet there are even exceptions to this rule. One thing is sure beyond a doubt. Their mandibles all overclose in a rearward fashion relative to the anatomical limits of the joint's tolerance. It makes no difference if the molars are Angle Class I or not. It makes no difference if the upper anteriors are torqued forward of cephalometric norms or not. When the sum total of all factors of bone position, size, and alignment, combined with whatever tooth angulations may be present, add up to force the condyle too far back at full occlusion, TMJ problems generally ensue. The joint works by feel in the dark. It can't look forward to see whether the occlusion has Class I molars or not. Thus, the removal of noxious stimuli such as occlusal interferences might possibly reduce symptoms temporarily, but the force vectors transmitted to the posterior areas of the joint via the head of the condyle will in time take their toll again. This is why the wearing of night guards to protect against the complicating problem of nocturnal bruxism also often meets with only temporary or incomplete success. Such measures only "pick up after" the symptoms of pain of structural imbalance that are accentuated by the bruxism but do nothing to directly attack and correct the cause. When viewed with an enlightened eye, the manifestations and even the causes in such structurally imbalanced patients are often glaring and overwhelmingly obvious: the history of headaches, neck aches, myofascial pains, clicking, the loss of vertical, retrusion of the mandible, and hence the superior and posterior displacement of the head of the condyle. This is not a list of signs and symptoms. It is a list of needs! And delineating a list of the patient's needs is tantamount to having the necessary treatment methods automatically spelled out for the clinician.

The most basic needs of the patient must be addressed first, followed only then by those of a less fundamental variety. When the most basic needs consist of advancing the mandible and increasing the vertical, those needs can and must be accomplished with the mandibular repositioning techniques of the FJO system. *Advancing the mandible* and *increasing the vertical* dimension with Bionator-type techniques places the patient in a position where the natural shock-absorbing effect of the joint is restored once again since, in time, the condyle is relocated down and forward in the glenoid fossa and is therefore often placed back on the disc. Once this is accomplished, it puts the working apparatus of the joint back into the rather wide-ranging "tolerant zone" once again where both the normal functional forces as well as those of minor occlusal interferences may be reasonably absorbed with impunity. It also puts the patient in a position where muscles are not being disharmoniously overcontracted or overworked at suboptimal conditions because the Class I proper vertical and orthopedic balance restored to the jaw relationships gives the muscles the chance to work at the proper lengths, in the proper directions, and to the proper levels of intensity for which the entire system was originally designed. These two factors alone, in the complete absence of any other form of corrective therapy, will go a very long way in reducing the TMJ symptoms that have chronically plagued the patient. Let us now take a closer look at just how these effects are implemented through the use of FJO techniques in the adult patient with TMJ pain-dysfunction.

Reversing the Order

The use of functional appliances and active plates in the treatment of structural imbalances in the adult patient with TMJ problems follows a somewhat slightly different course than that of their use in orthodontic treatment of the growing child or adolescent. The main difference is not in the clinical management of appliance technique but rather in the patient's age and biological response to its effects. Many patients with TMJ pain-dysfunction are biologically mature adults. And although many may still be late adolescents, an age during which interceptive TMJ therapy may be wisely instituted as a preventive and/or corrective measure during the growth years, a great portion of the body of patients with TMJ problems is unfortunately in the *fully matured adult category*, a time when any major growth potential at the condylar head and neck has long since been lost. But this does not preclude the use of the Bionator or Bionator-like appliances such as the Orthopedic Corrector I or III or the Biofinisher to treat such biologically mature individuals in order to correct vertical deficiencies or mandibular retrusion! We will now review how to use these functional appliances and their supporting cast of active plates and/or fixed appliances for TMJ treatment in the same order in which they were presented in the first part of this series of texts, starting with the discussion of the Bionator first, which is ironically the opposite order in which they are often used to treat the patient because the Bionator is almost always one of the last (and often *is the* last) of the appliances used in treatment sequences. The reason we shall discuss them in this therapeutically reverse chronological order is to stress the importance of setting the proper priorities on the most fundamentally important aspects of the FJO treatment philosophy. It also perchance is analogous to the reversed order of the actual process by which the patient's TMJ problems arose in the first place. The TMJ is by its very design highly adaptable to the various functioning condylar demands and is often the last anatomical component to surrender to the deforming influences brought on by the chronic disharmonious function of other components of the maxillofacial complex whose structural imbalance usually preceded its own. The individual arches are either collapsed or deformed in some manner first, followed necessarily by improper jaw-to-jaw alignment during function, which in turn is followed by adaptive muscular imbalances, myofascial pain, and joint disarticulation. The more innocuous and minor-appearing defects can easily accumulate to result in more profound problems on a far deeper biomechanical level. The function of malaligned and improperly formed jaws causes disarticulated joints. Disarticulated joints do not cause malaligned and improperly formed jaws!

The Bionator in Adult TMJ Treatment

In this review of the use of the Bionator/Orthopedic Corrector I (OCI) in the treatment of a hypothetical adult TMJ problem, we shall assume for the purposes of the discussion that both the upper and lower arches of our example patient are not in need of any major type of preliminary arch preparation but are already in reasonably good arch form. Clinically however, in most patients with TMJ problems this is seldom if ever the case. We will also assume that the structural imbalances that may exist are the following: a moderate to severe *loss in vertical* and a dental and *skeletal Class II relationship* between the upper and lower jaws (as a result of this mandibular retrusion there also will be accompanying *superior and posterior displaced condyles,* which are most often accompanied by an *opening and closing click*), and as our final qualification as mentioned before, the dentitions should already possess good arch form, thus obviating the need for arch preparation prior to Bionator insertion.

All the standard clinical and cephalometric criteria are applicable here for the verification of these conditions. Transcranial radiographs ensure that the condyles and fossa are of normal (or reasonably normal) anatomical shape, with the condylar head invading the posterior part of the fossa when the dentition is in the full intercuspation position. Ausculation of the joint with a common stethoscope confirms at least the presence of an opening and maybe even the closing click and the important absence of crepitus or "grating" noises during joint movement, which would lead one to suspect a torn, perforated, or otherwise damaged disc or ligament. If such is suspected, arthrography may be utilized if desired but is not necessary to obtain the information needed to initiate FJO treatment. Torn disc or not, the condyle still has to be brought down and forward in the fossa to eliminate compression of the posterior joint area. In our example case, we will simply assume that the disc is recapturable.

The Bionator (or Orthopedic Corrector most likely) is constructed in the usual manner* so as to address the needs of increasing the vertical, bringing the mandible forward, and decompressing and rearticulating the joint.[20] Thus the construction bite is registered in either the end-to-end or slightly past end-to-end incisal position at a 2- to 3-mm interincisal clearance. But the chronicity and severity of the mandibular retrusion may be such that full advancement of the mandible to the preferred end-to-end or slightly past end-to-end construction-bite mandibular position may be functionally impossible. Muscle soreness and/or trismus may be so intense that protrusion of the mandible to such an extent for any appreciable length of time is too painful for the patient. It may also be that at the

---

*For further information on the construction, usage, and adjustments of the Bionator and Orthopedic Corrector appliances refer to Chapter II of *Clinical Management of Basic Maxillofacial Orthopedic Appliances,* vol I, by Witzig and Spahl.

time of construction-bite registration, the patient seems to tolerate the degree of protrusion well only to show up several days after the insertion of the appliance with aching or even spastic muscles. This is a simple matter of too much too quick. In such an event the patient should stop wearing the appliance until the musculature is "normal" once again and then proceed to "break the appliance in" gradually over a period of 2 to 3 weeks so that the muscles have time to get used to all that stretch. This is where the use of the OCI comes into its full glory. If this appliance is to be used in such circumstances, the construction bite may be taken in as far forward a position of mandibular protrusion as the patient will seem to be able to comfortably tolerate. If there is reason for concern for the musculature, the mandible need not be protruded quite so far forward in taking the wax bite. A more conservative degree of advancement will do perfectly fine. Then the difference may be gradually eliminated as the appliance's side screws are opened and interproximal acrylic projection are removed to advance the lower cap, and mandible with it, in a manner confluent with proper OCI technique. The alternative is to simply use two (or more) consecutive Bionators. The first is constructed from a wax bite taken with the mandible as far forward as the patient may comfortably tolerate, and after a period of months, varying from individual case to individual case, a second Bionator is made from a wax bite in the fully advanced, normal construction-bite position since the now more relaxed and less painful condition of the musculature permits full mandibular advancement without patient discomfort. Analogously to using splints that impinge too much on the freeway space, when using Bionator/OCI-type appliances, you can't "yank 'em forward" too far, too quickly.

In the adult patient in reasonably sound periodontal health, the stimulation of the Bionator/OCI to increase the vertical will not only effect the "supraeruption" of teeth, albeit much more slowly in the posterior segments, as in the younger patient, but will also similarly stimulate an increase in the alveolar bone height along with it! This increase in alveolar bone height does not take place at an even par with the amount of eruption of the posterior teeth but rather straggles behind a little. Yet in time it may nevertheless still be observed.

But in the TMJ something a little different happens. We know from cephalometric studies that functional appliances like the Bionator stimulate (or at least facilitate) condylar growth in the growing child. But in the biologically adult patient, which we define in this case as courting the outer limits of about 25 years of age, this growth potential in the head of the condyle has nearly been lost. Yet, when some adult patients are cor-

---

Figure 5–12 (A) Orthopedic Corrector. **(B)** Side screws open to advance the cap, which results in greater protrusion of mandible when worn.

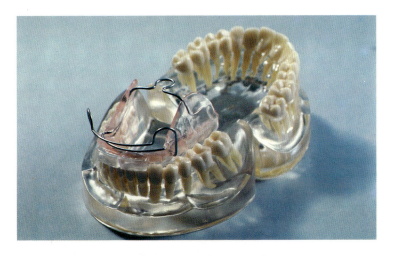

Figure 5–12(A)

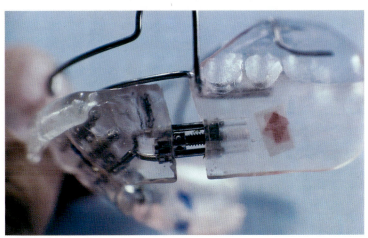

(B)

rectly treated for a sufficient period of time for compressed and posteriorly disarticulated joints, even if they have structurally deficient Class II mandibles, once the mandibular advancement, neuromuscular reprogramming, and increase in vertical dimension become complete, it is very difficult for even the most athletic of clinicians to force such repositioned mandibles back into an arc of closure similar to the path that was operative at the beginning of treatment. In those who do exhibit some retained tolerance for forcible retrusion of the mandible, it will be observed that the mandible still cannot be forced completely back all the way to its original pretreatment state of retrusion. If no condylar growth exists past the age of 25 years, what is responsible for this phenomenon? A number of major factors that can come into play to bring about this end result are (1) the newly acquired functional occlusion at its correspondingly new increased vertical dimension; (2) muscle length alteration, i.e., relengthening of what have become foreshortened muscles and conversely shortening of what have become overly stretched muscles; (3) new tissue formation, both hard tissue remodeling and soft-tissue proliferation; (4) temporal bone rotation and sutural decompression; and (5) other joint coalescence changes we do not yet fully understand.

The Bionator's ability to create a new occlusion   Prior to the insertion of the Bionator into a patient with a structurally imbalanced TMJ who is suffering from mandibular retrusion and SPDC, the muscles of mastication are usually overly strained. They try to adapt to this retrusive mandibular orthodontic/orthopedic relationship and as a result become programmed into the undesirable Class II neuromuscular reflexive arc of closure. This arrangement allows the head of the condyle to be forced posteriorly and superiorly into what we have referred to as the *"intolerant zone"* of the TMJ. But once the Bionator is inserted and *faithfully* worn, many changes begin to take place. First of course, comes the immediate decompression of the joint as the fit of the appliance in the mouth forces the entire jaw, condyle and all, down and forward, which in turn positions the condylar head desirably down and forward within the capsule of the joint. This action nearly always puts the condyle back on the disc (if in fact the disc actually is recapturable and reusable) since the disc by default has nowhere else to go to escape capture by the immediate action of appliance-induced capitular advancement. When such occurs, the disc can't be pushed any farther ahead due to the congestion of anatomy ahead of it. It can't be pushed medially because the petrous portion of the temporal bone and the mesiolateral portion of the eminential concavity of the tuberculum are highly uncooperative to mere cartilage challenging their osseous integrity. And it can't easily slip out laterally due to the tough and tenaciously dense cartilagenous fibers of the all-encompassing fibrous joint capsule. It stays in the only place it may, right smack between the opposing bony surfaces of the slope of the tuberculum and the now newly inferiorly repositioned and advanced capitulum of the condyle. But more importantly conceptually, this very favorable arrangement all takes place in the much more stable and satisfactory area of the joint that we have referred to in turn as the "tolerant zone." Functional stimuli, or stress if you will, are normal, healthy, and helpful to the maxillofacial complex as long as they are not indulged in excessively and *only* when the condyle-disc relationship abides in the tolerant zone with the condylar head cradled in the center of the disc. But these stimuli are *not* helpful when the disc-condyle relationship is put asunder with the head of the condyle up in the *in*tolerant zone and sliding off the posterior heel of the disc up into the bilaminar area. With the Bionator in place, the condyle-disc relationship in the tolerant zone, and the patient (and his facial muscles) unstressed and free of pain, the functional stimuli brought to the posterior teeth by the wearing of the appliance *slowly* brings about their vertical eruption, and the muscles definitely retrain to the newer, more satisfactory, and structurally balanced situation. Thus over the period of the treatment time of Bionator usage, it becomes increasingly easier and easier, as the teeth erupt and the muscles readapt, for the patient to "naturally" hold the mandible in the newer, more forward position.

Other considerations are that given the progressively increased period of time that the mandible is kept down and forward, muscles like the lateral pterygoid, which were formerly stretched due to excessive condylar retrusion on closing, no longer are forced to overstretch that far. Hence the phenomena common to all muscles that receive reduced amounts of stretch to full length takes place, and the muscle foreshortens a little due to myostatic contracture. Actually, this muscle-foreshortening only brings the lateral pterygoids back to what they would have been, had not the mandible become overly retruded in the first place. Nevertheless, it is one more factor theorized as being contributory to the resistance of the mandible to forcible retrusion to former pretreatment locations after a sufficient stint of Bionator advancement therapy.

Tissue proliferation also takes place within the joint after prolonged appliance wear. The articular portions and even the nonarticular portions of both the temporal bone and the condyle remodel to a certain degree. What is even more astounding is that recently it has been discovered that the entire temporal bone rotates down and forward en masse with attending decompression at the suture sites. This movement is not great; nevertheless, it is still present in some cases.

It must be remembered that the elongated ligaments damaged by excessive condylar displacement superiorly and posteriorly and compounded by anteromedial displacement of the disc never heal back 100% to their original ideal state. Healing of certain other forms of connective tissue damaged by condylar pressures does take place, however. It has been shown that capillary infiltration begins to occur into these damaged tissues, most of which are retrodiscal, as soon as 5 hours after the abuse of mechanical pressure from the condylar head stops. This is why patients may complain of increased pain at times in the earlier stages of the treatment plan when the Bionator/OCI is removed after a long period of

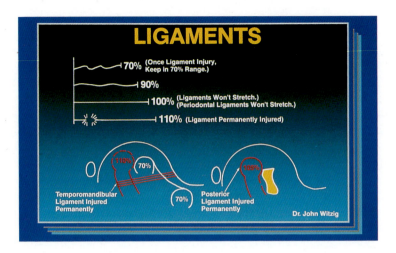

Figure 5–13 Elongated ligaments never heal back 100% to their original ideal state. Therefore in extremely severe TMJ cases the condyle should be finished well into the Gelb 4/7 position for safety, and extremes of functioning (wide opening, hard foodstuffs) and may have to be avoided in posttreatment use. (Courtesy of Dr. John Witzig.)

wear. There is also a type of coalescence of damaged and overstretched tissue that eventually takes place that is similar to what is observed in any other joint that is at first overstretched in some way and then reasonably immobilized to some degree for a period of time. This process, not totally understood, takes a while to manifest itself in the TMJ due to the fact that it is always moving. But given enough advancement of the condyle down and forward into the fossa daily over a long enough period of time during the treatment schedule, this process has the opportunity to contribute to the overall resistance of the joint to return of the condyle to its former pretreatment superior posterior state of displacement.

Changes occur also in vascularity, reorganization of connective tissue bundles, cellular proliferation, basement membrane structures, etc. But if the shrewd observer will carefully reflect on those clinical observations noted concerning the successfully treated adult patient with TMJ problems, he may instinctively perceive the faint whisper of reason in his ear suggesting that possibly the true core process involved in the reshaping of the TMJs during Bionator treatment designed and initiated to correct unacceptable mandibular retrusion is not in fact due to exceptionally sophisticated reconstructive healing or growth processes but ironically might well be due to an everyday and universally observed phenomenon that turns out to be as common as a shoe!

The human body is an amazingly elastic and adaptable organism. However, much of that adaptability is predicated on function, especially in the area of muscle, tendon, bone, and connective tissues. Take the well-known example of the young gymnasts of Olympic caliber. Due to repetitive stretching and exercising procedures, these athletes have their muscles and joints stretched and limbered to the point where they may easily contort their bodies in the most astounding manner. At the opposite extreme is the example of an individual with a broken limb. Once permanently set in a plaster cast, the immobility of the joints of the limb soon cause the tendons and connective tissues of such an immobilized joint to stiffen and atrophy to the point where after only several months of disuse the mobility of a joint so confined is seriously hampered and a great percentage of the full range of movement is lost until physical rehabilitation and physical therapy can be used to restore it to its normal range of movement once again. And should the cast remain in place for as little as 2 or 3 more months past this point, the joint will become so stiff and the tendons and connective tissue so rigid that attempts to force flexion of the joint would only result in out-and-out muscle and tendon tearing! After such long periods of disuse without proper reconditioning, the muscular and connective tissues would rather break than stretch!

Just exactly what goes on inside a TMJ that has been decompressed and rearticulated by means of Bionator therapy is not yet totally understood. But being that it is a joint made up of the same stuff as all other joints in the body, there is no reason to suspect it would not respond in the same way to similar circumstances. This is one of the many reasons faithful, daily compliance to the regimen of Bionator appliance wear is critical for the adult patient with TMJ pain-dysfunction.

The TMJs originally start out perfectly normal and symptom free in the young developing and growing child. "TMJ syndrome" is not a birth defect; it is a defect that results from chronic dysfunction, chronic misuse. The gradual transition from a normally articulated, anatomically correct joint to that of a compressed, disarticulated joint with the condylar head up in the intolerant zone during resting and/or full occlusion is the result of constant "stretching" and distortion of that joint (in the form of compression) by the head of the condyle in a manner and direction for which it was not designed: up and back! This condylar-induced stretching, even though it occurs over relatively short distances, eventually causes the ligaments and connective tissues to distort to the point where there is finally enough posterior joint space around the now-nonrestricted head of the condyle so as to allow it to reside up in this superior retruded position without being restricted from the area by external and internal capsular ligamentous and connective tissues. These have *now become flaccid, compressed, or overly stretched* tendonous and connective tissue–type material. The perpetual "use" or, actually, "*abuse*" of this articular tissue, that is, the repeated distortion of it by the head of the condyle during occlusion, keeps the tissues in a state of being slightly but nevertheless chronically elongated in a distorted configuration. The inability of the patient or clinician to manually effect pretreatment retruded positions of the mandible after an adequate period of protracted Bionator treatment is due to many factors to be sure. And one of them might be termed, in the broadest sense of the word, as *healing*. Vague and nondescript, the term *healing* tells us of only the result, not the method. Although it is based on clinical observation and inductive reasoning, it nevertheless emerges as an allur- ing notion to embrace the idea that part of the "healing" of TMJs receiv- ing Bionator treatment just might be due to the mere natural reversal of this chronic process of the functional disarticulation of the joint and the distortion of the posterior portion of its capsule. Instead of allowing the occlusion to force the mandible and condyle up and back, once Bionator therapy is instituted, the appliance in effect does the exact opposite—it forces the mandible and condyle down and forward. If it does this daily over a great enough period of time, the circumstances for common mech- anisms of the coalescence of the joint structures in the damaged area, as well as other functionally induced remodeling changes, soon have the po- tential to manifest themselves. It must be remembered that, in spite of the fact that the Bionator is not worn 24 hours a day by the adult patient with TMJ pain-dysfunction and although for that certain period during the day when the appliance is out of the mouth the mandible can function in the retruded position and allow the condyle to ride in the intolerant zone once again, correspondingly over a period of months the *occlusion* is in turn *changing* and *increasing the vertical*. This in turn gradually limits the degree of intrusion possible for the condylar head posteriorly and restricts this intrusion more and more as the occlusion and retrained musculature gradually hold the mandible and therefore the condylar head further and further down and forward for steadily increasing lengths of time. The more time the condylar head stays out of the retrocondylar intolerant ar- eas, the more time these areas have to regain original contours and also to adapt (which means reshape through decreased functional elasticity) to the progressively newer stereoscopic intracapsular relationships. It is be- lieved by astute observers of Bionator treatment for TMJ problems that just such a process is a major component of the posttreatment changes observed clinically in the action of the joints. This is why upon the com- pletion of Bionator treatment to increase the vertical dimension and ad- vance an improperly retruded mandible in an adult patient with TMJ problems it is often observed that even the most august attempts at man- ually attempting to force the mandible to its former pretreatment retruded position fail due to staunch resistance *perceived in the joint area!* Since it is commonly known that in the fully mature adult bony growth at the condylar head and neck ceases and cannot be stimulated to *increase* appre- ciably, the only remaining alternative that could be responsible for such seemingly permanent mandibular advancement and repositioning is that the size of the former pretreatment postcondylar area of unrestricted pen- etration *decreases*. This decreased range of motion or, more correctly, in- trusion is no doubt at least in part due to the decreased resiliency of cap- sular connective tissues. Such loss of elasticity of articular ligamentous tis- sues due to chronic immobility (or maybe more correctly, lack of chronic intrusion) is commonly thought of on a clinical level as true atrophy. This articular atrophy is a naturally occurring phenomenon seen universally in *all* the joints of the body that receive a chronically reduced range of movement. It is also often referred to as the process of "disuse atrophy." There may be other, more exotic forms of true healing that also take place within TMJs of the type that have been treated for their superiorly posteriorly displaced condyles by Bionators as well.

If this joint internal coalescence is in fact one of the contributing factors in the process that restores the joint during Bionator treatment, how it would ideally lend itself to what is going on in the dental arches out in front of the joint may readily be seen. As the vertical dimension of occlusion slowly increases or as its increase is augmented with Biofinisher-type technique and muscles readapt and redirect themselves at proper functional lengths, the jaw has not only less of a reason but also less of a capacity for closing in its former manner, a manner that used to drive the head of the condyle superiorly and posteriorly within the joint. Also, as these processes gradually take place, the disc-condyle assembly spends progressively more and more time down and forward in the tolerant zone of the joint. The pretreatment positioning of the condyle in the intolerant zone may be regained for short periods during meals because the patient habitually functions in that retruded position until the vertical increases become great enough and the muscle readaptation becomes sufficient enough that an increasingly newer functional occlusion holds the mandible in a progressively less retruded position. Concomitantly, the steadily increasing vertical dimension posteriorly makes overclosure less and less possible, and muscle readaptation due to the prolonged functional appliance wear makes a voluntarily retruded mandibular arc of closure progressively more and more difficult for the patient to obtain. The whole process makes the gradual transition over the period of treatment in a coordinated and amazingly self-regulated manner. After a sufficient period of faithful wearing of the Bionator/OCI, it will be noticed that the patient is able to function at a new and increased vertical, with the mandible in a more forward, naturally comfortable, and structurally balanced skeletal Class I position or, if need be, "super–Class I" or near–Class III position and this position is habitual. Function in this new found position will also generally take place in the complete absence of joint clicking. This combination will allow for as much atrophy, temporal bone remodeling, and other forms of internal joint readaptation less well understood to take place in the superior posterior retrocondylar area as Nature sees fit to induce. As time goes on, these tissues shrink and coalesce to the point such that since the condyle no longer has the capability of chronically distorting them, they will almost invariably assume their natural and proper anatomical configuration where possible as per the dictates of the genetic codes hidden deep within their cellular elements, codes that have always been present and are perfectly capable of redirecting things in their usual manner after being given the unobstructed opportunity to once again express themselves. The only things that may not fully return to normal are those ligaments of the joint that have been distorted and/or elongated beyond their ability to recover. This scenario represents the ideal in Bionator treatment for the patient with a structurally imbalanced TMJ, but as it turns out, it is not the only acceptable scenario.

One very important technique experienced operators employ is that of treating the patient to a slight (1.0–1.5mm) anterior open bite with the Bionator/OCI as a form of "overcorrection." By gradually thickening the cap, and with prolonged and diligent wearing of the appliance by the patient, the posterior quadrants can be allowed to erupt vertically towards each other to the point where they have actually "overerupted" enough to create a slight anterior open bite in the anterior incisor region. This is desirable whenever possible, because after the appliance is withdrawn, the bite will close back down again due to slight posterior quadrant "settling in." Bionator/OCI created increased posterior vertical dimension of occlusion can "settle back in" in certain cases, especially in adults. Correspondingly, Bionator/OCI created slight anterior open bites settle back in again upon appliance withdrawal and therefore should pose no concern for the treating clinician. Therefore the old axiom of "overcorrect slightly" holds true even with this procedure.

The second-best circumstance that might be a result of Bionator wear by the adult patients with TMJ problems is still totally acceptable, especially as far as the patients are concerned because all they are interested in is relief. Such would be the case where all of the above are effected by the Bionator except that a bit of a "dual-bite" situation might still remain. The patient habitually functions in the new post–Bionator treatment, Class I skeletal and dental relationship at the proper vertical dimension, free of clicking or discomfort, yet the clinician may still be able to manually force the mandible part of the way back to its old pretreatment retruded arc of closure, albeit usually not without some modicum of discomfort to the patient. In these types of cases there are other factors that enter and cause such circumstances to occur. The most common of these is a long T-TM distance (pterygoid vertical to C-point, Bimler) and/or the degree of severity of the deficiency of the diagonal length of the mandible (DLM; Bimler) of the individually involved structurally Class II mandible. When just such a combination of factors results in a cephalometric Class II mandible that has remained untreated during the growth and development stage of the patient's youth and then becomes involved as a major component of a larger group of etiological agents responsible for an "adult-onset" TMJ imbalance, the TMJ's distal position (long T-TM) and/or the mandible's usually diminutive skeletally Class II size, represented by a shorter DLM, increases the probability of observing the occasionally occurring post–Bionator treatment dual bite. But this in no way is an obstacle that should prevent treatment with the Bionator when indicated.

In the growing child, the shorter mandible is advanced through Bionator treatment and held in the newer more forward and vertically opened position by a combination of appliance wear, muscle retraining, and the increased vertical eruption of posterior teeth. In so doing, the condyle is also pulled down and forward within the joint, thereby creating a tension in the area along the condylar head and neck. In the growing child, this stimulates the growth centers of the condylar head to proliferate so as to seek out the former state, which in turn causes the head and neck of the condyle to lengthen to assume its former, nontensed, properly spaced anatomical stereoscopic position in the joint. This results in an overall larger DLM and changes the structural class of the mandible from skeletal Class II to skeletal Class I in the typical manner common to Bionator treatment.[21-36] But as previously stated, in the adult this growth potential is no longer as actively present. The condyle and condylar neck cannot lengthen regardless of how much they are tensed by the perpetual forward positioning brought about by Bionator wear. Chronically compressed joints also often exhibit a "bent-forward" condylar head and neck, which bears mute testimony to the degree the overall length of the mandible has been constricted by a locking occlusion. The best that may be hoped for in such a case is that a process possibly such as that of the aforementioned joint tissue coalescence of the postcondylar area will be sufficient to fill in the posterior joint space behind the condyle once that condyle is no longer being perpetually jammed into the bilaminar zone. Quite often, fortunately, this combination of factors discussed is all that is needed. But it must be noted that in the adult patient if the overall mandibular deficiency is great enough and the distance it must be translated to bring the mandible back to functional Class I position again is far enough, the condyle will be positioned relatively quite far down and forward in the glenoid fossa due to the adult mandible's short DLM. This "gap" retrocondylarly between where the capitulum resides, once the vertical is increased and muscle adaptation completed, and where it used to formerly reside up in the intolerant zone cannot always coalesce enough to prevent the forcible penetration of the condyle back up into the retrocondylar area. A residual elasticity may remain in this area to some degree. But with the occlusion now opened, the muscles readapted to the structurally balanced skeletal Class I position, and the condyle on the center of the disc in the tolerant zone during function (or if not on the disc because it is irretrievable, at least *out of* the bilaminar zone), patients will be entirely "rehabilitated" to this new and comfortable arrangement and would have no reason to forcibly retruded their own mandibles to their former undesirable pretreatment, retruded position. Since the undersized mandible was never "stretched" with Bionator treatment while orthopedic growth and lengthening was possible, although it has now been bodily repositioned, the patient is stuck with a mandible that is now in its proper place relative to its surrounding and opposing structures *on the front end* relative to the dental arch area, but one that also may be just a little orthopedically short and/or deformed in the condylar head and neck *on the back end*, hence the phenomenon of being able to be forced back up the slope of the tuberculum to its old ways of closure a little to produce the "Sunday bite." But the patient is happy and healthy and pain free, and so is the joint. With the advancement of the mandible and increased anterior nasal spine–menton (ANS-Me) lower face height, even the facial appearance looks better. The fact that such patients may still possess vestiges of their former retruded arc of closure that result in a "dual" bite is a phenomenon with which they are totally unconcerned. They are relieved of their pain and dysfunction and feel as if they have been "cured." And they have.

We must also honestly acknowledge that there will be instances when the clinician may be legitimately fooled into thinking that the patient is still within the boundaries of the scope of FJO treatment with a recapturable disc and an intact posterior ligament when in fact such is not the case. In these cases the concerned practitioner may not be able to advance the mandible far enough to recapture the disc completely or even at all, or when he does have the mandible positioned in a balanced position cephalometrically and structurally, i.e., increased posterior joint space and joint decompression, the disc may be so misshapened as to be utterly useless. These types of patients, although experiencing relief from decompression of the joint and reduction of the tension and pressure on the bilaminar zone (what's left of it), never really respond to treatment as fully as expected. Opening of the jaw may still remain somewhat limited, and the dual bite of forcible retrusion of the jaw to old ways and/or clicking symptoms may never completely disappear. Yet no harm is done by such honestly instituted attempts at conservative treatment because the therapeutically produced increased vertical dimension and habitually more advanced jaw position only restore to normal what should have been present bioarchitecturally in the first place, the lack of which was the major etiological agent that brought on the painful and destructive TMJ condition. If the patient is satisfied and pain free or at least shows dramatic long-term improvement at that point in the treatment sequence, the decision, after being fully advised, to consider the case as being "complete" is totally justified. If on the *rare* occasion such universally acceptable and correct conservative approaches to the management of such types of TMJ problems are insufficient to effect resolution, no criticism can be made of beginning first at the most conservative and fundamental of therapeutic levels. Many experts agree that only an extremely small percentage of patients will ever require surgery of the reparative variety due to things like frank ankylosis (tumors and acute trauma are, of course, another matter). Surgery, when questionable at the beginning as to its necessity, may always be called in when more conservative methods initially chosen in good faith and based on sound diagnostic principles prove inadequate. Such instances where surgery is needed may disappear altogether in the future, however, as our knowledge of FJO techniques grows vs. the problems we now see rising to the surface with the surgical approach. Sincere and heroic efforts to keep the patient from going "over the edge" in structurally imbalanced cases should never be deprecated but rather commended as long as there is a reasonable prognosis for success and especially since the "edge" so alluded to is that of the surgeon's scalpel!

> *"After a stronghold has been made*
> *of the bones, it is covered with*
> *flesh and blood, and there dwell*
> *in it old age, death, pride, and*
> *deceit."*
>
> Chapter IV, "The Dhammapada"
> 5th Nikaya of the Sutta,
> Second Tripitaka of the Buddhist Canon
> First century B.C.

ARCH PREPARATION IN TMJ TREATMENT: CORRECTION VS. DEVELOPMENT

Once it has been determined that posteriorly displaced condyles, loss of vertical dimension, and mandibular retrusion are major etiological contributors to a given patient's TMJ symptoms, the clinician may not necessarily be able to immediately begin Bionator treatment. In fact it is *rare* that the Bionator is the *first* appliance used. The same principles of arch preparation prior to the insertion of *arch-aligning* appliances such as the Bionator apply for the patient with TMJ problems as for the traditional orthodontic patient. This is simply because both types of patient are really one and the same and the FJO principles of orthopedics are what are being used to treat the main cause of the patient's TMJ condition. As with conventional orthodontics, a great deal of trouble may be avoided by aligning arches that are in fact true and proper in arch form and have adequate anterior arch length and compatible opposing arch width. Arch preparation almost invariably consists of first eliminating the anterior occlusal or incisal interference. If it is retroclined upper anteriors that are the initiators of the NRDM/SPDC phenomenon, they are developed labially to the relatively correct anterior clearance first by active place usage, taking advantage of the palliative splinting effect of the acrylic occlusal coverings of the maxillary Sagittal II active plate in the process to gain the "splinting effect" for relief of the TMJ symptoms. Sometimes the upper arch is collapsed bilaterally or in the fashion of a Gothic arch form requiring transverse or fan-type appliance arch preparation to pave the way so that the mandibular arch may subsequently be advanced with a Bionator or OCI. Sometimes irregular individual tooth malalignment must be corrected by leveling, aligning, and rotating the teeth with the common fixed appliance technique in order to facilitate the mandibular advancement that will follow. Sometimes both active-plate and fixed-appliance techniques are required to prepare one or both arches for the functional appliance phase of treatment. Once responsible orthopedic arch form is obtained, the teeth may then be moved around in an unstrained manner within them with simple fixed appliances. Thus it may be seen that in the use of FJO principles for the treatment of TMJ problems, the technique of arch forming, arch aligning, and mandibular advancement is being utilized and made to assume a dual role: (1) correcting the patient's jaw-deflecting malocclusion along with the attending structural and muscular imbalances and (2) thereby relieving and correcting the resultant temporomandibular pain-dysfunction by decompressing and rearticulating the joints into their proper state of biomechanical harmony. However, in the adult patient, active plate arch development, both laterally and AP, is obtained at a dear price. An old problem returns to haunt such necessary procedures—that of relapse!

This brings us once again to considerations of the difference between correction and development. These concepts were discussed in volume II of this series of texts. However, they are so important to the understanding of the problems associated with orthodontic therapeutics that a brief review of their implications would be appropriate here. As concepts, they must be categorized as generalizations, and as with all generalizations, some latitude is required in the interpretation of their meaning. They are both intimately related to the question of why some patients show a high propensity for relapse and some do not in spite of proper orthodontic technique and concerted efforts at posttreatment retention.

Correction implies moving a tooth or group of teeth back to the place where they originally erupted into the mouth but subsequently had been forced somewhere else. An example would be the correction of an upper anterior tooth that had erupted into a lingual crossbite with the lowers due to an inclined plane action of some sort acting to deflect its eruptive path. Another example germane to the FJO philosophy would be the distalization (correction) of posterior quadrants that have drifted forward to result in AP arch collapse and labially blocked-out cuspids. Extraction of second molars and distalization of the entire remaining posterior quadrants back to their original starting place with conventional Sagittal I or equivalent technique is a corrective procedure. Correction is always characterized by relatively high degrees of stability, all things considered.

Development on the other hand implies something quite different. It is used to denote the process by which a group of teeth and their supportive alveolar processes are moved to an entirely new location that they never did at any time yet occupy. Developing dental arches laterally and developing upper retroclined Division 2 anteriors and their surrounding premaxillary alveolar process forward are examples of development. And all cases that employ development are usually characterized by relatively high degrees of instability. Some of it just doesn't hold.

This also brings to light the question of the arch width indices of Schwarz and Pont and their true significance in treatment planning. It must be remembered that the normative standards these tables represent for the "ideal" arch width are merely mathematical averages.[37] This means that for a given proposed ideal arch width value, there will be a certain number of patients whose true individualized ideal width would be less and an equal number for whom it would be more. The amount of arch width a given patient will tolerate is a product of that individual's muscular limits of arch width. It is different from individual to individual and cannot be predicted. Only the average width for a given group can be predicted. It is similar to the relationship of fluoride to caries incidence. One cannot predict exactly which child will or will not get the cavity, only that the percentage of caries incident to a general sample population will decrease.

The indices of Schwarz and Pont for ideal arch width act as guides to average widths of a sample population. If a given individual's actual limits of tolerance of maximum arch width are less than the norm, efforts to keep them out past their own individual limits of tolerance will be frought with relapse problems. There seems to be only so much lateral development a given individual will take, and we cannot determine which patient will hold at the ideal width values of Schwartz or Pont and which will not, even when "hedging our arch-width-bets" with the modifying influences of facial type.

Therefore, development situations also involve considerations of the notion of directional decrowding. Also discussed in volume II of this series, directional decrowding implies several things, but relative to arch width problems, essentially it means "making peace with the muscles" as quickly as possible. In other words, do as much correction and as little development as the demands of the case will allow. If a patient is suffering primarily from AP arch collapse with blocked-out cuspids, etc., and only a slight modicum of lateral collapse, these principles state that it is better to eliminate that last little bit of crowding by a bit more distalization, which is stable, and forego the lateral development component, which is unstable, in order to decrowd the arch. A stable decrowded arch that is slightly less than the ideal indexed width and as a result may be a little longer and a little narrower than the norms claim as ideal would be a better compromise with Nature than would an arch decrowded to a more rounded arch form that might be "right on" indexed values but also may in the end turn out to be unstable.

Thus correction by distalization is preferable to development wherever possible. But development must often be employed, and when it is, concerted efforts at long-term retention must be made. The musculature draping over the upper and lower dental arches will tolerate only so much displacement by the teeth and alveolar processes before they start fighting back. The wise clinician gets good arch form to be sure, but he also accepts a compromise with Nature's preselected, "muscular environment–determined" arch length and width whenever possible.

In light of previous discussions on such topics as stress relief, the proprioceptive occlusal neuromuscular circuit, and splint usage, it may now be seen wherein lies the beauty of the Sagittal II or Transverse arch preparation appliances in the treatment of TMJ pain-dysfunction conditions. They also serve a dual role: first, that of arch preparers, and second, that of pain relievers! The active plate portion of these appliances do the work of correcting the patient's improper interferring arch form, while the occlusal acrylic coverings of these appliances provide a palliative "splint effect" for alleviation of the patient's symptoms. Of course, as with all arch development undertakings, it is best to remember the principles of "correction vs. development" at all times. However, in the case of the adult patient with TMJ problems, a facilitating compromise that can (and at times must) be added to the above principles is that of the extraction of a lower anterior incisor (preferably one that is crowded forward). This allows the lower arches to be shortened and constricted lingually via space closure and arch condensation procedures with fixed appliances. This in turn allows more mandibular advancement without the excessive forward development of interferring maxillary anteriors, which in adults are so prone to relapse. Nevertheless, Sagittal II and Transverse appliances are still often the appliances of choice for arch preparation prior to Bionator/Orthopedic Corrector therapy, even though they often imply lifetime night-only (or hours of sleep [HS]) retainers.

Both families of these appliances have these occlusal acrylic plates covering the upper posterior quadrants. This acrylic may be kept in a bilaterally balanced but smooth type of occlusion with the lower teeth in a manner identical to the "occlusion-eliminating" splints previously alluded to. The thickness of these acrylic occlusal coverings ranges from 1.5 to 3.0 mm, and this opens the vertical dimension of occlusion by the same amount, which in turn acts to decompress the joint slightly because complete overclosure to the occlusally deflected pretreatment level is impossible as long as the appliance is worn. Being that the acrylic pads have the capacity, if desired, to be ground smooth, the occlusion-eliminating aspects of these appliances offer relief to overworked muscles. During active plate wear, muscles do not have to overclose past their ideal physiological lengths, nor do they have to close the mandible to full occlusal contact in an excessively retruded fashion in order to avoid interfering anterior "misguiding planes." The occlusal coverings of the upper appliances take advantage of the proprioceptive reflexive neuromuscular "circuit breaker" effect identically to conventional TMJ flat-plane splint usage, the net result being that the patient often notices a great reduction in symptoms during the first month of wear of the appliance. And all this time the patient is making *positive* and *active* movements in the direction of actually correcting the problem structurally rather than just "sitting passively" in a splint. There even exists the possibility that additional relief of overstrained musculature may come from the fact that, at the newer increased vertical caused by the thickness of the occlusal acrylic of the appliance and the smooth occlusal interfacing surface that can be provided against which the lowers make contact, the muscles can close the mandible in just about any manner AP and/or laterally (to correct midline shifts) that they desire. This alone will account for a certain percentage of patients exhibiting the ability to bite farther forward naturally on the appliance as if the mandible were waiting to be unlocked so it can "spring forward" on its own. This would naturally be more comfortable for the muscles as well as the joints. One will be surprised how often one observes this phenomenon once locking and interfering anterior teeth are "cleared out of the way." Yet, some patients will still be seen to struggle in this phase of treatment.

It has been observed clinically that for some patients with a high degree of sensitivity to occlusal irregularities or for patients with more severe and chronic TMJ pain-dysfunction conditions, there is a benefit to be derived from the balancing and preparation of the biting surfaces of acrylic over the posterior quadrants of the Sagittal or Transverse appliance to a smooth occlusal surface in a manner confluent with full-coverage, maxillary flat-plane splints. If the acrylic is thick enough as a result of the construction-bite thickness, the Sagittal may be trimmed and adjusted so that the normal indentations of the lower cusp tips in the upper bite pad acrylic are all but eliminated. Sometimes putting a glossy finish on the smooth biting surfaces of acrylic after such adjustments seems to add to the comfort of some very sensitive patients (usually females). If the occlusal acrylic is initially too thin to permit reduction to a flat-plane level without making the acrylic weak or subject to excessive perforations, cold-cure acrylic may be added in a thin coat over the posterior pads and the mandible tapped into it as it is setting to provide a posterior thickness of acrylic of about 2 mm between the cusp tips of the posterior teeth. This added thickness may then be ground flat as desired to produce a posterior interocclusal pad that is both smooth, balanced, and of sufficient thickness so as to resist the forces of occlusion without fracture. Some prefer making active plates like Sagittal II appliances by means of the more sophisticated Levandoski technique, with the occlusal acrylic pads either left as per the locking bite of the Levandoski method or ground flat but produced his way to allow for any variance needed between one side of the plate and the other as per the dictates of an asymmetrical posterior vertical or a mandible longer and/or more retruded on one side over the other. However, leaving occlusal indentations of a locking nature as per the Levandoski technique is only permissible on Sagittal II appliances. Flat-plane occlusal coverings are required for Transverse or fan-type appliances. Yet other practitioners merely use the Sagittal or Transverse in the conventional manner: it is constructed on a construction bite taken without any transcranial compound bite direction or manual guidance of the patient's mandible by the clinician at all. The patient is merely allowed to bite ad lib into the wax. The purpose behind this method is to deliberately obtain the cusp tip indentations on the bite pads. These are thought to act as an aid in anchoring the appliance during occlusion and thereby facilitate transmission of the expanding forces of the expansion screws to the teeth and alveolar tissues as the plate is activated. These cusp tip indentations, which are a product of standard bite registration, may also be "forward ground." That is, the mesial portion of each indentation in the acrylic pad made by the opposing lower cusp tip is tapered forward with acrylic denture adjusting burs while the posterior portion of the indentation is left unadjusted. This encourages the mandible to slide forward slightly as the cusp tips of the lower teeth occlude with the acrylic occlusal pads of the upper plate. This, in conjunction with the increased vertical provided by the thickness of the acrylic of the occlusal pads of the active plate, is felt by many to be just enough to bring about adequate decompression of the joint and eventually effect a great deal of myofascial relief of discomfort. In either case the patient will usually note relief over about the first month of wear. The method selected is usually a product of the patient's level of sensitivity (i.e., the rapidity of response to the conventional Sagittal as it is normally used) and the personal preferences of the particular practitioner.

The Role of the Sagittal Appliance in TMJ Treatment

By far the most classic example of profound TMJ symptoms brought on by a structurally imbalanced malocclusion is in that of the Class II, Division 2, deep-overbite, adult dentition case. Actually, all functionally induced TMJ problems are very akin to this type of malocclusion, at least conceptually anyway. It is here where the Sagittal appliance (sometime referred to as a sagittal splint) "shines" in its dual role as both a corrective orthodontic device and a palliative TMJ splint. The Class II, Division 2, deep-bite condition is most likely the singularly most destructive situation with respect to the integrity of the articular components of the TMJ. It is this jaw-to-jaw occlusally induced relationship that brings the maximum effect of the NRDM-SPDC phenomenon to bear on the disc-condyle-fossa relationship. The combination of muscular vertical overclosure needed to effect posterior quadrant contact and the incisal interference caused by the lingually torqued and retroclined upper incisors against the lower incisors, which in turn causes the mandible to be driven back from its normal orthopedically guided path of closure to one of an extremely retruded type, makes for a double-edged combination that is devastating to both the patient's musculature and even more importantly the intracapsular joint structures themselves. And if this isn't enough, quite often there is attending lower anterior incisor crowding in the mandible. Even when slight, if the lower crowding is such that it should perchance force a lower central incisor out labially, this greatly accentuates the NRDM-SPDC phenomenon and worsens the untoward effects on the muscles and especially the joints. The mandible, were it to have its way, would close on an arc of physiological closure far more forward than the lingually torqued upper incisors of such a Division 2–type arrangement will permit. Upon closure, the lower incisal edges slide right up the lingual surfaces of the upper retroclined anteriors as the reflexive neuromuscular actions of the closing muscles, spurred by the information provided by the exquisitely sensitive proprioceptive neural fibers of the periodontal ligament, are forced to guide the mandible posteriorly. The deeper the bite, the more accentuated is this process. The primary corrective considerations here must be directed toward moving the upper anteriors out of the way labially so that the vertical may be increased and the mandible may be free to close more normally—and for a trapped mandible in such a situation, that means *forward!* Assuming that the upper arch is already on or near the corrected indices of Schwarz or Pont for arch width at the bicuspid *and* molar regions, thereby obviating any possible locking effect of a Gothic-shaped upper arch, the Sagittal II may be inserted and balanced in the manner of all upper TMJ splints if need be.* It then may be activated so as to impart the sorely needed labially directed movement to the offending maxillary anteriors. Expansion screw activation does take a slightly different level of frequency in adults due to the harder, nongrowing maxillary bone. Usually one turn of the screws every 4 to 5 days is well tolerated, but sometimes it must be slowed to once per week to avoid patient complaints of discomfort. Nevertheless, once activated and faithfully worn for a major portion of the day, the appliance will definitely move the teeth. They may be moved forward to at least the McNamara limits (facial surface of the upper central within 4 to 5 mm anterior to the A perpendicular, provided of course that the A point is correctly located relative to its own reference point, the Na perpendicular), or preferably even slightly beyond these limits, since there is a high proclivity for teeth so moved to relapse lingually. Overcorrection (to compensate for what modicum of relapse will occur during the Bionator phase of treatment) and long periods of retention (HS, or night only) at the completion of treatment (often lifetime) are part of every TMJ treatment plan where upper anteriors must be advanced prior to the unlocking of the mandible

---

*For further information on the construction and use of the Sagittal appliance refer to Chapter IV of *Clinical Management of Basic Maxillofacial Orthopedic Appliances,* volume I.

with follow-up Bionator technique. Sagittal II technique for arch preparation for the patient with TMJ problems is a *development* situation, and that means serious concerns for retention. An HS retainer is a small price to pay for a lifetime of freedom from TMJ-related pain. Patients have no problem dealing with such requirements, neither should their clinicians.

Such actions as these are standard fare for classic Class II, Division 2, deep-bite TMJ conditions, but they also serve surprisingly well for patients who are borderline or exhibit what may appear as only slight Division 2 tendencies. Here the upper anteriors may show only a slight degree of lingual version or be nearly vertical in the appearance of their clinical crowns and may not be the true primary culprits in the generation of the NRDM/SPDC mandibular retrusion but merely serve the role of "accessories to the crime." Here it may be the crowded, forward, labially protruding, lower central incisors that act as the primary agents. Or the case may deceptively appear on the surface as a full skeletal and dental Class I both cephalometrically and according to Angle's molar classification. But a slightly retruded maxilla, a slightly longer than normal mandibular DLM (Bimler), a barely detectable retroclination of the upper anteriors, a maxillary anterior tooth rotation, slightly overly proclined lower anteriors, or an endless variety of combinations of all of the above can all add up to initiation of the NRDM/SPDC phenomenon. Once the condyle becomes posteriorly displaced during function, a compromised TMJ results. The combination of the above factors as well as others may be so subtle as to be clinically all but undetectable. But the combination of pa-

---

Figure 5–14 The sagittal "splint" appliance. **(A)** The conventional Sagittal II appliance serves as both a TMJ splint and an orthodontic appliance. **(B)** The acrylic occlusal coverings act as a bite guard and produce the splinting effect that relieves TMJ discomfort. **(C)** The screws may be activated every 4 to 7 days to advance interfering retruded upper anterior teeth forward prior to Bionator/OCI advancement of the mandible, which would follow. (Courtesy of the Ohlendorf Co, St Louis.)

Figure 5–15 **(A)** Anterior incisal interference often begins the process of TMJ degenerative arthrosis by causing an overly retruded mandibular arc of closure that drives the condyle up and back too far off the disc into the area of sensitive nerves and arteries behind the condyle. **(B)** Eliminating anterior incisal interference often requires sagittal appliances (splints) that both relieve pain (occlusal acrylic pad, splint part) and move the teeth forward (expansion screw, orthodontic part) to free up the mandible and its arc of closure so that the mandible-condyle unit may operate in the correct (down and forward) physiologically stable location. Eliminating the distal-driving anterior incisal interferences eliminates the NRDM/SPDC phenomenon. Then the pain ceases. (Courtesy of Dr. John Witzig.)

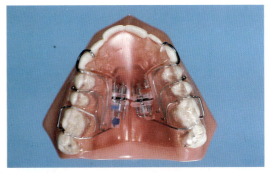

Figure 5–14(A)

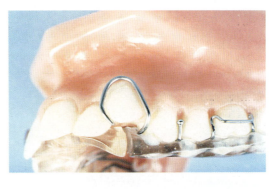

(B)

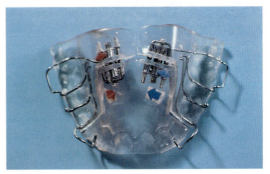

(C)

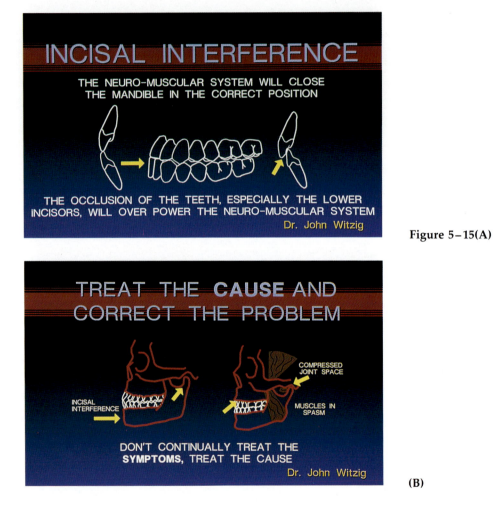

Figure 5–15(A)

(B)

tient anamnesis and transcranial radiographic findings still remain definitive regardless of how Class I the case may appear! For the patient with functionally induced TMJ arthrosis, as far as Nature is concerned, the net effect or sum total of the occlusion on the action of the mandible during function turns out to be the same: the incisal interference anteriorly causes a retruded mandibular arc of closure to full interdigitation, a compressed joint with invasion of the condylar head into the intolerant zone, strained and overworked musculature, reciprocal clicking, and resultant classic myofascial headaches and TMJ-type associated pain. Here again the same principles of treatment apply. Although the lower arch may be corrected orthodontically to eliminate the protruding lower anterior (sometimes by means of the previously described technique of judicious lower anterior incisor extraction and anterior arch contraction with reciprocal space closure), it must also be remembered that the posterior vertical must usually still be opened, any interfering upper anteriors cleared forward out of the way with a Sagittal II, and the mandible advanced by Bionator treatment so as to retrain and readapt the Class II retrusive type musculature that has developed over the years as a result of the incisally induced retruded arc of closure. Being that they are such creatures of habit, the muscles supporting the mandible may not permit full decompression of the joint by autoadvancement of the newly unlocked mandible once the incisal interferences have been removed anteriorly. The muscles of mastication may have to be "forced to forget." The constant and properly managed wear of the Bionator allows the healing and reorganization processes previously discussed to take effect in the joint, which, along with the retrained musculature and the gradually shifting occlusion, progressively helps prevent condylar intrusion posteriorly into the intolerant zone. Thus it may be seen that the eventual joint readaptation acts as a process that also helps the muscles "forget." As previously mentioned, in the instance a lower arch may not be practically perfected orthodontically in traditional fashion for various reasons, the offending crowded forward lower central (or lateral) incisor may have to be sacrificed, after which the space is closed reciprocally (relieving the anterior crowding in doing so) and the case may be prepared and finished in the normal manner confluent with Sagittal II/Bionator combination treatment. The reason for such seemingly radical treatment as lower incisor extraction in cases of certain types of lower anterior crowding turns out to be threefold. First, it is quite a bit more difficult to distally drive the lower first molars to any appreciable extent in the hard mandibular bone of the adult patient, even with the benefit of second molar extraction, although with time and diligent effort it can be done. Usually slightly more sophisticated fixed appliance mechanics are enlisted, or else diligent unilateral efforts with the Sagittal I, "gang-up–kick-back" technique with the Crozat appliance, or unilateral distalization techniques with Wilson appliances may be employed. This requires more cooperation over a longer period of time from the patient. Sometimes this extended treatment time of itself becomes a problem. This brings us to a second reason lower anterior single-tooth extraction might be the treatment of choice—simple expediency! This second reason is right out of the philosophy of directional decrowding. After assuming the maxillary dentition can be made compatible with the lowers if such an extraction were carried out, which it almost always will, the great deal of time and therapeutic effort saved for both the adult patient and the clinician faced with an extremely difficult orthodontic arch preparation problem more than justifies any slight technical imperfections in the final alignment of teeth. It is the alignment of the jaws that counts. Third, and this is really a quite unexpected surprise, such techniques as this that remove the offending source of NRDM/SPDC in the lower anterior area sometimes allow for the occurrence of a truly remarkable phenomenon, autoadvancement of the mandible by none other than Nature Herself, even without the benefits of functional appliances!

However, sometimes all that is needed to generate the NRDM-SPDC phenomenon with its attending TMJ problems is the combination of a deep overbite and high interincisal angle *in the complete absence* of a protruding lower incisor. In such high interincisal angle cases where deep overbite also exists, the conditions are often right to combine to have the same effect on the TMJ as do the more classically profound Class II, Division 2 varieties. The deep overbite anteriorly combines with the effects of a more vertical upper incisal angle (Bimler) to cause just enough incisal interference upon mandibular closure to initiate the NRDM-SPDC phenomenon. The proof diagnostically that such reflexive posterior retrusion and/or overclosure is in fact taking place in such a case is the appearance of the telltale TMJ signs and symptoms clinically and posterior condylar displacement observed radiographically via transcranial films. Therefore, increased vertical dimension and mandibular advancement are needed *regardless* of how much in confluence radiographically the anterior arrangement is to the cephalometric norms or how clinically "normal" the dentition may appear to the eye. Looks can be deceiving, but TMJs don't lie! Sometimes a nearly perfect appearing upper arch with only the slightest excess of overbite and with first molars in "ideal" dental Class I position is in fact orthopedically retruded just far enough as to initiate the anterior incisal interference NRDM/SPDC phenomenon and produce TMJ pain and chronic headache-type myofascial discomforts. Even if advancing the mandible would result in a dental "super Class I" or near Class III in the molar region, so be it. The joints must have their way. If such Class III–type posttreatment dental alignments were to occur, the patient was most likely a borderline skeletal Class III in a Class I disguise anyway. A simple advancement of the mandible in such "close" cases to the "as if" position of an end-to-end bite or, if need be, postincisal end-to-end bite (divulging the severity of retrusion of the upper anteriors and hence the mandibular arc of closure) will show the patient as well as the clinician whether this NRDM/SPDC phenomenon is in fact occurring. With the patient opening and closing to the "as if" incisal end-to-end position, the joint clicking in a vast majority of cases will be seen to instantly disappear, thus indicating that the condyle is riding once again at the center of the disc in normal fashion somewhere down in the tolerant zone of the joint once again. This would also clearly demonstrate for both patient and doctor that an increase in the degree of maxillary incisor protrusion or mandibular incisor retrusion followed by Bionator advancement with (or in some cases possibly without) an increase in vertical dimension is entirely indicated. However, the degree of involvement of each of these factors is usually slight in these "close" cases because the angulation of the upper anteriors is not excessively severe to begin with. Such conditions are verifiable cephalometrically. But it must be remembered that slight advancements of the anteriors past cephalometric limits anteriorly are very easily well tolerated esthetically because 1 or 2 mm either way does not exert much of an effect on appearance when weighed against the total appearance of an object as large as the human face, but it certainly has a big effect on the function of something as small as the highly sensitive post-condylar space of the joint. Back there 1 mm equates to a mile!

There may also be the less frequent occasion where the opposite distalizing action of the Sagittal I appliance may be required. Anterior crowding, unilaterally or bilaterally, may exist in the anterior segments, which may already be protrusive enough. Since in these types of Sagittal I cases the entire posterior portion of one or both quadrants of the upper arch has drifted unduly forward unilaterally or bilaterally, the maxillary anteriors may not be able to be protruded much farther past their existing anterior limits because they are already quite protrusive. To relieve crowding and to obtain proper arch form, transverse or fan-type Gothic arch correction (if needed) followed by distalization techniques for relief of any remaining forward crowding of the upper posterior quadrants is indicated. For in this type of case, if forward drifted molars are left "undistalized" to their proper location, the correct amount of mandibular protrusion needed to decompress the joint might not allow the lower molars to "catch up" to the excessively forward drifted upper molars, which would only result in cusp tip-to-tip occlusion posteriorly or some otherwise unacceptable occlusal table situation. Once the mandible with its lower arch of teeth is properly positioned forward as per the dictates (needs) of the joint, any remaining Class II molar malalignment from the AP aspect is obviously due to excessively forward drifted upper molars by default. In such rare cases as this, after careful deliberation and when all other alternatives have proved to be unacceptable, removal of the second molar(s) may be required to secure proper and uncrowded arch form for the upper arch. Such patients are informed of the problem, and as always, the decision to treat or not to treat is theirs. Patients will do surprisingly well on only one set of upper molars in uncommon circumstances as those just described that mandate upper second molar removal. They will certainly do far better with only one upper molar if need be than if left untreated, which will only result in further joint degeneration and intensification of symptoms. The upper arch must be secured into a "stronghold" of cephalometrically structural and orthodontically proper arch form. For it is against this stronghold that the entire thrust of the Bionator that follows is anchored. This all-important maxillary anchorage provides the foundation for the forces that bring about muscle readaptation, vertical dental eruption, and decompression of the strained TMJs, all of which are effected by wearing the Bionator and all of which are needed for proper resolution of the problem. The alternative of clearing the upper anteriors as needed, advancing the mandible, and leaving upper posterior quadrants somewhat crowded forward with blocked-out cuspids or other forms of anterior crowding and slightly Class II molars posteriorly may be acceptable if the joint is decompressed and the less than ideal occlusion manages to somehow keep it that way. Patient choice and clinical judgment must prevail here.

In many of the TMJ cases treated with FJO technique, the social or work-related problems of wearing the Bionator all day compromise its 24-hour use. In these circumstances the Sagittal then not only acts as its own retainer, keeping upper anteriors forward (when Sagittal II technique has been used), but also gives some "splint effect" relief to the joint and musculature from the not quite fully revamped occlusion during the day. There is also enough flex to the Sagittal appliance across the open expansion screws to absorb the changing effects of the occlusion as the posteriors gradually erupt vertically. When the occlusion changes enough in the later stages of treatment with the Bionator such that the Sagittal II no longer fits adequately to act as its own retainer for the periods of the day (optimally, short periods) when the Bionator isn't worn, a simple Hawley retainer may have to be constructed and temporarily used in its place. As always, at the completion of any case where the upper arch is developed either laterally or anteroposteriorly, the use of upper retainers during sleep for the remainder of the patient's life is a frequent condition to successful treatment. Patients readily accept and adapt to such compromises in order to remain pain free just as readily as they accept and adapt to a lifetime of wearing eyeglasses, hearing aids, or pacemakers. Just ask them!

Come forth into the light of things
Let Nature be your teacher.

"The Tables Turned"
William Wordsworth, 1770–1850

Treatment Triptych for TMJ

The application of FJO techniques to the treatment of the structurally compromised TMJ patient has followed three basic pathways in the efforts to decompress the joint. The first major form of treatment consists of the traditional Sagittal/Bionator combination, which may or may not include a little fixed appliance therapy for esthetic reasons. This type of treatment process usually implies that some sort of retroclined upper anteriors are extant in the pretreatment state. They may be actual Division II angulated uppers or uppers that for some reason, such as a short maxillary (AT Bimler) length or a severe rotation, result in the equivalent to a "Division II effect" on the mandibular arc of final closure to occlusion, which then, of course, initiates the NRDM/SPDC phenomenon and pushes the condyle back up off the disc. Occasionally a fixed appliance is needed for correcting severe rotations of an anterior tooth or group of teeth that act as a source of anterior incisal interference. However, usually the Sagittal II appliance with its palliative splintlike effects of the occlusal coverings is the most frequent appliance used to initiate treatment for TMJ pain-dysfunction patients with trapped mandibles as a result of Division II effect coming from anterior incisal interference.

An interesting and not infrequent phenomenon that sometimes accompanies Sagittal II arch-lengthening procedures in TMJ pain-dysfunction patients with posteriorly displaced mandibles is the previously alluded to, gradual autoadvancement of the mandible as the upper anteriors are moved out of the way. This seems especially true when the rest of the arch form is fairly good and the patient is still an adolescent or young adult. As the upper anteriors are progressively advanced by the action of the appliance, the mandible in such patients autoadvances such that when the occlusion is checked periodically with the appliance out the lower incisors may be seen to continue to tuck themselves right in behind the uppers, in spite of the fact that the uppers have been moved labially, as signified by the opened spaces of the appliance. This is most likely due to the body's desire to seek out its own naturally programmed levels of structural balance. All it sometimes needs is a free hand at it. This will cut down on the amount of work that the Bionator will have to do and, on certain fortunate occasions, may obviate the need for it altogether. However, this scenario would be predicated upon the preexistence of adequate vertical.

Another thing that cannot be overstressed is the need for timely and adequate forms of retention any time maxillary anterior segments are *developed* forward. This generally takes the form first of a brief period of 3 to 5 months of stabilization with the expanded appliance (or a substitute retainer) at the end of the Sagittal phase of treatment. Second, the problem must almost always be overcorrected slightly, and no fears should haunt the clinician that overly advanced upper anteriors will remain too far for-

CASE HISTORY

PATIENT: Age 50 years, 1 month

MAIN PROBLEM:
1. Frequent, reoccurring headaches, so severe that patient was going to stop working.
2. Pain in right TMJ.
3. Constant discomfort.

FINDINGS:
1. Right TMJ very painful to palpation.
2. Right and left TMJs locked.
3. Class II/Div. II malocclusion.
4. Incisal interference forcing the mandible posteriorly in occlusion.

RADIOGRAPHIC FINDINGS:
1. Right TMJ - Posterior superior displaced condyle.
       - Flattening of condyle.
       - Large bone spur on condyle.
2. Left TMJ - Posterior superior displaced condyle.
       - Flattening of condyle.
3. Right TMJ arthrogram
   a. Disc perforation.
   b. Severe degenerative change.
   c. Late stage internal derangement.

DIAGNOSIS: Internal derangement with degenerative arthritis, both left and right TMJs, advanced stage. Right TMJ has a documented perforation.

TREATMENT:
1. Sagittal splint (Sagittal II appliance) - 8 months.
2. Transverse splint (Transverse appliance) - 6 months.
3. Orthopedic Corrector I - 6 months.
4. Retainer splint - Wear at night indefinitely (to prevent upper anterior teeth to returning to former position.)

RESULTS:
1. Terrible headaches eliminated.
2. Patient said, "I don't have headaches anymore."
   Patient said, "I feel good with my lower jaw biting forward."
3. No pain or problems.
4. Mary was examined and TMJs x-rayed, 6½ year post treatment.
   a. No headaches, pain or problems.
   b. Wears retainer when sleeping.
   c. Opening: 39½ mm.
      Left lateral: 11¼ mm.
      Right lateral: 12½ mm.
   d. TMJ x-rays showed condylar remodeling.
   e. TMJ x-rays showed condyles are no longer posterior-superior displaced.

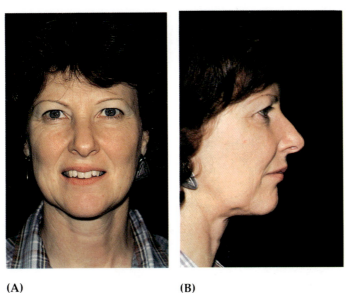

(A)   (B)

Figure 5–16   The Gothic arch trap. **(A and B)** Pretreatment facial views. **(C–E)**
Pretreatment models. **(F)** Note the Gothic arch appearance of the outline of the
maxillary arch that forces the slightly wider mandibular arch to close further
back to where upper and lower arch widths coincide, another form of the
NRDM/SPDC phenomenon (neuromuscular reflexive displacement of the
mandible causing superior posterior displacement of the condyles). **(G)**
Transcranial radiograph of the left TMJ before treatment. There is a 2.8-mm
posterior joint space at rest, but a 0.8-mm posterior joint space at full
intercuspation. **(H)** Tomogram of the right TMJ pretreatment at full intercuspal
occlusion. **(I)** Arthrogram with dye initially injected only into the lower
compartment of the right TMJ. Note how the dye has gone through the
perforation in the posterior attachment to fill the upper compartment (white). **(J)**
Sagittal II appliance to (1) move the front teeth forward out of the way of the
future advanced mandibular arc of closure and (2) act as a TMJ splint by virtue
of occlusal coverings of acrylic over the upper back teeth. **(K)** Next a transverse
appliance (splint) was used to develop the upper arch laterally. A wider upper
arch would allow eventual advancement of the currently wider lower arch and
still permit proper dental interdigitation of the upper posterior teeth with the
newly advanced lowers. Wire (cut at midline) on the appliance helps prevent the
newly advanced upper anteriors from relapsing in lingually again during the
transverse appliance phase of treatment. Acrylic coverings of the transverse
appliance help prevent TMJ pain and headaches in a splintlike fashion similar to
the action of the acrylic occlusal coverings of the sagittal (splint) appliance. **(L)**
The patient is wearing a splint and is free of TMJ pains or headaches. **(M)**
Orthopedic Corrector I (OCI) appliance to increase the vertical permanently and
reposition the mandible down and forward as per standard OCI technique. **(N)**
Mandatory HS (hour of sleep) bite guard and retainer worn at night only during

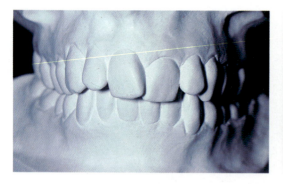

(C)

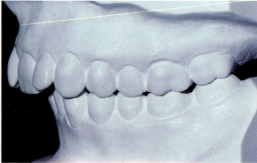

(D)

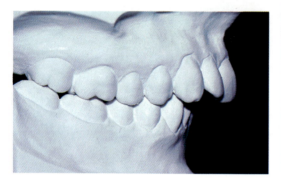

(E)

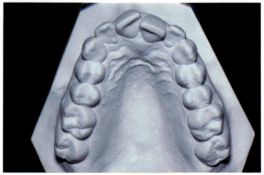

(F)

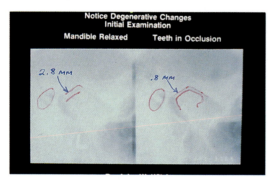

(G)

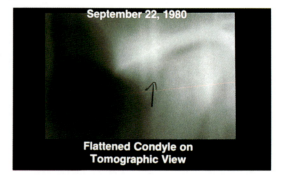

(H)

sleep indefinitely. **(O)** Six and one-half years posttreatment, on a transcranial radiograph, note the large posterior joint spaces as compared with pretreatment films. **(P)** At 6 ½ years posttreatment there are no myofascial pains, headaches, or TMJ problems. (Courtesy of Dr. John Witzig.)

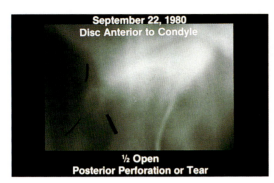

(I)

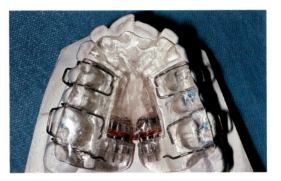

(J)

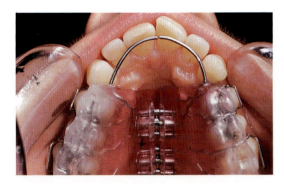

(K)

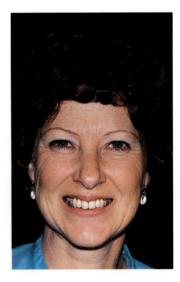

(L)

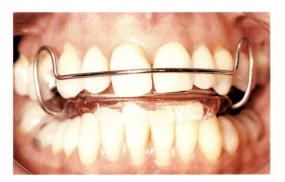

(M)

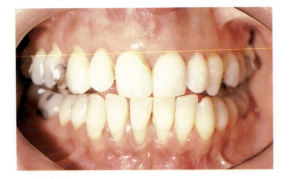

(N)

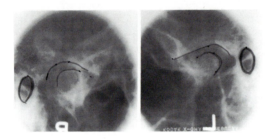

(O)

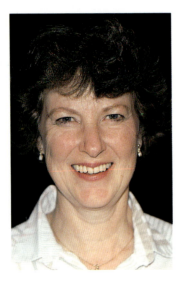

(P)

ward. They relapse back entirely on their own, sometimes with the most alarming rapidity. And it must also be remembered that there is an enhancement of that effect represented by the Bionator itself that follows the Sagittal II phase of treatment against which the lingual retention wire of the Bionator is only partially effective. Third, the use of lifetime night-only retainers are quickly becoming the rule of thumb for adult patients with TMJ problems who have had anterior development with Sagittal II appliances.

The Gothic Arch Trap

Closely associated with this first major group, i.e., the Sagittal II/ Bionator-type patient, is the patient requiring some form of preliminary lateral arch development, be it either equilateral or fan type. In the case of the need for fan-type development of the upper arch in the bicuspid region, the shape of the Gothic or pointed upper arch can of itself be a source of the NRDM/SPDC phenomenon since the mandible is forced back to a more distal and therefore wider part of the upper arch for proper interdigitation of its non-Gothic lower arch upon closing. In the pretreatment state this principle is easily seen by having the patients advance their mandibles forward to the "as if" position where the incisors are at or near end-to-end relationship. This puts the mandible orthopedically in the proposed posttreatment position similar to what it would be like at the end of the Bionator phase of treatment. With the arches in this relationship, one will observe that the upper bicuspids and maybe even mesial buccal cusps of the upper first molars of the narrower Gothic upper arch are in a buccal cusp tip-to-buccal cusp tip relationship to the lowers, a highly unstable and impossible functional relationship. Thus preliminary arch preparation consists of a 3- to 6-month active stint with a fan-type appliance of some sort to round out the arch. This will allow for proper intercuspation once the mandible is finally advanced out of its Class II retrusive position. Often fan-shaped upper arches have Division 1 angulated upper centrals. Therefore, proper adjustment of lingual acrylic and use of the labial bow retracts these flared-forward teeth nicely. Of course, one would want to avoid overretraction of the upper anteriors for fear of initiating any unwanted anterior incisal guidance of the mandibular arc of closure distally. The key point to remember here is that, as with anterior development with Sagittal II appliances, lateral development with either fan-type or Transverse appliances in the adult patient with TMJ problems mandates timely and adequate amounts of retention. This takes the form of a stabilizing period of continued appliance wear before going to the next appliance, slight amounts of overcorrection, and quite possibly perpetual use of retainers HS once treatment is completed. One must always keep in mind the difference between correction and develop-

CASE HISTORY

PATIENT: Age 20 years, 2 months

MAIN PROBLEM:
1. Frequent headaches.
2. Painful TM joints.

FINDINGS:
1. Severe, loud clicking in both TMJs.
2. Opening of 37 mm.
3. Class II occlusion.
4. Upper first bicuspid extractions, fixed appliances to close spaces, plus headgear.

RADIOGRAPHIC FINDINGS:
1. Left TMJ - Posterior superior displaced condyle.
                    - Bone spur.
                    - Degenerative bone changes.
2. Right TMJ - Posterior displaced condyle.
                    - Flattening of condyle.
                    - Bent-over condyle with advanced degenerative arthritis.

DIAGNOSIS: Internal derangement with advanced degenerative arthritis.

TREATMENT:
1. Upper sagittal splint (Sagittal II appliance) = eight months.
2. Orthopedic Corrector II appliance at home, upper sagittal splint at work = 1 year.
3. Upper Brackets - 3 months
4. Wore upper invisible retainer for 6 months, until 3–4 mm first bicuspid spaces were restored with bonding.

RESULTS:
1. No headaches.
2. 47.2 mm opening.
3. Left TMJ has some pain on wide opening.
4. No clicking.

Figure 5–17   Post–bicuspid extraction treatment of NRDM/SPDC. **(A and B)** Pretreatment facial view of a 20-year-old TMJ pain-dysfunction patient with a history of upper bicuspid extraction and headgear treatment. **(C and D)** Transcranial radiography reveals bilateral degenerative bone changes with a bone spur (osteophyte) on the left condyle and flattened, bent-over right condyle. Both condyles are posteriorly displaced. **(E and F)** Pretreatment models, note the retrusion and vertical angulation of the upper anteriors. Occlusion of the teeth in such a bite as this generates the NRDM/SPDC phenomenon. Notice that the previous orthodontic treatment left the patient finished in dental and (as the joints revealed) skeletal class II. **(G)** The Sagittal II appliance serves two functions: (1) screw activation moves the front teeth forward as per standard

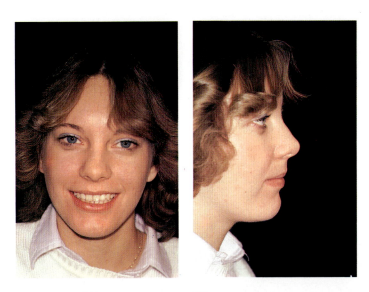

Figure 5–17(A)   (B)

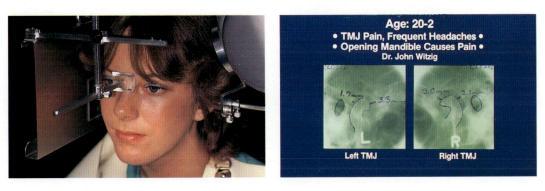

(C)   (D)

Sagittal II techniques, and (2) occlusal acrylic pads produce a splint effect to relieve headaches and TMJ pains. This appliance is also referred to as a "sagittal splint" when used in patients with TMJ problems to stress the pain-relieving splinting effect of the occlusal acrylic pads. **(H)** Note how occlusal coverings of the appliance prevent full closure of the teeth. **(I)** Sagittal appliance in the mouth. **(J)** Since the vertical dimension of occlusion was adequate prior to treatment, an Orthopedic Corrector II appliance was selected by virtue of that appliance's ability to advance the mandible without increasing the vertical. **(K)** Note the interocclusal acrylic pads of the appliance that prevent the supraeruption of the upper and lower posterior teeth that would result in increased vertical. **(L)** The mandible is advanced through muscular retraining of

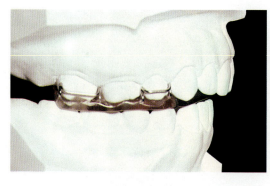

(E)

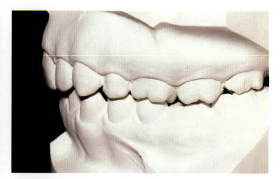

(F)

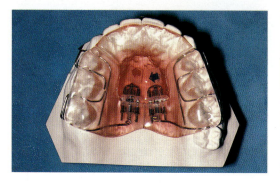

(G)

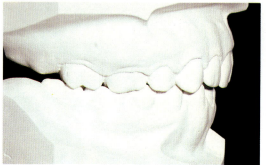

(H)

the class II neuromuscular sling in stepwise increments of advancement as per usual Orthopedic Corrector technique; as the screws are opened, the lower acrylic is relieved to allow the lower teeth and mandible to advance in an unobstructed fashion. **(M)** Straight-wire bonded brackets used for 3 months to level, align, and rotate the teeth. **(N)** Patient 6 months after removal of the brackets. **(O)** Notice the spaces in the first bicuspid area after moving the front six teeth forward (out of the way). **(P)** Spaces closed by bonding on the mesial portion of the second bicuspids. **(Q and R)** Facial views 6 months past treatment. Note the fuller facial profile as compared with the pretreatment profile due to advanced mandibular position. HS maxillary arch retainers are a safeguard against posttreatment lingual migration of upper anteriors. (Courtesy of Dr. John Witzig.)

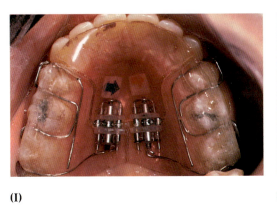

(I)

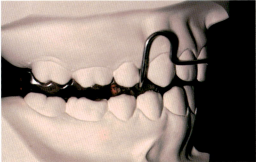

(J)

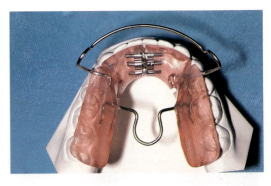

(K)

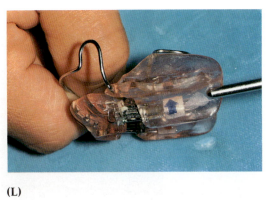

(L)

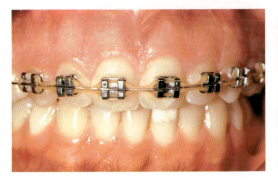

(M)

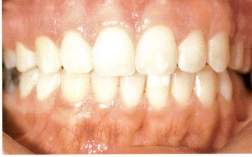

(N)

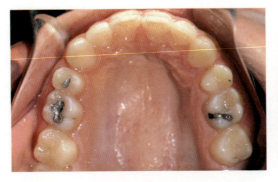

(O)

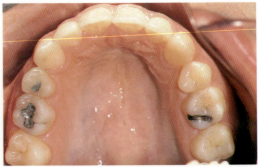

(P)

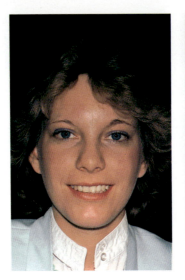

(Q)

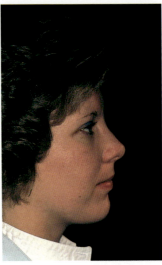

(R)

ment and remember that development means retention.

A second major category of patients who may be treated for their TMJ problems with FJO technique are those who have had a previous history of orthodontic therapy involving the extraction of four bicuspids. Even though the posttreatment arches are smaller and orthopedically retropositioned, they are still in fairly good arch form as a result of the previous orthodontic treatment. Of course, the mandible is retruded, and the effects of the NRDM/SPDC phenomenon, due to the anterior incisal interference represented by the condensed anterior segments, are in full force. This represents the major problem that the patients face in the operation of their stomatognathic system. In these types of cases the first appliance of choice is almost universally the Sagittal II. Since the arch form is usually good to start with and since the upper cuspids are usually retracted somewhat as a result of the mechanics required to close the bicuspid spaces, an important little modification is made to the Sagittal II appliance. Small-wire finger springs are placed distal to the upper cuspids so that as the appliance expands and moves the anterior teeth forward the cuspid support wires move forward also (because they are embedded in the anterior third of the appliance), thereby helping the cuspids keep pace with the advancement of the rest of the anteriors. This allows the anterior segment to be advanced as a unit, helps reduce the chances of excessive diastema formation between the upper anteriors, and allows the space to appear instead between the distal part of the cuspid and mesial portion of the remaining bicuspid. Here, around on the sides of the upper dental arch, aesthetics are much less of a problem. Also the space can easily be closed by a variety of operative methods, depending on the size of the space. It is seldom a space that causes serious concern for patients suffering from chronic TMJ myofascial pain. Even if left untreated, a small space between a cuspid and bicuspid doesn't bother them. Painful headaches do. As with other types of patients for which anterior development is required, stabilizing periods before Bionator insertion, slight overcorrection, and what are jocularly referred to as "pajamas for the teeth," or HS retainer usage, helps prevent relapse lingually once the treatment is complete. However, it has been observed that there appears to be less of a problem with upper anteriors relapsing lingually in patients who have had traditional four-bicuspid extraction–oriented orthodontics. It's as if the anterior segments are more content to remain in their newly regained advanced position. It is theorized that the "perioral muscle tension brace," as Bimler calls it, is less offended by such actions because the advanced teeth are merely being brought "home" to their original pretreatment position, which they happily occupied before being overretracted in the hapless effort to close the space of a man-made bicuspid extraction site! However, caution should always be exercised in the form of HS retainer availability. This case scenario takes on more of the aspects of *correction* as opposed to development.

The third, newest, and most highly controversial method of applying FJO technique to TMJ pain-dysfunction patients involves the previously mentioned technique of extraction of a lower central incisor. In cases where the occlusion and the orthopedics are such that the patient is very "tight," i.e., the upper incisors are quite steep, and a lower central incisor or lateral is crowded forward, the functionally high interincisal angle and the crowded forward lower anterior incisors combine to create an anterior incisal guidance or interference upon full occlusion to initiate the NRDM/SPDC phenomenon. In this specific example, however, although several factors might well be responsible, the crowded-forward, lower central incisor is as guilty a culprit as any. Extracting it can help the patient both from an orthopedic standpoint and an orthodontic standpoint in a variety of surprising ways! It also is a most sound application of the compromises grouped together under the notion of directional decrowding.

First and foremost, extracting a crowded lower anterior eliminates one of the critical agents in the action of the anterior incisal interference that is responsible for deflecting the mandible back upon closure. With the offending lower central (or sometimes it's a lateral, but the effect is the same) out of the way, the mandible is no longer forced posteriorly upon closure due to an inclined plane action of the offending lower incisor against the lingual surfaces of the uppers. Second, it relieves the crowding in the lower anterior area via reciprocal space closure, and realignment with basic fixed appliance–type technique (full-arch power chain) aligns the three remaining incisors very nicely between the cuspids for a greatly improved aesthetic result. Third, the resultant lower anterior arch is condensed lingually and is somewhat smaller after the three remaining teeth are realigned into the extraction site, and in effect the mandibular *dental* arch becomes shortened on the AP plane. This correspondingly allows the mandible to be advanced in efforts to decompress the joint without the lower anteriors immediately colliding with the uppers in final closure.

There are other very important advantages to this technique also, not so much in areas of what must be done, but ironically in areas of what does not have to be done. First, if the amount of artifically created overjet is great enough after the offending lower incisor has been extracted and the remaining three teeth "straightened" and if the upper anteriors are perchance far enough forward "out of the way" to permit proceeding directly to the Bionator phase of treatment, the entire Sagittal II phase of treatment and its lingering penchant for relapse may be avoided. This is, of course, predicated on the fact that the space available, i.e., that overjet resulting from the extraction and lingual condensation of the lower front teeth, is great enough orthodontically to permit the mandible to be advanced far enough orthopedically to properly reposition the condyle so as to eliminate clicking and TMJ-type headache pain. Experimenting with the "as if" position in the usual manner at times may indicate if such is possible. Transcranial radiography may also be used. If it is, avoidance of the Sagittal II phase of treatment greatly enhances the stability of the case and obviates the need for the perpetual use of an HS retainer. If not enough space for forward advancement of the mandible results from this lower incisor extraction technique, it may still be used in combination with accompanying Sagittal II technique on the uppers to pick up the difference. This also would then mean that the uppers need not be advanced as far labially as they would have to be if the Sagittal II technique were used alone. But it must be remembered that this technique works best when lower *crowding* is present in the incisor region and one of those lowers is crowded out labially. Thus it may be seen that in the future, aligning the midlines anteriorly can have a dual meaning. For some patients it might mean vertical alignment of the embrasure between the upper centrals with that of the lower centrals. Yet for others it could mean the vertical alignment of the embrasure between the upper centrals with the exact dead center of the clinical crown of the middle one of the three remaining incisors. Aesthetically, it is a result far more pleasing to the eye than are four teeth that are crowded. Physiologically, it is a result far more pleasing to the body than chronic headache, neck ache, and myofascial pains are. But there is more.

The final phenomenon to be mentioned here may also be categorized as yet another "thing that might not have to be done" when using the lower incisor extraction technique and turns out to be the most surprising of all. In fact, it might just be the most stunning finding elucidated in this entire series of texts. It is that of the aforementioned autoadvancement of the trapped mandible after lower incisor extraction, even without the aid of a Bionator! After treating a number of cases of this type, Dr. John Witzig discovered that about 75% of the time the mandible will autoadvance just enough over a period of months, after condensing the "three-incisor" lower arch, to allow just enough decompression of the joints to eliminate TMJ-type symptoms! This phenomenon is predicated on the existence of adequate vertical dimension and severe crowding in the lower anterior region so as to cause a lower incisor to be quite well labially blocked out. After a 3-month period of "muscle prepping" with the Witzig splint, the lower "crowded-forward" incisor is extracted, the remaining teeth realigned, and the lower anterior arch correspondingly shortened and ultimately condensed with fixed appliances. A conventional straight-wire or similar type appliance with an elastic power chain is all that is required to close the space in 4 to 8 months' time. The crowns tip into the empty space first, followed by uprighting of the roots secondarily. But once the offending tooth is removed, due to the muscle preparation effected by the 3-month stint with the Witzig splint and because of the newly available artificially created "reverse" overjet resultant of the lower arch condensation, the trapped mandible has the possibility of

CASE HISTORY

PATIENT: Age 14 years, 8 months

MAIN PROBLEM:
1. TMJ Pain.
2. Headaches.

DENTAL HISTORY: Pain started during orthodontic treatment in a Minneapolis orthodontic office. Patient wore Class III elastics during orthodontic treatment, to move the mandible back. Patient also wore mid-line correction elastics.

After patient finished her orthodontic treatment and was suffering pain and headaches, her mother, being a general dentist in Minneapolis, treated Carla with splint treatment. This eliminated the TMJ pain and headaches as long as the splint was worn.

The mother then asked Dr. Witzig to finish the treatment, so her daughter would not have to wear a splint for the remainder of her life.

FINDINGS:
1. Opening - 36½ mm.
2. By removing the flat plane splint, the mandible closure was in a forward position.
3. Painful TMJs.
4. Incisal interference.
5. Incisal misguidance.

RADIOGRAPHIC FINDINGS:
1. Right TMJ
   a. Posterior displaced condyle
   b. Bone spur on condyle where external pterygoid muscle attaches.
   c. Degenerative arthritis changes of condyle.
   d. Compressed posterior joint space.
2. Left TMJ
   a. Posterior-superior displaced condyle.
   b. Bent-over condyle.
   c. Compressed posterior-superior joint space.

DIAGNOSIS: Incisal interference (misguidance) causing internal derangement of both TMJs (NRDM/SPDC).

TREATMENT:
1. Flat plane splint (by patient's mother) to relieve pain.
2. Lower incisor removal, straight wire appliance on lowers to close space and retract anterior teeth.
3. Lower retainer - 6 months.

RESULTS:
1. No headaches or pain.
2. Does not wear any splints or appliances.
3. Mandible bites in a more forward position than previously (due to autoadvancement and elimination of anterior incisal interference or the NRDM/SPDC phenomenon).

THREE YEARS AFTER RETENTION:
1. No headaches.
2). No pain

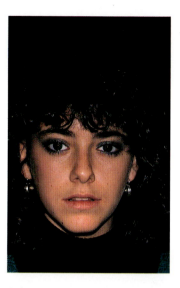

(A)

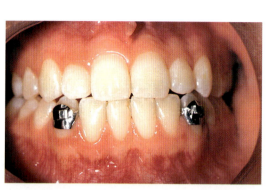

(B)

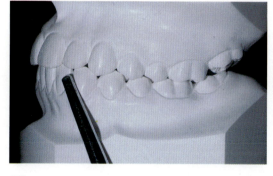

(C)

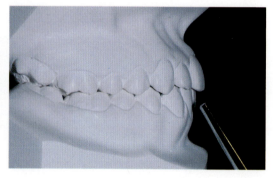

(D)

Figure 5–18   Lower incisor extraction and mandibular autoadvancement. **(A)** Pretreatment. **(B)** After completion of previous orthodontic treatment with class III elastics. Note the tight incisal interference. **(C and D)** Pretreatment models (after previous orthodontics and Class III elastics). The maxillary anteriors are already torqued forward at or slightly past the cephalometric limits. Incisal interference with the mandibular arc of closure initiates NRDM/SPDC. **(E and F)** Transcranial radiographs showing joint compression and degeneration. **(G)** Maxillary Witzig splint. **(H)** Brackets to close the spaces after extraction of the lower central incisor. This also condenses the remaining lower anteriors back lingually. **(I)** Lower retainer. **(J)** Mandibular arch after space closure. **(K)** Completed case, mandible autoadvanced without the benefit of the Bionator/OCI phase of treatment once the NRDM/SPDC phenomenon was eliminated. **(L)** Three years posttreatment, there are no signs or symptoms of TMJ problems. (Courtesy of Dr. John Witzig.)

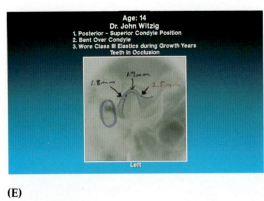

(E)

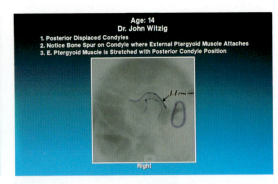

(F)

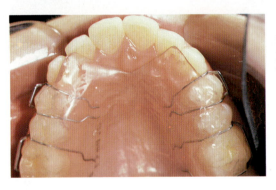

(G)

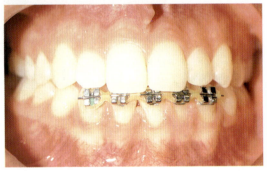

(H)

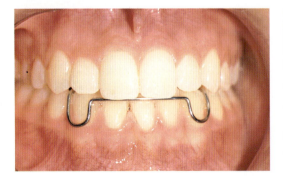

(I)

(J)

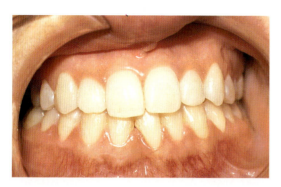

(K)

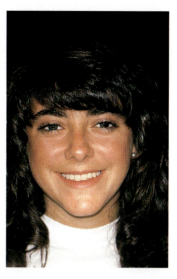

(L)

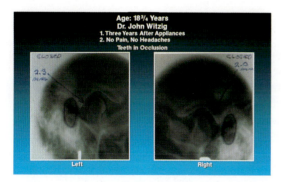

(M)

bringing itself forward on its own. Evidently there is enough leeway in the Class II neuromuscular sling in a certain number of individuals to permit the minimal amounts of autoadvancement necessary to decompress the joint and relieve the patient's TMJ symptoms. If these avant-garde procedures are not enough on their own to effect the desired result, one can always reenlist the more conventional services of the Bionator to finish the job. Using the "as if" position prior to initiation of treatment will sometimes aid in determining whether enough room would exist for autoadvancement with the upper incisors in their pretreatment state. However, it must be noted that this may not always serve as a completely reliable guide. The point in all this is that there appears to be a large percentage of posteriorly locked mandibles that have a limited ability to spring forward on their own once the anterior incisal guidance that ultimately forces them back is removed. This makes the business of advancing the mandible and retraining the Class II neuromuscular sling all the easier if and when Bionators or Orthopedic Correctors are employed in efforts to decompress compromised TMJs. Nature often seems to want to tell us what is needed by Her actions. If only we will listen!

Round-Tripping

This point cannot be overstressed. Hence it bears repetition. For all its greatness as a technique for solving the complex problems of functionally induced TMJ arthrosis, the discipline of FJO is not without its own share of attending problems. The biggest problem that arises when the technique is used to treat an adult patient with TMJ problems is that of "round-tripping." At its most basic of levels, FJO treatments for TMJ pain-dysfunction patients generally consist of first preparing the maxillary arch in such a fashion that it no longer deflects the mandible posteriorly. This is followed by deliverance of the now-unlocked mandible to a mandibular arc of closure and state of final occlusion that locks the mandible/condyle unit down and forward in a more orthopedically and physiologically correct location. Yet the appliances used in the second phase of this scenario have a tendency, by virtue of their design, to effect the unwanted trait of constricting the anterior portions of the maxillary arch back in lingually again. This, of course, is undesirable in a case where, say for example, the upper anteriors have just been pushed forward in a "Class II, Division 2 effect–type" case of anterior incisal interference (NRDM/SPDC). The lateral development of the maxillary arch seems to hold fairly well in adults once the Bionator/OCI appliance is inserted because these devices by virtue of their design naturally resist lateral arch collapse. But the same cannot be said for holding the newly gained development of the arch anteriorly. True, the snug fit of the lingual "retention" wire of the Bionator/Orthopedic Corrector appliance resists the drift of the upper anteriors back in lingually again. Nevertheless, some modicum of relapse in a lingual direction of newly advanced upper anterior teeth during functional appliance advancement of the mandible is unfortunately inevitable. Yet measures may be taken by the treating clinician to keep this untoward action, which is especially petulant in adults, to a minimum.

First and foremost, patients must eat with the active-plate appliance that precedes the functional appliance phase. Function is the key to much of what is accomplished by the FJO method, and eating is the prime intention for which the stomatognathic system with all its components is designed. Full-time wear of the active plate, be it Sagittal II, Transverse, fan, or whatever, in conjunction with eating with the appliance in the mouth obtains the best results from Nature and appears to "really help sock in" the teeth in their new, advanced (or widened) locations. Wearing the appliance all the time and *not* eating with it allows the teeth to be moved also, but they appear more mobile (unstable) in their new locations as treatment progresses. They also appear to relapse much more quickly than do teeth moved under the additional functional stimuli of mastication. It must be remembered that part of Nature's design intent for the stomatognathic system is to be able to adapt to the demands of function, specifically *masticatory* function. It is commonly known from decades of observations of teeth being moved with fixed appliances that the best (healthiest) way to move a tooth with a brace, i.e., the best way to prevent walking a tooth through an alveolar cortical plate or causing a labial gingival dehiscence, is to move that tooth under naturally occurring steady function—and that means tooth-to-tooth masticatory function. Tooth-to-acrylic bite pad masticatory function amounts to the same thing as far as Nature is concerned. Dr. Albert Wiebrecht, George Crozat's chief disciple, was right when he said, "Function is our greatest ally."

Other methods of combating a relapse of anteriorly developed upper incisors during mandibular advancement mechanics is to be sure that the lingual wire of the Bionator/OCI is snug against the cingula of the teeth. Some clinicians are fond of having this wire processed into the appliance with little helical loops bent into the wire where it comes out of the body acrylic of the appliance so that the wire may be adjusted to just the right tension so as to impart a gentle but adequate force to the upper incisors in a labial direction. Cutting the lingual retention wire at the midline is another way to accomplish this, although such methods offer less versatility to this type of adjustment. In this technique only the free ends of the cut wire are movable. The wire still remains fixed where it comes out of the acrylic. Of course, both methods could be combined by cutting a lingual wire at its midline that has helical loops bent into it at its exit points out of the appliance.

As with any arch development technique, slight overcorrection in the active-plate arch preparation phase of treatment to compensate for such impending relapse is also indicated here. The fear of overdevelopment of upper anteriors labially is unrealistic since in the adult patient the upper front teeth almost invariably want to relapse back in lingually again once the appliance is withdrawn. In adult orthodontic/TMJ problems, moving the teeth out too far labially is not the vexing issue; it's keeping them there. This brings us to our final point. Once the mandible has been adequately advanced and the mandible/condyle unit is relocated and locked down and forward where it should be, lifetime night-only (HS) retainers are all but mandatory. Patients accommodate to a lifetime of other health care augmentation devices such as glasses, hearing aids, or pacemakers. The streamlined little "sleep-only" maxillary retainers designed to keep upper front teeth far enough forward (or upper back teeth far enough sideways) to keep the "big MAC," the mandibular arc of closure, free to operate forward in joint-structure–dictated fashion are the easiest of all such devices to accommodate to. Should any excessive anterior maxillary arch development remain at this point (once mandibular advancement is adequate), a controlled relapse may be allowed to gradually take place without retainers until the desired location of these teeth is reached and the holding action of night-only retention once again becomes necessary.

The worst-case scenario is that in the middle of a treatment segment with a Bionator/OCI to advance the mandible/condyle unit and increase the posterior vertical dimension, the lingual (or lateral) relapse will become manifested enough to require cessation of the functional appliance phase of arch alignment and force a return to the arch preparation (development anteriorly and/or laterally) active-plate phase of treatment. This does not happen regularly, but if it does in a given case, so be it. Such things can tax the clinical judgment and occasionally fool even the most experienced of clinicians. Knowledge that such phenomena occur, careful planning and preparation, and timely monitoring of the patient during treatment help keep such problems to a minimum.

Figure 5–19 **(A)** Cutting the lingual retention wire of the Bionator/OCI allows for active pressure to be applied to the lingual surfaces of recently advanced upper anteriors to combat the strong tendency for lingual relapse. **(B)** Bonded lingual upper cuspid-to-cuspid retainers may prove useful during the Bionator/OCI phase of treatment. Distal extensions off the cuspid bonding metal pad brace against the mesial portion of the bicuspids and hold the front six teeth forward but do not prohibit eruption of the bicuspids vertically. The lingual retention wire on the Bionator/OCI then becomes redundant and must be removed. **(C)** The simple Hawley retainer worn HS may well be the symbol of lifelong defense against lingual relapse of the upper anterior teeth and a recurrence of NRDM/SPDC-type TMJ problems. (Courtesy of the Ohlendorf Co, St Louis.)

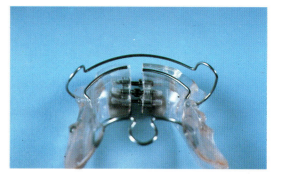

Figure 5–19(A)

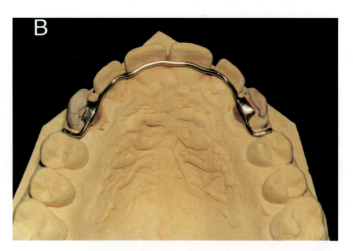

(B)

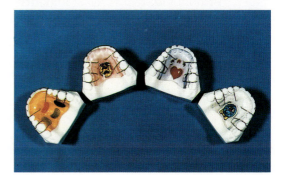

(C)

One exception to this process that is observed with a modicum of frequency is the treatment of the aforementioned post–four-bicuspid extraction, orthodontic-type TMJ cases. Sometimes the upper anteriors will "stick" fairly well after advancement. This is because they are merely being returned to their original (and correct) "genetic osseous beds" anyway. But if there is any doubt whatsoever that stability is anything but ensured, HS retention should be employed. This applies to cases of lateral development as well as anterior development.

Sometimes the resolution of the problem merely revolves around increasing the posterior vertical and advancing the mandible down the lingual slope of the extant anterior arch with or without the correction of a rotation or lingually verted upper central or lateral. In such cases HS retainers may not be needed.

In light of the above, it may now be seen why there are advantages to the technique involving extraction of the labially crowded forward lower central or lateral incisor. Condensing the remaining three incisors into the already diminutive lower anterior arch space in effect condenses the lower anterior teeth back lingually (as well as give the appearance of "straight teeth"). This artificially creates the liberating overjet between the upper and lower anterior arches that allows mandibular advancement to proceed unobstructed by anterior incisal interferences. The uppers remain untouched, stable in their muscularly and physiologically neutral (stable) location. This obviates the problem of combating incessant lingual relapse of upper anteriors with HS retainers.

But sometimes circumstances are not favorable for the lower incisor extraction method, and compromises in the form of maxillary arch development laterally and/or anteriorly must be made. This is not a reflection of failure of the system, as some of its detractors would like to believe, but merely represents the circumstances of Nature that prevail. It has oft been stated in this series of texts that diagnosis and treatment planning in orthodontic/TMJ cases is a matter of determining and directly addressing the patient's orthodontic (occlusion) and orthopedic (TMJ) needs. Sometimes those needs include prolonged or even lifetime periods of "pajamas for the teeth," i.e., HS retainers. It's a small price to pay indeed for a headache-free life.

"Do you hear the children weeping,
Oh my brothers,
Ere the sorrow comes with years?
But the child's sob in the silence curses
deeper,
Than the strong man in his wrath."

"The Cry of the Children"
Elizabeth Barrett Browning, 1806–1861
English poetess

PEDIATRIC TMJ CONDITIONS

One of the more astounding and disturbing findings to come out of clinical practice in recent years has been the discovery of a high incidence of functionally induced TMJ problems in the pediatric patient. A surprising number of children in the 9- to 11-year-old age group will exhibit classic TMJ symptomatology similar to those of the adolescent and adult. Although clicking in the usual sense may be present, the clicking of the joints that these young patients are more likely to exhibit is not as profound as that of the older patient. Instead of a sharp crack, click, or pop of the condylar head traversing over the heel of the disc into the central concavity, a more muffled sound is detected. It often requires the use of the most acute stethoscopic technique and may sound more like a mere audiosensation of motion. This type of clicking can be detected in children as young as 5 years of age. As with the more mature joint, pediatric joints simply should not make noise. When they do, the joint sounds almost invariably indicate improper internal joint relationships. However, joint sounds may not necessarily be present when other common TMJ symptoms of headache, neck ache, myofascial pain, and muscle tenderness to palpation are present. The young joints have not always developed enough to exhibit an audible click. But they are always developed enough to suffer the pains of posterior condylar displacement if the occlusion up front is sufficient to initiate routine NRDM/SPDC-type mandibular retrusion.

The history of headache becomes an extremely important and revealing finding in dealing with the pediatric TMJ patient. Such findings carry great diagnostic weight for a number of reasons. First, the joints of these patients are still quite underdeveloped from an osteological standpoint, and as a result their lack of calcification makes routine imaging with conventional transcranial projection techniques difficult. Tomographic techniques are often required for better evaluation of condyle-fossa relationships. Second, the findings of headaches in the younger child are strongly indicative of functionally induced TMJ problems because most of the other general systemic problems have already been ruled out. Young children receive a higher degree of medical attention due to the concern of parents for fulfilling the requirements of good post-natal care. General medical evaluations are required prior to entering school; for participation in school athletics, gym class, etc.; and for proper maintenance of immunization records. Chances are that any general systemic pathology that could be responsible for recurrent headaches and neck aches would have been previously diagnosed prior to the patient's orthodontic/TMJ evaluation. It is therefore reasonably safe to assume that if no other general medical problems exist in the young child who complains of recurring headaches, functionally induced TMJ problems related to the occlusion may be considered the chief etiological agent until proved otherwise! Headaches will be the chief complaint of the patient. They usually are temporal, emanating from the origins of the anterior portion of the temporalis muscle. They may not be as frequent an occurrence as those of the adult, and it may take careful questioning of both the child and his or her parents to uncover such a history. Without meaning to, parents may at times be indifferent to the complaints of young children concerning headaches. Often the parent feels that such complaints are merely the result of the child being tired or in need of a little extra attention. Incidentally, it has been observed that if the child fabricates a complaint of a physical malady for the sake of attention and psychological stroking, he usually complains of stomachaches, not headaches. Often, the parent will assume the child's complaints of headaches are a result of a need for eyeglasses. Sometimes unfortunately, adults simply do not believe the complaints until they become persistent enough that the parent truly believes that something is wrong. However, often this only signals the beginnings of more problems to come for the child and parent.

When headache complaints become severe enough, seeking medical attention is usually the first and, for the well-meaning parent, most logical course of action to pursue. Physical examinations with family physicians, blood and urine tests, neurological evaluations, otolaryngological evaluations, ophthalmic examinations, and even sophisticated imaging procedures such as computer-activated tomography (CAT scans) or magnetic resonance imaging (MRI) procedures may be employed. And through all this, the frail and often frightened child bravely follows the bidding of the adults in charge. The failure to detect a culpable etiological agent in all this can bring about high levels of frustration for the clinician and increases the emotional burdens of fear and worry in both the parent and the child. Wellsprings of complete and total faith in the ability of the adults in their lives to properly care for them, the young child suffering from TMJ problems bravely and hopefully endures the ordeal of such investigations and ends up confronting their painful condition with resigned acceptance. Resigned acceptance may be acceptable for the helpless patient and the troubled parent, but in light of what we now know concerning the diagnosis and treatment of this condition, it is inexcusable for the treating clinician.

Along with careful recording of the history and anamnesis of these patients, examination should also include the usual auscultation of the joints during opening and closing as well as the usual simple muscle palpation procedures. Children with functional TMJ problems often exhibit muscle tenderness to palpation in the area of the third and fourth cervical vertebrae. They may also occasionally complain of earaches, although temporal and/or frontal headaches are by far the chief complaint. Due to the tremendous vitality of the growing young tissues, muscle tenderness to palpation may not be quite as acute as that of adults. When it is, the TMJ condition (and the headache pain) is usually quite severe.

The joints should also be imaged in some fashion. Compressed joint spaces and even condylar flattening and other regressive remodeling changes can be detected. The minor arthritic degenerative changes of the condylar head that might be present often require tomographic imaging to detect. But due to the "green" and growing characteristics of the condylar head at this young age, treatment of the usual variety that unlocks the condyle, advances the mandible, and increases the vertical results in complete repair of the damaged osseous components of the joint in as little as 6 to 12 months. The same basic principles of joint kinematics apply to the pediatric joint as they do to the adult joint with the exception that the pediatric joint has an enormous capacity to heal itself once the distal-driving occlusion is eliminated and the joint is properly decompressed. The unbounded growth potential of early youth is a tremendous ally.

The occlusion of the pediatric patient is analyzed in the same manner as that of the adult. Anything that could act as a source of locking occlusion or posterior deflection of the mandible must be corrected. This includes retroclined upper anteriors with or without accompanying deep overbite. Severe anterior rotations, which may indicate anterior incisal interference problems with lower anteriors, or any other combination of maxillary skeletal and/or dental retrusion might combine with any form of mandibular dental protrusion to result in the initiation of the NRDM/ SPDC phenomenon. The maxillary posterior crossbite is also an indication of a high likelihood of damage to the young joint. This relationship is so consistently observed that it has prompted one nationally known orthodontist and TMJ authority to state, "Show me a posterior crossbite, and I'll show you a damaged joint!"[38]

The disadvantage of not always being able to obtain an ideal image of the joint by conventional transcranial methods in very young TMJ pain-dysfunction patients is more than compensated for by the advantage of how rapidly these patients respond to simple joint decompression– type treatments! The advantage in this, of course, is that if the clinician is uncertain of his diagnosis of functionally induced TMJ arthrosis in the pe-

Figure 5–20 Pediatric TMJ condition. This 11-year-old girl had a history of frequent TMJ-type headaches and "tired jaw muscles" for over a year. No clicking existed in the TMJs yet. Transcranial radiographs showed slightly compressed superior and posterior joint spaces. Steep angulation of the upper anteriors and the high interincisal angle in the pretreatment state were strongly indicative of anterior incisal interference trapping the mandible back too far upon closure (NRDM/SPDC) and causing condylar compression in the joint. Treatment consisted merely of several months of Sagittal II appliance activation to move the upper anteriors forward out of the way. The appliance was then worn as its own retainer and as a TMJ splint for about 6 months afterward. The mandible autoadvanced without the use of further appliance treatment. The patient noticed relief of TMJ symptoms and headaches the first week of appliance wear. "I can feel the pressure is gone back by my ears already," she said after the second day of wearing the Sagittal II (splint) appliance. **(A)** The pretreatment profile appears normal. **(B)** Pretreatment occlusion. Note the tightness of the anterior incisal interference. **(C and D)** Pretreatment transcranial view at bite and rest positions. At the bite position the superior joint space is 2.5 mm in the right joint, 2.0 mm in the left joint. **(E and F)** Pretreatment occlusion exhibits a tight anterior incisal interference that forces the mandible back. **(G)** Insertion of the Sagittal II (splint) appliance. **(H)** Note how the acrylic pads of the appliance help "splint" the occlusion open. This provides relief of TMJ and facial muscle pains and headaches. **(I)** Appliance opened, upper anteriors moved forward. **(J)** Note the increased overjet due to appliance advancement of the upper anteriors. **(K)** The mandible autoadvanced once the occlusion unlocked, and once again the lower anteriors are coupled with the uppers. **(L)** Sometimes the amount of advancement of the upper anteriors needed to unlock a distal-driving occlusion is not great. **(M)** Posttreatment right TMJ with a superior joint space of 3.0 mm. **(N)** Posttreatment left TMJ with a superior joint space of 2.7 mm—all entirely due to autoadvancement. **(O)** Pretreatment Steiner cephalometric analysis. **(P)** Posttreatment Steiner cephalometric analysis 5 months later. Note that with only a millemeter or so of condylar autoadvancement in the back the amount of change cephalometrically in the front is difficult to detect because the change there is not great. However, note the change in the interincisal angle and the angle of the upper central to the NA line; this indicates forward movement of the upper anteriors "out of the way." Pretreatment vs. posttreatment values were as follows: WITS, 0.7 vs. 0.9 mm; 1 to NA distance, 3.7 vs. 3.2 mm; 1 to NA angle, 11.9 vs. 19.3 degrees; interincisal angle, 147 vs. 134.5 degrees; ANB angle, 2.5 vs. 2.9 degrees; SNB angle, 77.5 vs. 78.3 degrees. 1 = upper central incisor. (Courtesy of Dr. T.J. Spahl, St. Paul, Minn.)

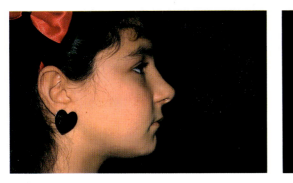

Figure 5–20(A)

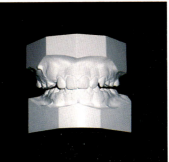

(B)

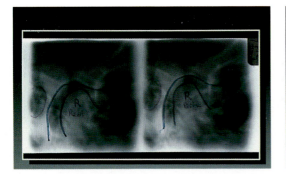

(C)

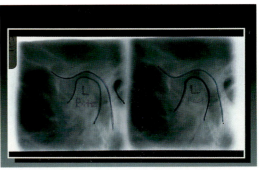

(D)

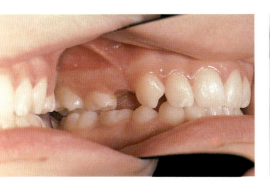

(E)

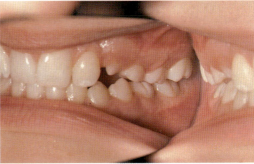

(F)

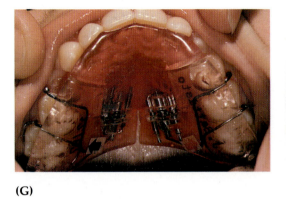

(G)

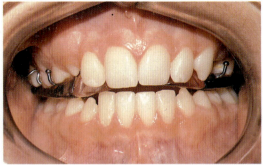

(H)

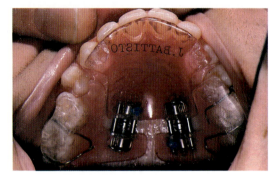

(I)

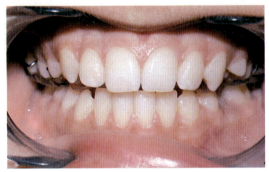

(J)

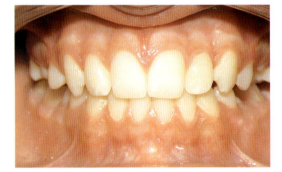

(K)

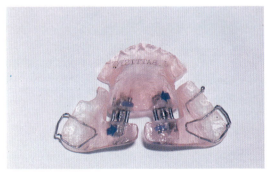

(L)

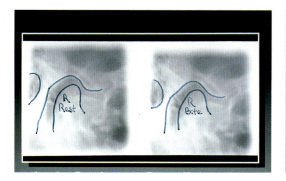

(M)

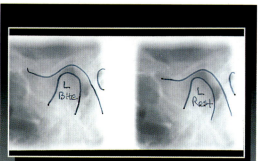

(N)

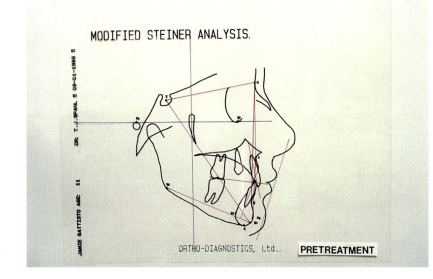

(O)

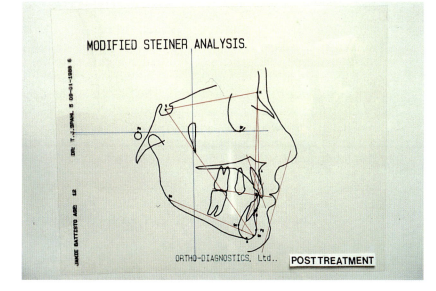

(P)

diatric patient, the construction and insertion of a simple balanced flat-plane splint of either the Sears pivotal or Witzig type soon settles the issue. Such palliative procedures will produce dramatic relief for the more severely involved pediatric patient in as little as 24 to 48 hours! The young growing mandible is figuratively "begging" to be freed from its locking and/or distal-driving occlusion. Once that freedom is effected by the intervening acrylic pads of a splint or initial active-plate–type orthodontic appliance such as the Sagittal II, the mandible all but "springs" forward on its own. The resultant joint decompression that this represents, as slight as it may be, is all that Nature needs to get on with the pain-free business of making bones, joints, ligaments, and muscles grow in a physiologically and biomechanically balanced fashion once again. The resilience of the younger patient is nothing short of amazing. Nature is kind in that She routinely "stacks the physiological deck" in favor of Her little ones.

It will be commonly observed in pediatric patients of this type that once interferring upper anteriors are cleared out of the way in an anterior direction, the mandible will autoadvance out of its posterior state of retrusion. Of course, major structural Class II mandibular retrusions and deep overbites will have to be delivered via conventional Bionator technique once the usual arch preparation procedures have been accomplished. But all this being equal, quite often the Sagittal II appliance will be all that is needed to correct a pediatric TMJ case. The forward movement it imparts to the upper anteriors is often all that is needed to allow inhibited natural growth forces to decompress the joint. The acrylic bite pads of the Sagittal appliance will also effect rapid and dramatic relief of the patient's symptoms while treatment is being rendered.

The Class II, Division 1 malocclusion in the very young patient in the mixed dentition stage of development can also be a source of TMJ problems. The "Gothic arch effect" must be considered here. The upper arch can become constricted laterally and pointed in the anterior incisor area, and this results in the classic Gothic arch outline of the upper teeth. This is often the result of airway constriction and related breathing problems. The narrower Gothic upper arch cannot accommodate the normal Roman arch–shaped lower dentition at the proper arch-to-arch (i.e., maxilla-to-mandible) AP relationship because in this state the transarch width at a given point on the upper arch is narrower than the corresponding transarch width of the lower arch. The only way the upper arch can accommodate the lower arch is if the lower arch moves farther back to a wider part of the upper. This is in fact what happens, and the trapped mandible functions too far posteriorly, which results in posterior condylar displacement. Correction of the upper arch outline to a wider, more proper Roman arch shape facilitates and encourages mandibular advancement and proper AP alignment orthopedically. This, of course, is what is needed for the compressed joint.

The ease at which the child's symptoms may be ameliorated with even the simplest of splints makes the aggressive pursuit of complaints of recurring headaches with these techniques one of the most gratifying aspects of all FJO. Child or adult, the same basic joint kinematics takes place in both, and the same fundamental treatment methods apply. When upper anteriors are advanced, they should be overcorrected slightly and/or properly retained to prevent excessive unwanted relapse lingually. When the occlusion is cleared, if the mandible does not spring forward spontaneously as a result of autoadvancement principles and released growth potential, appropriate appliance therapy must be enlisted to finish the job. If clearing the anterior teeth out of the way allows for mandibular autoadvancement, all the better. But once that mandible is advanced, if there are gaps in the occlusion due to an insufficient posterior vertical, etc., the case is more than a simple matter of unlocking the occlusion by pushing a few retroclined upper anteriors out of the way. Yet this is no problem either, for correcting these basic types of problems is the main forte of the entire spectrum of FJO.

It may now be seen that the clinician with an understanding of the basic principles of TMJ function and pathofunction must examine for it. This includes examining even the younger patients for such problems. Often the first and most important step in this examination is to ask the right questions. Ask both patient and parent: "Do you ever have headaches? Does your child ever complain of headaches? If so, how often? Where, when, how does it hurt?" To gently pursue such a course of inquiry and, if need be, initiate corrective action for the sake of the pediatric patient may prove a source of initial uneasy feelings in a few. But in view of the plight of the young child in pain, who may go undiagnosed and untreated, to know that help and relief may be obtained and to fail to endeavor in one way or another to effect it should prove a source of a writhing conscience in us all.

"Though you drive Nature out with
a pitchfork, she will ever return."

Epistles I
Horace
Roman poet, 65–8 B.C.

FINISHING

Finishing Bionator treatment of a TMJ problem is a matter of individual circumstances. A fixed appliance may be applied for aesthetic and functional perfection of both the posterior and anterior segments and/or

CASE HISTORY

<u>PATIENT:</u> Age 11 years, female

<u>MAIN PROBLEM:</u>
1. Both TMJs clicking. Mother very concerned, as she herself had traditional orthodontic treatment that left her with TMJ problems.
2. Mother did not want bicuspid extraction orthodontic treatment for her daughter
3. 13 mm overjet

<u>FINDINGS:</u>
1. Class II/Division I malocclusion
2. Very deep overbite
3. Both TMJs clicking
4. Lower incisors biting into upper soft tissue in roof of mouth.
5. 13 mm overjet

<u>RADIOGRAPHIC FINDINGS:</u>
Left TMJ (pre-treatment)
1. Left condyle displaced to a posterior-superior position
2. 1 mm posterior joint space (abnormal)
   1.9 mm superior joint space (abnormal)
3. Condyle head bent over at the neck of the condyle
Right TMJ (pre-treatment)
1. Posterior-superior condyle displacement
2. .9 mm posterior joint space (abnormal)
   1.3 mm superior joint space (abnormal)

<u>TREATMENT:</u>
1. Orthopedic corrector I appliance—14 months.
2. Upper straight wire appliance with elastic power chain to close anterior spaces—9 months.
3. Upper retainer—3 months.

<u>RESULTS:</u>
Left TMJ
1. No clicking.
2. 3.0 mm posterior joint space.
   4.3 mm superior joint space.
3. Condyle moved downward and forward, from mandibular correction of Class II to Class I, plus increased vertical dimension to correct the deep overbite.
Right TMJ
1. No clicking.
2. 3.1 mm posterior joint space (abnormal).
   3.7 mm superior joint space (abnormal).
3. Condyle moved downward and forward, from mandibular correction of Class II to Class I, plus increased vertical dimension to correct the deep overbite.

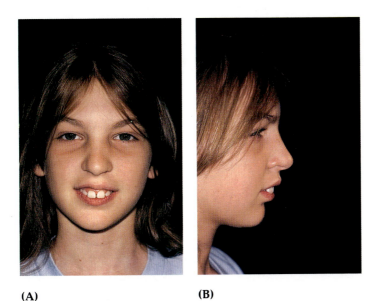

(A)   (B)

Figure 5–21   Pediatric TMJ condition. **(A and B)** Pretreatment facial views. Note the typical Class II profile. **(C)** Pretreatment intraoral view showing a deep overbite. **(D and E)** Pretreatment study casts. Note the large 13-mm overjet. **(F)** Left transcranial view of the TMJ at the relaxed (rest) and biting positions. **(G)** Right transcranial view of the TMJ. Note how in both joints the condyles are driven too far up and back at full intercuspal occlusion. **(H)** The OCI appliance was worn for 14 months. **(I)** Side screws of the OCI opened to increase the amount of mandible advancement. **(J)** Brackets and an elastic power chain were used to condense the interdental spacing. **(K)** One year after completion of treatment. **(L)** Posttreatment transcranial views of the TMJs. The posterior joint space during full intercuspation is 3.0 mm for the left joint and 3.1 mm for the right joint. **(M and N)** Posttreatment facial views. Note the improvement in facial profile due to mandibular advancement. **(O)** Pretreatment Functional Orthopedic cephalometric analysis computerized tracing. **(P)** Pretreatment data printout of the cephalometric tracing. **(Q)** Posttreatment Functional Orthopedic cephalometric computerized tracing. **(R)** Posttreatment printout. Note the relapse of the upper anteriors out labially again, due to the failure of this patient to properly wear final retainer. (Courtesy of John Witzig.)

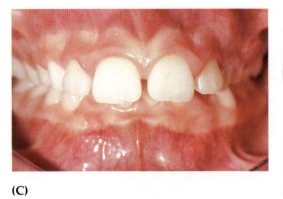

(C)

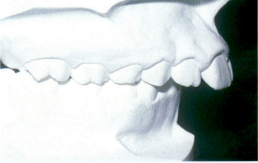

(D)

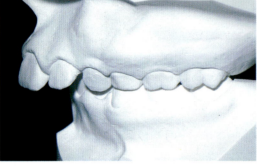

(E)

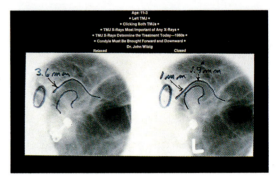

(F)

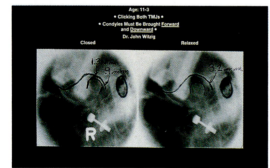

(G)

(H)

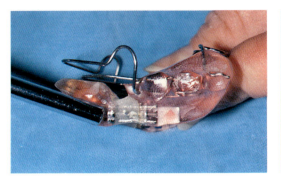

(I)

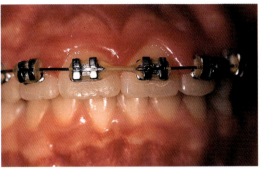

(J)

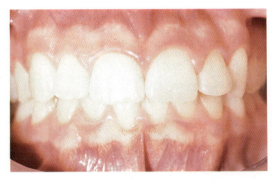

(K)

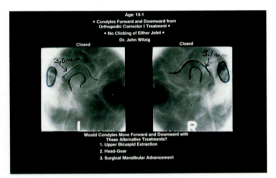

(L)

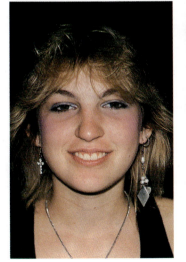

(M)

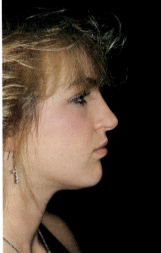

(N)

FUNCTIONAL ORTHOPEDIC ANALYSIS.

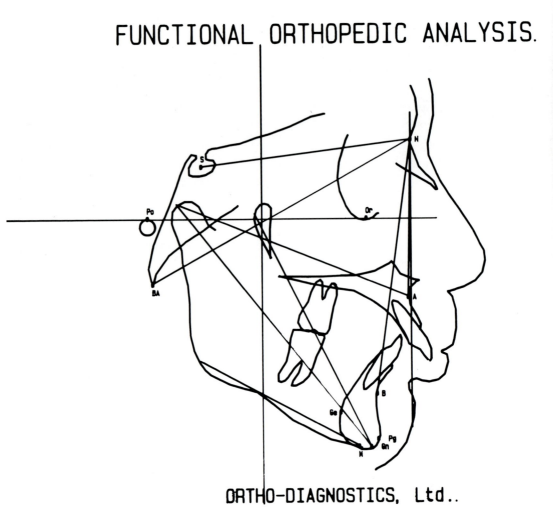

ORTHO-DIAGNOSTICS, Ltd..

(O)

FUNCTIONAL ORTHOPEDIC ANALYSIS

MEASUREMENT	NORM	ACTUAL	COMMENT
A. RELATING THE MAXILLA TO THE CRANIAL BASE			
A Pt to N Perp	-2.0mm to 2.0mm	-1.2mm	
B. RELATING THE MANDIBLE TO THE MAXILLA			
Eff. MAXILLA Lgth	***	94.4mm	
Eff. MANDIBLE Lgth	119.6mm to124.6mm	117.8mm	SHORT MANDIBLE
Diff=MAX-MAND Lgth	***	22.2mm	
Lower Facial Ht[Vert Dim]	66.4mm to 71.1mm	67.3mm	
C. RELATING THE UPPER INCISOR TO THE MAXILLA			
Up1 to A Perp	4.0mm to 6.0mm	8.7mm	
D. RELATING THE LOWER INCISOR TO THE MANDIBLE			
Low1 to A-Pg Line	1.0mm to 3.0mm	0.8mm	
E. MANDIBULAR POSITION			
Pg to N Perp	-5.4mm to -1.6mm	-12.9mm	POSSIBLE RETRUSION
F. OTHER USEFUL CEPHALOMETRIC MEASUREMENTS			
SNA	80.0° to 84.0°	81.4°	
SNB	78.0° to 82.0°	74.8°	RETROGNATHIC MANDIBLE
ANB	0.0° to 4.0°	6.7°	SKELETAL CLASS II
Interincisal Angle	120.0° to140.0°	115.5°	POSSIBLE BIMAXILLARY PROTRUSION
Mandibular Plane Angle	20.0° to 30.0°	26.9°	
Facial Axis (Ricketts)	86.5° to 93.5°	93.2°	
WITS	-2.0mm to 2.0mm	6.5mm	SKELETAL II

(P)

ORTHO-DIAGNOSTICS, LTD.

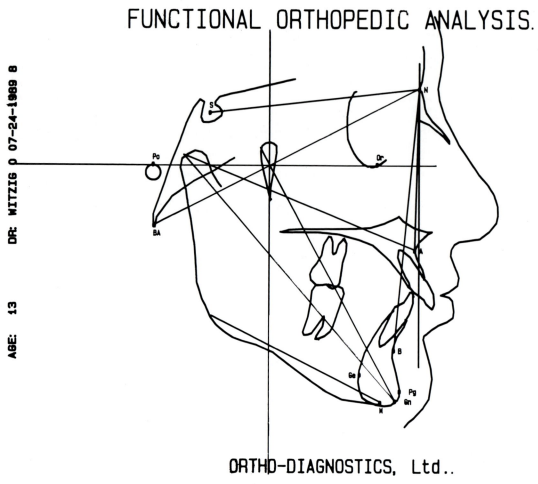

FUNCTIONAL ORTHOPEDIC ANALYSIS.

ORTHO-DIAGNOSTICS, Ltd..

DR: WITZIG □ 07-24-1989 8   AGE: 13

(Q)

FUNCTIONAL ORTHOPEDIC ANALYSIS

MEASUREMENT	NORM	ACTUAL	COMMENT
A. RELATING THE MAXILLA TO THE CRANIAL BASE			
A Pt to N Perp	-1.0mm to 3.0mm	-1.7mm	UNDERDEVELOPED PRE-MAXILLA
B. RELATING THE MANDIBLE TO THE MAXILLA			
Eff. MAXILLA Lgth	***	98.0mm	
Eff. MANDIBLE Lgth	125.5mm to130.5mm	127.5mm	
Diff=MAX-MAND Lgth	***	27.9mm	
Lower Facial Ht[Vert Dim]	68.9mm to 74.1mm	70.7mm	
C. RELATING THE UPPER INCISOR TO THE MAXILLA			
Up1 to A Perp	4.0mm to 6.0mm	7.7mm	
D. RELATING THE LOWER INCISOR TO THE MANDIBLE			
Low1 to A-Pg Line	1.0mm to 3.0mm	1.5mm	
E. MANDIBULAR POSITION			
Pg to N Perp	-4.6mm to -0.4mm	-7.5mm	POSSIBLE RETRUSION
F. OTHER USEFUL CEPHALOMETRIC MEASUREMENTS			
SNA	80.0° to 84.0°	81.9°	
SNB	78.0° to 82.0°	78.0°	
ANB	0.0° to 4.0°	3.9°	SKELETAL CLASS I
Interincisal Angle	120.0° to140.0°	121.5°	
Mandibular Plane Angle	20.0° to 30.0°	25.0°	
Facial Axis (Ricketts)	86.5° to 93.5°	89.5°	
WITS	-2.0mm to 2.0mm	2.2mm	SKELETAL II

(R)

for residual rotational or alignment problems. However, the teeth are sometimes put in a straight-wire appliance prior to the insertion of the Bionator in lieu of a Sagittal II when only slight crowding or slight labial flare is needed. Here rotations act as the culprits in the anterior incisal interference model of the problem, which the fixed appliances more easily correct. A severely rotated upper tooth in the anterior area when struck by the incisal edge of a lower incisor can have the exact same effect as a crowded-forward lower incisor or lingually placed upper incisor when it comes to initiating the NRDM/SPDC phenomenon. Anything that drives the mandible back upon closure must be corrected one way or another before the mandible can be properly advanced.

It may also be conjectured that a considerable amount of equilibration to balance the occlusion may be required once the new Class I, increased vertical occlusion is attained. This quite often proves to be surprisingly not the case. It must be remembered that as the posterior teeth vertically erupt to their new occlusion, they do it gradually and *functionally*. Thus they seek their own level in a manner similar to the common methods of posterior teeth erupting into the mouth during natural growth and development stages. Therefore, any prematurities that might occur often automatically level themselves out as the entire pair of upper and lower posterior segments move occlusally toward one another in self-seeking, functionally guided, and functionally induced unison. It must be remembered that this is a much slower process in the adult as opposed to the child or adolescent patient, thus making the "cap-raising" technique *mandatory*. At about the 3- to 4-month stage of Bionator/OCI wear, the cap may be thickened on its upper biting surface, where it is struck by the upper incisors, by adding cold-cure acrylic at the rate of 1 mm/mon for 3 or 4 months, which increases the vertical eruptive process posteriorly. And once the joint has regained its physiologically correct position again in the tolerant zone, the naturally built-in shock-absorbing condyle-disc assembly of the joint comes into play once again and combines with this "autoleveling" effect of the teeth as they gradually "erupt" toward one another to produce an occlusion that is very biocompatible with the patient. As the occlusion progressively "settles in" more and more, this combination of phenomena reduces the need of posttreatment equilibration to the level of an infrequently performed adjunct to the primary form of orthodontic/orthopedic therapy. Should one be concerned such may be needed, simple checking of the occlusion by natural arc of closure methods as well as observance of lateral excursive movements will easily reveal the need for any minor reduction of any balancing-side or working-side interferences or centric prematurities. There are as surprisingly few! And or course, posttreatment transcranial radiography in the full-occlusion position confirms that the condyle has in fact been advanced down and forward, thus decompressing the posterior joint space and its accompanying, highly sensitive bilaminar zone.

TREATMENT TIME FRAME AND SEQUENCING
IN ADULT TMJ CONDITIONS

It may be safely assumed for the most part, although not in all cases, that correction of malocclusions that act as the chief etiological agents in the generation of TMJ problems in adults requires *longer* treatment times than do similar treatments in the growing child. This may be attributed to a variety of reasons. First is the general all-around increased density of bone in the adult vs. the child. Usually the patient's own individual limits of tolerance will dictate the frequency of expansion screw activation in active-plate usage. Some will indeed still be able to expand the plate once every 4 days or even twice a week while others will experience jaw pains, headache pains, or excessive tooth sensitivities if such frequency of screw activation is used and therefore may be forced for the sake of both comfort and appliance fit to drop back to as little as one turn per week. Another complicating factor in this area is the decreased amount of appliance wear that adults may be forced to experience due to social or work-related requirements. As with more conventional active-plate treatment in the younger patient, slight overexpansion anteriorly with the Sagittal II technique is always a sound procedure because a relapse of the upper anteriors lingually is difficult to prevent entirely. Yet when properly advanced and retained by means of a combination of continued Sagittal appliance wear and the secure fit of the lingual wire of the Bionator following Sagittal appliance usage and, of course, nighttime retainer wear once the treatment is complete, the upper anteriors can be made to stay at their proper interincisal angle, especially once the mandible is advanced and the uppers receive the support of the lower anteriors against their lingual surfaces during full occlusion. Should the patient be unable to wear the Bionator during the day due to the previously mentioned social or work-related demands, the Sagittal appliance can be used as its own retainer, or a series of more streamlined retainers may be substituted. If the Sagittal appliance is used, the open spaces may be filled with quick-cure acrylic between the expanded sections of the appliance for the sake of hygiene and patient comfort. However, if the increase in vertical required is more than just a slight amount, some practitioners prefer to leave the plate "unfilled in" with acrylic since the inherent flex of the plate across the wide-open screws facilitates better fit of the appliance as the occlusal table shifts during vertical-increasing procedures effected by the Bionator. The splint effect of the acrylic occlusal coverings of the plate act to sustain the initial palliative relief for the patient until the occlusion is opened enough and the mandible advanced enough to act as their own combined source of joint decompression. This might take some time if the Bionator is being worn for only a reduced part of each day. (At least 16 hours per day is mandatory.) Thus the Sagittal appliance once again serves a dual role. Once the mandibular advancement and increased vertical start to become great enough to decompress the joint to the point where the Sagittal is no longer needed for palliative purposes and is therefore subsequently withdrawn, any excess labial crown torque (or tip if you will) that might still remain will usually return (relapse) during the "Bionator-only" phase of treatment. Should the lingual wire of the Bionator/OCI act as an interference to any desired movements of this nature, it can be easily cut and adjusted out of the way. This is generally unnecessary because the upper anteriors work their way back all too easily on their own. The slightly excessive labial positioning of these teeth will always make them seek their own level in returning to a more lingual placement as the amount of Bionator wear wanes during the later stages of that phase of treatment. More often than not the uppers have a proclivity to "overrelapse," much to the consternation of the clinician, rather than remain in their new found, overprotruded, Sagittal appliance–effected position. The importance of continued nighttime retention for the severe Division 2 case cannot be overly stressed.

Since Sagittal development, especially in a posterior direction, is always more stable and more arch "decrowding" than lateral development is, even in the growing child, *extreme caution* must be exercised when approaching any major efforts in *lateral* development in the *adult* patient for either orthodontic or TMJ treatment purposes. The principles of "directional decrowding" should be employed whenever possible. Should an adult TMJ pain-dysfunction patient exhibit a bilateral posterior crossbite in conjunction with mandibular retrusion, final HS retainers become all but manditory. This is due to the fact that bilateral posterior crossbite correction in adults, even young adults, has proved over the years to be an extremely precarious undertaking frought with a relatively high percentage of relapses and eventual failure. The Europeans have long known this since the days of Schwarz (at the University of Vienna), who was the founding father of active-plate–effected lateral development. It is commonly accepted among the European orthodontic community that correction of such types of crossbites should not be attempted past the late teens! This is why this series of texts lists the bilateral posterior crossbite in the young growing child as an "urgency case" to be treated as soon as the diagnosis is made and the cooperation of the patient will allow. The more long-standing such cases are, the more difficult they are to correct *permanently*. Such procedures that are either radical or surgically augmented, such as the Epker-Wolford procedure discussed in a previous volume, may shed some new light on this age-old orthodontic nemesis, but until further information and evidence of consistantly higher percentages of success becomes available, attempts at treatment of severe crossbites in adults should be labeled with only a fair prognosis at best! If the chances for a successful outcome appear reasonable on marginal cases and attempts at correction are initiated by means of such appliances as the Transverse, it should be done with the full knowledge and consent of the patient and the caveat that perpetual nighttime appliance retention may be needed or eventual complete relapse may be imminent.

PATIENT RESPONSE TO TREATMENT

TMJ arthrosis is a permanent condition. Once the level of involvement has become great enough that the ligaments have become elongated, bone has become sclerotic, deformed, or otherwise reflective of osseous arthritic breakdown, once discs or posterior attachments have become perforated, once trigger points have not only formed but also have become deeply ingrained into the musculature, even after successful and proper treatment, "scars" remain. Sometimes they are true forms of physical scar tissue. Sometimes the scars are more conceptual in nature. Nevertheless, they remain. The more long-standing the condition has been and the greater the level of severity of the intracapsular arthrosis, the more likely are the chances that the patient will exhibit some form of posttreatment evidence that damage has been done. This may often manifest itself as a persistent or recurrent click during joint function. It may manifest itself in the form of adequate yet nonetheless somewhat restricted ranges of motion. It may also manifest itself in the form of occasional reoccurrence of headaches or myofascial discomforts. Although a great many patients respond to the treatment with complete elimination of all signs and symptoms, a small percentage of the more severe cases may report only a 90% reduction in symptoms. Yet this is still very acceptable to both patient and clinician. For both can only be expected to work with the "physiological hand that fate has dealt them."

The same might be said for the way patients respond to treatment during the active periods of appliance wear. The manner in which symptoms subside, as might be guessed, follows the general axioms that the younger the patient and, to a certain extent, the less severe the levels of initial damage, the quicker the symptoms will subside once treatments begin. Patient sensitivity also is a factor here. Some respond favorably when appliances are inserted that are made from construction bites of average thicknesses. Others on less frequent occasion will respond only fairly for a while to the active-plate phase of treatment because they require more exacting levels of jaw positioning before muscles and joints completely "settle down." If the response is not as favorable as desired in the initial active-plate phase of treatment (and rare indeed is the patient who will not show at least some form of improvement during this period), once the Bionator or Orthopedic Corrector is inserted, the remaining symptoms readily subside. It must be remembered that it has been shown that splints do not always adequately decompress the joint. Hence the "splinting effect" of the occlusal coverings of Sagittal II or Transverse appliances may not always be sufficient to reduce the patient's headache and myofascial pain symptoms completely. The mandibular advancement and condylar decompression capabilities of the Bionator/Orthopedic Corrector may be needed for that. The patient's signs and symptoms generally are seen to be reduced on average by about 75% to even 90% the first month or two of treatment. Some even exhibit this favorable level of response the first several weeks! But is must be remembered that the patient's signs and symptoms have appeared as the result of years of untoward function and abuse of the joint and its musculature. They cannot be expected to subside overnight.

As the treatment approaches completion, the patient will steadily exhibit increased vertical dimension of occlusion and a more forward repositioning of the mandible. The amount of adult wear of the Bionator will often be for a period of at least 12 months as a safety measure for the sake of the assurance that not only have the teeth and the joints been fully addressed during treatment but also the musculature. A lifetime of altered function of the orofacial musculature in the form of the Class II neuromuscular sling may need a longer period of retraining and readaptation in the adult. Once completely corrected to more conventional "Class I musculature" by proper Bionator usage, the muscles of mastication act as a formidable force in *keeping* the mandible permanently repositioned down and forward regardless of what is happening intracapsularly within the joint. In its altered state that same Class II muscular sling was a major etiological factor in permanently *keeping the condyle riding off* the disc up in the intolerant or bilaminar zone, even during nonfunctioning or rest positions. So too, the musculature, once corrected by functional appliance treatment, becomes a major factor in holding the condyle and the entire mandible in a more forward correct position and *keeping the condyle riding on* the disc back down in the tolerant zone once again, even during nonfunctioning or rest positions.

The importance of the Bionator phase of treatment during TMJ rehabilitative efforts cannot be overemphasized. It is important for at least three major reasons. It can change not only the teeth (vertical) and bone (condylar position) but also the musculature. It is very important to cor-

---

Figure 5–22 Adding acrylic to cap of the Bionator/OCI helps speed eruption of the posterior teeth. Remember that the lower posterior teeth will not erupt if the curve of Spee is too deep. This locks the lower teeth in place because they would have to erupt into each other's own pathway of eruption due to angulations brought about by a deep curve of Spee.

Figure 5–23 **(A)** The Biofinisher of Dr. Jack Lynn. **(B)** Close-up view of vertical elastics. **(C)** Overlay prosthesis (Part A courtesy of Dr. John Witzig; parts B and C courtesy of the Ohlendorf Co, St Louis; part D courtesy of Hermanson Dental Laboratory, St Paul, Minn.)

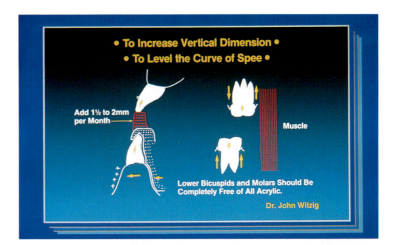

Figure 5–22

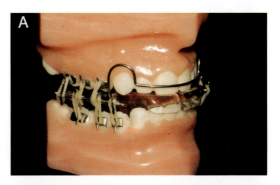

Figure 5–23

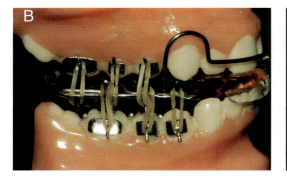

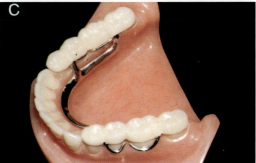

rect errant musculature by some means. The Bionator and Orthopedic Corrector are the best and most efficient muscle lengtheners, muscle retrainers, and muscle readaptors in the entire FJO repertoire of appliances. The Levandoski "super splint" is also capable of delivering "Bionator effect" as far as the musculature is concerned. Reestablishing proper muscle balance with devices like these usually requires about 6 months of faithful cooperation on the part of the patient, i.e., wearing these appliances as much as possible during a 24-hour period. It has been observed that 16 hours per day is the absolute minimum amount of wearing time that still proves effective, albeit barely so. Of course, treatment times stretch out as a result of reduced daily wearing of the appliances also.

In more difficult cases where symptomatic problems seem to wax and wane with recurrent exacerbations of myofascial, cephalalgic, and cervical pains periodically throughout the course of treatment, it has been found that the Bionator itself makes an excellent HS retainer. In more extreme cases it may even have to be used as a lifetime HS retainer. Severe joint damage from the trauma of unsuccessful joint surgery or advanced levels of osteoarthritic breakdown are candidates for the use of a functional appliance as a long-term HS retainer. If there is concern that the vertical might increase too much due to overeruption of the posterior teeth because of the nighttime wear of a Bionator, acrylic may be added to the appliance in the posterior areas similar to that of a conventional Bionator III appliance. This will hold the posteriors (as well as anteriors) at a constant vertical. However, overeruption of posteriors is seldom if ever a problem in TMJ treatments. More often it is a problem of not being able to effect enough posterior eruption or, more correctly, not being able to effect it quickly enough that bothers both the patient and treating clinician. Erupting the posterior quadrants with functional appliances is the time-consuming portion of any TMJ treatment plan. Therefore, several modifications to the conventional way this is done have evolved that assist greatly with this problem.

The first is, of course, the traditional way of speeding the eruption of posteriors in standard Bionator technique by increasing the thickness of the anterior bite cap with acrylic. In the adult TMJ pain-dysfunction patient, caution may have to be exercised in just how quickly the cap is thickened on its biting surface because too rapid a change in vertical by such means may be too great a shock for the musculature and result in muscle splinting or frank myospasm problems. Deep curve of Spee problems also act to inhibit eruption of lowers. Hence these things should be corrected also before eruption can be expected to take place in the posterior quadrants.

The second modification of the basic Bionator technique with respect to enhancing the speed of eruption of posteriors is, of course, the use of vertical posterior elastics in the manner of the Biofinisher technique as described by its developer Dr. Jack Lynn. Alternation of this style of treatment during nighttime wear with conventional Bionator/active-plate wear during the day turns out to be a combination that is both efficient and practical for the patient. A modification of the Lynn Biofinisher–type appliance involves the use of removable rakes for more comfortable use of the appliance when not being worn in conjunction with the little-vertical elastics.

The third method involves the use of fixed or cast removable restorations of a variety of types to "instantly" correct posterior open bites once the clinician is assured that the muscles have been retrained and the condyle properly repositioned as a result of the functional appliance phase of treatment. It's a simple matter of putting the jaw in the right place and filling in the empty spaces with crowns, onlays, or an overlay cast prosthesis of some sort to keep it there. Patients, given the choice, find the savings in time worth the increased expense, especially in severe deep-bite cases or in cases where the posterior teeth could use the restoration work anyway due to the deteriorating conditions of large amalgams, etc.

The teeth, the bones, and the musculature in their altered state all have a role in the generation of TMJ pain-dysfunction problems. All three must be addressed, each in its own way as per the dictates of its own needs, to effect total and permanent resolution of the TMJ problem. Clinicians in possession of the knowledge of fixed appliance, active-plate, and functional appliance techniques are in the best position to treat TMJ problems. For such "heavily armed" practitioners have the power to change the altered state of not only the teeth but now also the bone and the musculature and their relationships to one another to a more favorable level of structural balance for the sake of the patient. The basic rudiments of the knowledge needed by the main body of treating clinicians to effect such treatment is at hand. The techniques and methodologies have been made known and accessible. Now it simply becomes a matter of will. Some egos will struggle, resent, and even rebel, but the truth will always triumph eventually.

"And in green underwood and cover
Blossom by blossom the spring begins"

"Atlanta in Calydon"
Algernon Swinburne, 1837–1909
English poet

References

1. Perry HT, Marsh EW: Functional considerations in early limited orthodontic procedures, in Gelb H (ed): *The Clinical Management of Head, Neck and TMJ Pain and Dysfunction.* Philadelphia, WB Saunders Co, 1977, pp 262–263.
2. Bell WE: *Temporomandibular Disorders: Classification/Diagnosis/Management.* Chicago, Year Book Medical Publishers, Inc, 1986, pp 242–243.
3. Gelb H: Personal communication, March 1985.
4. Gelb H (ed): *The Clinical Management of Head Neck and TMJ Pain and Dysfunction.* Philadelphia, WB Saunders Co, 1977, pp 314–320.
5. Clark GT, Beemsterboer PL, Solberg WK, et al: Nocturnal electromyographic evaluation of myofascial pain dysfunction in patients undergoing occlusal splint therapy. *J Am Dent Assoc* 1979; 99:607–611.
6. Goharian RK, Neff PA: Effect of occlusal retainers on temporomandibular joint and facial pain. *J Prosthet Dent* 1980; 44:206–208.
7. Nel H: Myofascial pain-dysfunction syndrome. *J Prosthet Dent* 1978; 40:438–441.
8. Shore NA: *Temporomandibular Joint Dysfunction and Occlusal Equilibration,* ed 2. Philadelphia, JB Lippincott, 1976, pp 193–205, 237–249.
9. Tanner HM: The Tanner mandibular appliance, in *Continuum '80, Journal of the L.D. Pankey Institute.* New York, Science and Medicine Publishing Co, 1979, pp 23–34.
10. Weinberg LA: Treatment prosthesis in TMJ dysfunction-pain syndrome. *J Prosthet Dent* 1978; 39:654–669.
11. Whatmore G, Kohli D: *The Physiopathology and Treatment of Functional Disorders.* New York, Grune & Stratton, 1974.
12. Sheer W: Personal communication, Las Vegas, June 26, 1981.
13. Christensen C: A rational articulator. *Ash's Q Circ* 1901; 409–420.
14. Christensen C: The problem of the bite. *Dent Cosmos* 1905; 47:1184–1195.
15. Gysi A: The problem of articulation. *Dent Cosmos* 1910; 52:148–169.
16. Snow GB: Articulation. *Dent Cosmos* 1900; 42:51–55.

17. Snow GB: The philosophy of mastication. *Dent Cosmos* 1900; 42:531–535.

18. Bonwill WGA: Scientific articulation of human teeth as founded on geometrical, mathematical and mechanical laws. *Dent Items of Interest* 1899; 21:617–636, 873–880.

19. Bonwill WGA: The geometrical and mechanical laws of articulation of the human teeth: The anatomical articulator, in *American System of Dentistry*, vol 2. W.F. Litch Publishers, 1887, p 487.

20. Witzig J, Spahl TJ: *The Clinical Management of Basic Maxillofacial Orthopedic Appliances.* Littleton, Mass, PSG Publishing Co, 1987, pp 35–149.

21. Grude R: The Norwegian system of orthodontic treatment. *Dent Rec* 1938; 58:529–551.

22. Engh O: Treatment with the Andresen activator. *Trans Eur Orthod Soc* 1951; 200–208.

23. Bjork A: The principles of the Andresen method of orthodontic treatment, a discussion based on cephalometric x-ray analysis of treated cases. *Am J Orthod* 1951; 37:437–457.

24. Korkhaus G: Present orthodontic thought in Germany. *Am J Orthod* 1960; 46:270–287.

25. Brown RW: *Cephalometric Study of Mandibular Length Change During F.J.O. Treatment* (thesis). University of Michigan, Ann Arbor, 1959.

26. Moss JP: Cephalometric changes during functional appliance therapy. *Trans Eur Orthod Soc* 1962; 327–341.

27. Meach CL: A cephalometric comparison of bony profile changes in class II, division 1 treated with extra-oral force and functional jaw orthopedics. *Am J Orthod* 1966; 52:353–370.

28. Marchner JF, Harris JE: Mandibular growth in class II treatment. *Angle Orthod* 1968; 36:89–93.

29. Freunthaller P: Cephalometric observations in class II, division 1 malocclusions treated with the activator. *Angle Orthod* 967; 37:18–24.

30. Ahlgren J: A longitudinal clinical and cephalometric study of 50 malocclusion cases treated with activator appliance. *Trans Eur Orthod Soc* 1972; 48:285–293.

31. Demisch A: Effects of activator therapy on the craniofacial skeleton in class II division 1 malocclusion. *Trans Eur Orthod Soc* 1972; 48:295–310.

32. Hausser E: Functional orthodontic treatment with the activator. *Trans Eur Orthod Soc* 1973; 427–430.

33. Reey RW, Eastwood A: The passive activator: Case selection, treatment response and corrective mechanics. *Am J Orthod* 1978; 73:378–409.

34. Wieslander L, Lagerstrom L: The effect of activator treatment on class II malocclusions. *Am J Orthod* 1979; 75:20–25.

35. Cohen AM: A study of class II, division 1 malocclusions treated by the Andresen appliance. *Br J Orthodont* 1981; 8:159–163.

36. Stoeckli P: Personal communication, Annual Meeting of the European Orthodontic Society, Barcelona, Spain, 1979.

37. Witzig J, Spahl TJ: *The Clinical Management of Basic Maxillofacial Orthopedic Appliances.* Littleton, Mass, PSG Publishing Co, 1987, pp 282–293.

38. Marteney J: Personal communication, Minneapolis, Advanced TMJ Seminar, Oct 16, 1988.

CHAPTER 6

Prosthodontics for the Edentulous Patient With Temporomandibular Joint Pain-Dysfunction: Science Imitating Life

TREATMENT: THE PROSTHODONTIC APPROACH

The discipline of functional jaw orthopedics (FJO) is predicated upon the presence of a complete dentition. Its most fundamental principle of operation centers around correction of imbalances in the teeth, bones, and muscles, the three legs of the maxillofacial triangle that are responsible for the state of the patient's malocclusion. The orthopedic side of the triangle includes addressing not only maxillary and mandibular arch form problems in the apical bases, anteroposterior (AP) maxillomandibular relationships, and vertical dimension of occlusion discrepancies, but also functional imbalances and irregularities within the temporomandibular joint (TMJ)—the most important orthopedic relationship of all.

Some of the most significant orthopedic imbalances exist in patients with incomplete dentitions. For instance, in the case of a patient with a few missing key posterior teeth bilaterally and remaining upper and lower teeth, the lower anteriors could just as easily slide up the lingual surfaces of the uppers in such a case and cause superior posterior displacement of the condyles as they could in the most Classic Class II, Division 2, deep-bite malocclusion in the full dentition. Worse yet is the pa-

412

tient with upper and lower anterior teeth present but no posterior teeth in either arch. With no vertical stops whatsoever in the posterior areas, even if the vertical and AP alignments were initially adequate, such a case would be highly susceptible to posterior displacement upon full closure.

The principles set forth in the FJO approach to treating malocclusions in the full dentition also apply to the TMJ pain-dysfunction patient who possesses a less than complete dentition. The occlusion, regardless of how it is fabricated, should recreate the proper anterior and posterior vertical dimension, the proper transverse alignment, and proper AP alignment of the mandible so that at full occlusion the condyles are on the disc in the physiological position (condyle slightly down and forward), or "tolerant zone," of the joint. If the disc cannot be recaptured due to excessive anteromedial displacement with ligament elongation, that prosthetic occlusion should still support the condyles in the physiological position within the joint so as to at least be out of the intolerant zone. The muscles should also be rehabilitated such that even at rest they support the mandible in the physiological position so the condyle doesn't ride in the intolerant, retrodiscal bilaminar zone. They should also be able to work at a proper length, a length for which they were genetically preprogrammed. This length is reflected in the balanced, uninvolved, "non-TMJ" patient as the amount of vertical exhibited by the patient and the amount of freeway space present. These principles universally apply to the patient in possession of a full dentition, to patients who may have upper and lower removable partial dentures, and patients who may have no teeth at all and must wear full dentures. Ironically, the full-dentition concept of FJO, when applied to patients with missing dental units, forces the treating clinician to become aware of a uniform insight that governs and coordinates the various disciplines. This represents what some have referred to as "a general unification theory" in dentistry.

The prime impetus for the application of the above principles to the discipline of prosthodontics has been as a result of the truly spectacular work of one of the great prosthodontists of this century, Dr. Ronald Levandoski of Erie, Pennsylvania. His work on the development of the Levandoski mandibular repositioning appliance and the development of a three-dimensional articular that is fully adjustable to the dictates of transcranial (or tomographic) directed condylar repositioning needs and other cephalometric radiographic parameters has been monumental and will no doubt serve as a turning point in the development of TMJ-oriented prosthetic dentistry and a major step in the development of a unification theory.

As previously stated in an earlier chapter, the Levandoski mandibular stabilization prosthesis represents a sort of hybrid link between splints and functional appliances. As a splint, it can act to interrupt the occlusal neuromuscular circuit and is capable of altering both anterior and, most importantly, posterior vertical dimensions of occlusion. It also has the characteristics of a functional appliance in that, given a sufficient length of time of wear (6 to 9 months), it appears to reestablish correct muscle balance, which in turn is what is responsible for helping the mandible assume a more advanced and stabilized posture with the condyles in the physiological position at rest. By virtue of its technique of construction, when using the Levandoski vector analysis from a transcranial or tomographic image, lateral and AP cephalometric films, and the three-way fully adjustable Levandoski articulator, the Levandoski mandibular stabilization prosthesis (splint) is capable of delivering positive and precise control of condylar position without guesswork. It specifically limits lateral excursive movements, which are universally hard on healing TMJs and as a result also provides the big thing as far as the patients are concerned, positive control of their signs and symptoms.

The contributions Levandoski has made to the coordination of TMJ treatment techniques with prosthetic techniques has been nothing short of visionary. Yet ironically, they involve principles that are familiar territory to the profession of dentistry as a whole. No new players on the board—just the same old chess pieces, but cleverly rearranged and unified in a totally new and highly creative game plan. The basic "occlusion-condylar–stabilizing" type of splint technique that forms the structural basis for his stabilization prosthesis utilizes the "Christensen phenomenon," previously described, whereby the posterior vertical dimension of occlusion opens faster than does its anterior counterpart as the mandible is advanced (especially in deep-bite cases). This observation, nearly a century old, has until recently been just another interesting ripple in the general dental consciousness because of the lack of definitive instrumentation to use this information therapeutically.

Typically, the prosthesis is inserted, and the patient will wear it for 6 to 9 months. When the mandible has been muscularly advanced to restore proper condyle-fossa position, the patient will clearly exhibit a posterior open bite. This open bite may represent the lack of posterior eruption, compensatory intrusion in cases where the vertical dimension of the

---

Figure 6–1 **(A)** Lack of posterior vertical dimension of occlusion goes hand in hand with functionally induced TMJ problems of the NRDM/SPDC type (neuromuscular reflexive displacement of the mandible resulting in superior posterior displacement of the condyle). **(B)** Once the "class II neuromuscular sling" has been retrained to hold and habitually operate the mandible-condyle unit in the physiologically stable position (Gelb 4/7) after the first 4 to 7 months of Bionator/OCI mandibular advancement treatment or Levandoski "supersplint" treatment, even though the muscles want to hold the mandible in the correct orthopedic position, the patient is routinely left for the moment with an unresolved posterior open bite. This final problem may be solved either with continued orthodontic or prosthodontic techniques.

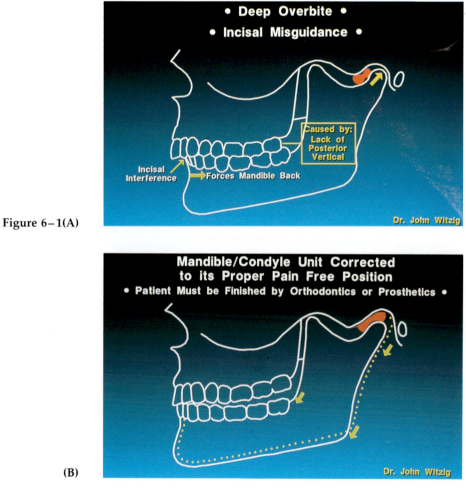

Figure 6–1(A)

(B)

TMJ has decreased due to a dislocated disc, intrusive orthodontic treatment, unrestored partial or total edentulism, or any of a number of other reasons. Any attempts to retrude the condyles or walk them back to the original position after orthopedic neuromuscular balance has been achieved will cause renewed joint instability and an acute "flare-up" of the patient's original symptoms.

The restoration of that posterior open bite (the old "bite-raising" techniques of the 1940s) with cast overlay, removable partial dentures or even eventually crowns or onlays is also a technique with which organized dentistry has long been familiar. Even the concepts of repositioning a superiorly and posteriorly displaced condyle down and forward in the joint to decompress compromised bilaminar zones and relieve TMJ-type symptomatology have a long track record in TMJ therapeutics. But the techniques of the transcranial vector analysis and the ideas of building a three-dimensional articulator designed to accept these vectors, thus bringing the methodology of repositioning the condyles out of the realm of educated guesswork and placing it squarely in the realm of exact science, are Levandoski's unique contribution to dentistry. His creativity combined with his incisive insights as to the true nature of the TMJ problem allowed Levandoski to obtain the most extraordinary effects from the most common trappings of the TMJ theater of operations. Another example of this talent is his approach to analyzing the common panographic radiograph.

LEVANDOSKI PANOGRAPHIC ANALYSIS

As an adjunct to clinical and radiographic analysis of the patient with TMJ problems, Levandoski developed a unique system for analyzing the common panoramic film. His analysis is based on the comparison of various linear measurements taken from the film. The absolute values, of course, are not significant because there is a considerable amount of magnification associated with the panographic film, but rather it is the relative comparison of those values with each other that Levandoski feels gives insights to the case that are unobtainable from the conventional cephalogram or transcranial radiographs.

The Levandoski panographic analysis, like any of the other radiographic analyses for transcranial or cephalometric views, demands that the film be properly oriented and of diagnostic quality. The palatal line (or as a substitute, the dark space between the upper and lower teeth) should be parallel to the horizontal edge of the film, i.e., it should not be "smiling" or "frowning." If it is smiling, it means the patient's head was down on his chest too far when the film was exposed. If it is frowning, it means the patient's head was extended too far back during exposure. The condyles and the fossae should be clearly visible. The exposure should also be of sufficient levels of intensity that the cervical vertebrae do not obliterate the image of the upper and lower central incisors. Although various levels of magnification and focal distances change from machine to machine, the analysis considers only comparative values, *not absolute* values. Therefore, it is all relative anyway. (Note: The image produced by the older S.S. White machines does not qualify for the techniques of this analysis due to the delay in the positioning of the chair when imaging the opposite side of the patient. This produces an image that is divided into two sections.) Levandoski stresses that the individual become thoroughly familiar with the idiosyncracies of his own machine to help facilitate interpretations of this analysis. It is as follows:

1. Like all radiographic analyses, the Levandoski analysis is predicated upon the construction of a series of base reference lines. The first reference line constructed is the maxillary vertical midline (line 1). By placing the point of a compass at the end of the maxillary tuberosity (or the distal height of the contour of the second molar if the third molars are in the way of a clear view of the tuberosity area), a small arc is scribed in the nasal septum about 3 to 5 cm long. The point of the compass is then transferred to the opposite maxillary tuberosity area at an equivalent location (or to the distal height of the contour of the opposite upper second molar if that technique is being used), and a second arc is scribed in a similar manner. The two points at which these two arcs cross represent the two points of a straight line, the maxillary vertical base reference line. It is drawn between these two points and extended to below the symphysis. This line should pass through the nasal septum.

2. A line is then drawn perpendicular to the maxillary midline tangent to the *highest* condyle (line 2). This line is extended horizontally to the opposite condyle. By default, if the opposite condyle is not symmetrical in height so as to also be tangent to this line, it will be below it.

3. The ramal lines are drawn along the posterior edge of each ramus (line 3).

4. A line is drawn bilaterally from the point where the midmaxillary vertical base reference line crosses the lower border of the symphysis of the mandible in each direction to the ramal line through the gonion (line 4).

5. Lines are drawn from each condylion (the most superior posterior point on the anterocurvature of the condylar head) to a point in the contact zone between the maxillary central incisors and the mandibular central incisors (lines 5 and 6). The actual vertical location of these points between these teeth is somewhat arbitrary, which in the case of these particular lines and the purpose for which they are used is perfectly acceptable.

6. Lines are drawn from the gonion to the condylion and from the gonion to the tip of the coronoid process on each ramus (lines 7 and 8).

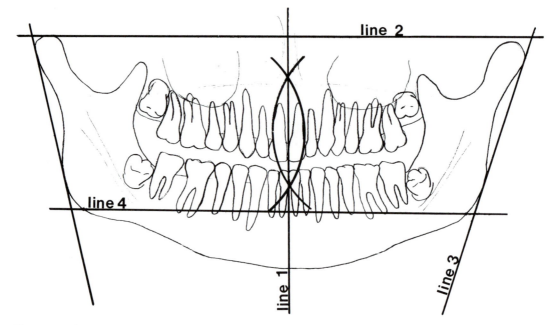

Figure 6–2(A)

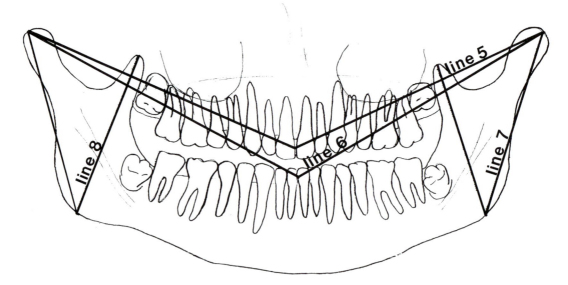

(B)

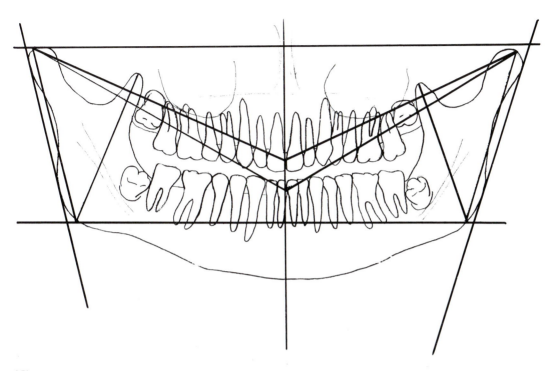

(C)

Figure 6–2 Levandoski panographic analysis. **(A)** Lines 1 to 4; **(B)** lines 5 to 8; **(C)** completed analysis.

In interpreting the measurements of his panographic analysis system, Levandoski again stresses that the absolute values are not important but that it is the comparison of values from one side to the other that is significant. The information gained from the panographic analysis supplements information gained from the other components of the examination, particularly the cephalometric analysis. After comparing right-side to left-side measurements from the panographic analysis, a number of factors come to light that are unobtainable from other radiographic analyses such as the cephalogram, the transcranial radiograph, the tomogram, or even the arthrogram.

One of the first things to be noted is whether or not there is a short condyle. It might be observed that the lines depicting the length of the coronoid processes are relatively equal (line 8), whereas the lines depicting the relative lengths of the condyles (line 7) are different by more than 3 to 4 mm. The shorter condyle will also usually show a shorter gonion. This key observation can be used to determine which gonial angle is higher on a cephalometric tracing. This relationship may be deceptive on the cephalometric radiograph in norma lateralis. Usually one would expect the outline of the inferior border of the mandible closest to the film to be the higher of the two images on a lateral view of the cephalogram. However, if one line is seen, it may be assumed that, given that the patient's head was properly positioned in the cephalostat, the side farthest from the film would be the shorter of the two, thus allowing for such a superimposition of images to take place. But if two lines are seen, i.e., two lower borders of the mandible and two gonions appear, then conceivably, if the side farthest away from the film were to be short enough (or conversely, if the side of the mandible closest to the film were long enough), the image of the farthest side could actually appear higher on the lateral view. The comparison of lines 7 and 8, the length of the coronoid process, and the condylar lengths from right to left should settle the issue one way or the other.

Levandoski also believes that there is great significance to a discrepancy in the lengths of the coronoid processes (line 8). He feels that a long coronoid process (a discrepancy of 3 to 4 mm) is usually highly indicative of osteophytic changes secondary to degenerative arthritis in the joint of the ipsilateral side with concomitant condylar shortening. This condylar shortening would be associated with chronic shortening and spasm of the medial pterygoid, masseter, and temporalis on the ipsilateral side. This chronic muscle shortening could lead to muscle hypertonicity, muscle splinting, myospasm, and other chronic myogenic-type problems. Such chronic muscle tension problems as these can manifest themselves in the form of uneven tensions placed on the coronoid process of the involved side, which has been shown to cause changes in its external morphology such as osteophytic maladaptive lengthening. Levandoski also believes that this can also result in osteophytic changes at the gonial angle, i.e., muscle tension can cause increased accentuation of the antegonial notch. This is most common in Class II, Division 2 cases. Levandoski even goes so far as to propose that any significant form of antegonial notch that is present on the inferior posterior borders of the mandible is a sequela of "functional maladaptation" and is not a naturally occurring genetic manifestation.

In conjunction with studying the lengths of the condyles and coronoid processes from one side to the other, Levandoski also examines the panograph to see if it may be deciphered as to which fossa is the higher of the two. This often correlates with the observation of one eye being higher than the other from a frontal view.

Referring back to the very first lines drawn for this analysis, Levandoski compares the "effective lengths" of the maxilla from one side to the other. It must be remembered that these measurement lines (line 9), originating from the point of the compass location that was used to draw the arcs that determined the maxillary midline, must be drawn perpendicular to the maxillary midline (line 1). A difference in linear lengths of these two lines of more than 2 to 3 mm could mean that the maxilla is rotated in the direction of the shorter line about a vertical axis through the midpoint of the midpalatal suture. However, care must be exercised here if the maxillary dental midline does not closely coincide with the orthopedic midline. The maxillary dental midline could vary from the orthopedic midline by a considerable degree due to something like a congenitally missing upper lateral incisor, bicuspid, or unerupted and impacted cuspid. Yet if the maxilla is also rotated to that same side, as a whole, it will make the dental midline appear on the tracing farther away from the orthopedic midline than it actually is. Conversely, if the maxilla should perchance be rotated in the opposite direction, it would make the dental midline appear closer to the orthopedic midline on the tracing than it actually is.

Closely associated with this portion of the analysis is the consideration of the cant of the occlusal plane from a frontal aspect. This consideration, however, does not concern itself with a comparison of the linear lengths of two lines or with checking the effective maxillary lengths for rotation of the maxilla as a whole, but rather it concerns itself with where the two lines drawn perpendicular to the maxillary orthopedic midline (line 1) happen to meet (or fail to meet) with respect to vertical approximation. When measuring the maxillary lengths right and left, the measurement line is originated at the place where the point of the compass was placed at the end of the maxillary tuberosity and drawn perpendicular to the maxillary midline. A slight variance of compass point location right side to left with respect to the horizontal plane will have very little effect on the arcs constructed, the maxillary midline drawn through the two intersecting points of those arcs, or the perpendicular lines drawn from the compass point location to the maxillary midline. These two lines are analyzed for comparative linear values. They usually will not meet at the exact vertical location up and down along the maxillary midline (line 1). However, this is not important because all we are interested in is comparative linear lengths. But in the analysis of the cant of the occlusal plane, two different lines are drawn in what at first may appear as a similar manner, but they are quite different, and although their mathematical linear values are of no consequence, the point at which they meet at the maxillary midline is. To construct these lines, a point is selected on the distal height of the contour of the maxillary first molar (or second molar if it is in function) on each side and a line drawn perpendicular to the maxillary midline (line 1). Care must be exercised that equivalent points on the distal heights of the contour of these teeth are used. If the cant of the occlusal plane *from a frontal aspect* is reasonably horizontal, these two lines will either meet or approximate each other quite closely at the maxillary midline. If not, it would be strongly indicative that the occlusal plane is canted toward the side of the short condyle, thus indicating a greater relative degree of lack of the posterior vertical dimension of occlusion on that side.

The dental midline of the mandible may also be measured in a similar manner. Again, this is a comparative linear measurement to check for the mandibular incisor midline shift. The lines for this are constructed from the condylion to the midline between the mandibular incisors (line 6). The maxillary dental midline, it must be remembered, may be analyzed with respect to the maxillary orthopedic midline (line 1), provided any rotational effects represented by discrepancies in effective maxillary lengths (line 9) are also taken into consideration. But to analyze the mandibular dental arch midline with respect to the mandible itself, one cannot compare the mandibular dental midline with the maxillary orthopedic midline (line 1), but rather one should compare it with the mandible itself. This is done by comparing the linear lengths of lines running from the condylion on each side to the mandibular dental arch midline embrasure between the lower centrals (line 6). The two lines should be equal. A short condyle is short vertically (usually due to some sort of condylar degenerative changes or unexpressed growth), but this will not affect midline measurements made in such fashion to any appreciable degree, for these measurements are made on a mostly horizontal plane.

When one compares the mandibular dental midline with the mandible itself, one may then compare that point (or small vertical line, if you wish) with the maxillary dental and orthopedic midlines and with the actual occluded models of the patient to see whether the mandible is being deflected more to one side of the other. Merely analyzing dental midlines of upper and lower study models of the patient alone without the benefit of the Levandoski panographic analysis may give a false impression of what is really happening in the case regardless of how the upper and lower dental midlines align on the hand-held plaster.

In an "ideal" case analyzed from a panographic standpoint, the following is optimal:

1. The fossae should be of equal height.
2. The condyles should be of equal height (line 7).
3. The coronoid processes should be of equal height (line 8).
4. The gonial angles (cephalometric) should be equal.
5. The effective maxillary lengths should be equal, which indicates that the maxilla is not rotated as a whole (line 9).
6. The cant of the occlusal plane should be level as indicated by lines 9 meeting at the same location vertically on the maxillary midline (line 1).
7. The mandibular dental arch midline should be centered over the mandibular body as indicated by equal values for line 6.
8. The maxillary orthopedic midline (line 1) should coincide with the maxillary and mandibular dental arch midlines (lines 5 and 6).

Notable findings from this analysis may be the following:

1. If the maxilla is bodily rotated as a whole about a vertical axis through the midpalatal suture, the effective maxillary lengths (lines 9) will be unequal by more than 2 to 3 mm, with the maxilla rotated to the side of the shorter length.

2. The occlusal plane will be canted with respect to the horizontal *from a frontal aspect* if lines 9 fail to meet perpendicularly at the maxillary midline (line 1), with the side of the upper and lower dental arches in most need of extra posterior vertical dimension of occlusion being represented by the higher of the two lines.

3. The rotation of the maxilla must be considered (if present) when analyzing a discrepancy between the maxillary orthopedic midline (line 1) and the maxillary dental arch midlines (lines 5).

4. A short condyle may be easily detected (line 7).

5. A long coronoid process may be easily detected (line 8).

6. A dental arch midline shift in the mandible is easily detected (lines 6).

7. A comparison of the dental midline shift on the study models between the upper and lower arches may be analyzed radiographically by the above method to see which member is at fault or whether both contribute and to what relative degree.

When added to the information obtained from clinical and other radiographic sources, not only does the Levandoski panographic analysis increase the clinician's overall understanding of the case, but it also provides information unobtainable by any other means.

LEVANDOSKI METHODS OF APPLIED CEPHALOMETRICS

Levandoski also applied his diagnostic insights to the more commonly traveled paths of roentgenocephalometrics with some very interesting and important results. Looking at the discipline of traditional cephalometric analysis from a TMJ point of view, Levandoski realized, as did others in the FJO camp, that most of the cephalometric analysis systems in use in the United States were developed before the 1970s. As a result, they fail to fully appreciate the orthopedic capabilities of functional appliances and their abilities at altering the maxillofacial relationships of the teeth, bone, and muscle and that most important of entities, the TMJ. With the appearance of these European-developed techniques on the scene, not only did the cephalometric analysis systems being used to aid in the diagnosis of the case have to be able to relate the teeth to one another, but they also had to consider the locations of the maxilla and mandible to the cranial base and how the locations of all three, the teeth, the maxilla, and the mandible, worked together at full functional occlusion. Most importantly, they also had to consider how their alignments during that full functional occlusion affected the TMJs. The major portion of traditionally trained orthodontists were on the whole slow to grasp this overall relationship. For Levandoski, even after having come from primarily a prosthodontic background, the significance of these relationships quickly became glaringly obvious.

Of the newer generation of cephalometric analysis systems, Levandoski is most fond of the McNamara and Sassouni analyses. (The workings and interpretation of these analyses are adequately covered in volume II.) One of the advantages of the more orthopedically oriented McNamara analysis is that it allows one to determine the correct relative anterior nasal spine–Menton (ANS-Me) lower anterior facial height, even in edentulous patients, something in which prosthodontists are very interested. Levandoski realized that this particular analysis, when coupled with evaluation of transcranial radiographs (or tomograms) and study models properly mounted on the fully adjustable Levandoski articulator (Logic I), could provide unparalleled accuracy in evaluating the true pretreatment status of a given case. It also allows for even better construction of stabilization prostheses (Levandoski's "supersplint"), removable restorative prostheses (partial and full dentures), and full-mouth "rehab" fixed restorative prostheses (crowns, bridges, and onlays).

The Sassouni plus analysis, originally developed by Dr. Viken Sassouni at the University of Pittsburgh during the late 1950s and early 1960s and expanded somewhat by Dr. Richard Beistle of Buchanan, Michigan, is another orthopedically oriented cephalometric analysis system that is useful for its ability to aid in determining the AP status of the maxilla. Levandoski is fond of this particular analysis since it confirms his findings that the maxilla is often the main etiological culprit in posteriorly deflected, retrusive mandibular TMJ problems and frequently needs forward development, especially in children. The coordination of information obtained from these two analyses in conjunction with the transcranial vector analysis allows the clinician to more precisely determine the true nature of the patient's maxillomandibular relationships. It also allows for a more scientific (i.e., mathematical) method of determining the anterior vertical dimension of the ANS-Me lower face height. This has been clearly manifested in yet another contribution to the diagnostic process, the Levandoski proportional analysis.

LEVANDOSKI PROPORTIONAL ANALYSIS

After carefully studying the works of McNamara and Harvold, Levandoski soon observed the relationship of the lengths of the maxilla and mandible to the ANS-Me lower face height. Therefore, he constructed a simple yet extremely handy graph for determining the proper lower face height as a product of those lengths. The graph consists of a horizontal x axis upon which is represented the diagonal linear length of the mandible (condylion to pogonion, or the McNamara effective mandibular length) starting at 85 mm and extending to 140 mm. The vertical y axis represents the maxillary length (condylion to A point, or the McNamara effective maxillary length) and extends vertically from 70 mm, at its intersection with the x axis, to 105 mm. A third straight line representing the linear values of the ANS-Me lower face height that would be a function of the maxillary (y axis) and mandibular (x axis) effective lengths is then constructed with values plotted along its length extending from 50 mm at its origin to 75 mm. This third line is called the z axis. Not only will this z axis line reveal the proper anterior lower face height for a given maxillary or mandibular effective length, but it also forms the third side of a triangle formed by the linear value lines for those lengths when the maxilla and mandible are disproportionate. For example, if the effective maxillary length is 100 mm (as it would be in the average adult male), then the proportional effective mandibular length should be 130 mm. If a maxillary length y axis value of 100 mm is drawn as a vertical straight line and a mandibular x axis value of 130 mm is drawn as a horizontal straight line, they would meet at the 70-mm mark on the lower face height z axis. Thus a 100-mm maxillary length and its correspondingly proportional 130-mm mandibular length would require an ANS-Me lower facial height of 70 mm to be balanced. Well, almost. Levandoski admonishes clinicians to "judiciously" add 6 to 8 mm extra facial height to the z axis values in adults. Thus, in adults, the z-axis values according to Levandoski would represent more of an acceptable minimum rather than ideal values. His feeling is that the fully mature adult can not only easily tolerate but actu-

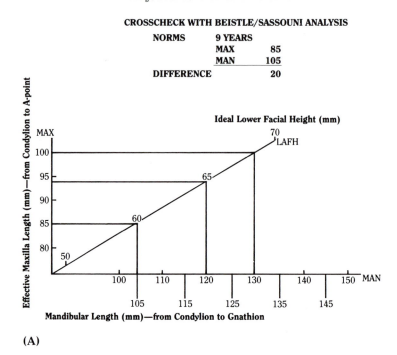

(A)

Figure 6–3 Levandoski proportional analysis graphs. **(A)** Adult dentition scale. **(B)** Primary/mixed dentition scale.

Levandoski Proportional Analysis (after Harvold)

Ideal Lower Facial Height (mm)—from Anterior Nasal Spine to Menton

Adult Dentition Scale

CROSSCHECK WITH BEISTLE/SASSOUNI ANALYSIS

NORMS		ADULT MALE		ADULT FEMALE
	MAX	100	MAX	94
	MAN	130	MAN	120
DIFFERENCE		30		26

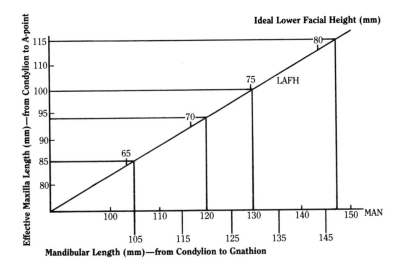

Figure 6-3(B)

ally require a bit more lower face height than the mathematical ratios represented by the graph actually indicate.

However, if these two lines fail to meet at the same point location along the linear lower facial height z axis, they will form a small triangle with each line—the x axis line, the y axis line, and the z axis line—forming a side. This will be due to a disproportionality between the maxilla and mandible. There is no way to tell which is the incorrect member merely by the way the triangle is formed either above the z axis or below it from the Levandoski proportional analysis alone. If it is above it, it might be because the mandible is too small in proportion to the maxilla. If it is formed below the z axis line, it might be because the maxilla is too small in proportion to the mandible. It is critical that the diagnostician realize that these relationships are predicated upon a previous knowledge of which member, the maxilla or mandible, is the more disproportional of the two to begin with. However, this is not difficult. Cephalometric analysis such as the Sassouni plus would reveal a retruded maxilla, etc. In our previously mentioned example, if the maxilla were in a "Class II" relationship with the mandible as in a case of a 100-mm effective maxillary length but an effective mandibular length of only 115 mm, one would not be able to tell merely from the Levandoski proportional analysis graph if the case were one of a normal maxilla and an undersized mandible or a normal mandible and an oversized maxilla. The same would be true for a "Class III" numerical relationship. With a maxillary length of 85 and a mandibular length of 117, would the maxilla be too short or the mandible be too long? Obviously, other data from the case such as the age and sex of the individual concerned and cephalometric analysis would clearly determine which is which in the above examples. The Levandoski proportional analysis graph merely shows what the proper lower anterior face height linear measurement (ANS-Me) should be for the more correct of the two components, be it the maxilla or mandible. Again, it must be remembered that for the mature adult Levandoski advises a 6- to 8-mm addition to the ideal z-axis lower face height reading determined from the graph. Thus it may be seen from the above material that setting the vertical dimension of occlusion for patients with full or partial dentitions, or even in fully edentulous patients, becomes a scientifically and mathematically determined matter of getting the mandible in the right place on its back end and with respect to the needs of the joint and the dictates of the Levandoski transcranial vector analysis as well as getting it in the right place on its front end as per the needs of the facial appearance and the vertical dictates of the Levandoski proportional analysis. Transcranial radiographs (or tomograms), cephalometric radiographs, and panographic radiographs are required to provide the previously discussed information and therefore, due to the fundamental and basic nature of the techniques involved, should be a part of the diagnostic analysis procedure of every major TMJ, orthodontic, and full-mouth restorative case.

APPLICATION OF THE LEVANDOSKI METHODS
TO THE FULL DENTITION

As previously discussed in an earlier chapter, children are just as susceptible to functionally oriented TMJ problems as a result of malocclusion as are adults. However, the treatment of these problems is tantamount to treatment of any other type of malocclusion in children and invariably results in the employment of FJO-type orthodontic technique. This, as also previously discussed in volume I, not only consists of the use of functional appliances but also incorporates the use of active plates and fixed-appliance technique as per the dictates (needs) of the case. Therefore, in the pediatric or adolescent TMJ patient, although the diagnostic process is the same and utilizes the same analytical methods, the therapeutics involved usually bypasses the splint stage of treatment and immediately engages the techniques of the corrective type of orthodontics needed. However, now the information needed to program the occlusal pad area of any Sagittal appliances that may be used can now be generated from the records and analyzed and applied to casts mounted on a Levandoski (Logic I) articulator if desired.

In the more mature adult, however, although the same maxillofacial orthodontic/orthopedic techniques may still pertain, albeit in a slightly modified fashion, the adult status of the individual (and usually the severity of certain aspects of the case such as insufficient vertical) allows for the occurrence of several optional methods of finishing the case that employ techniques other than orthodontics. This is where Levandoski's "supersplint" comes into play.

In the case of an adult TMJ pain-dysfunction patient with a full dentition who is suffering from functionally induced TMJ problems of the sort concerned with neuromuscular reflexive displacement of the mandible causing superior posterior displacement of the condyle (NRDM/SPDC), once the occlusion is cleared and the mandible is advanced, there almost invariably remains the problem of erupting buccal teeth and treatment of the attending posterior open bite. The posterior open bite reflects joint and muscle stabilization and may result from either the end stages of a 6- to 9-month stint with a Levandoski mandibular stabilization prosthesis or the point in an orthodontic treatment plan where the anterior occlusion has been cleared, one way or another, and the Bionator or Orthopedic Corrector I has been worn about 5 to 6 months. At this point the muscle-retraining and -relengthening effects of the appropriate appliance wear have caused patients to be desirous of closing their mandibles in the more orthopedically proper advanced position. However, in their desire to do so, the posterior molar support is not yet fully present, and if the pretreatment deficiency of posterior vertical has been great enough, it will be a considerable time before it arrives due to eruption of the posterior teeth. Posterior molar support is necessary to keep the mandible advanced even during function. Here is where the options become available.

Adults in demanding life-styles are often willing to trade economics for expediency. The time frame involved in closing the posterior open bite in an adult whose mandible has been "muscularly advanced" with a Levandoski splint or functional appliance may not be compatible with that particular patient's life-style (or in some cases "work style"). The increased time of Bionator or Orthopedic Corrector I wear, in spite of the cap-raising techniques designed to speed up the increase in vertical, may not be popular with certain patients. Some patients also find adjustment to the use of Biofinisher technique with its lateral rakes and vertical elastics very difficult. In these instances when the degree of posterior open bite is considerable and the vertical is slow in changing due to things like the distance the teeth must erupt, the age of the patient, or any "eruption-inhibiting" deep curve of Spee problems (which should have been corrected prior to advancement via arc-lengthening development techniques), the patient may opt for treating the posterior vertical open space between the upper and lower molars and bicuspids with a variety of prosthetic techniques.

There are also patients with problems that are beyond the scope of current dental therapeutics. The patient who has had four bicuspids extracted followed by intrusive orthodontics may have a complete "open" bite (lack of posterior *and* anterior vertical dimension which actually leaves them overclosed in an orthopedic sense at full occlusion). Eruption of anterior teeth intruded with utility arches in most cases is irreversible, and thus an overlay partial denture with anterior incisal and posterior occlusal pads is indicated. The patient who has had postsurgical condylar shortening may be impossible to stabilize and unable or unwilling to cope with functional appliances. The patient with several missing key teeth who cannot afford or is unwilling to invest the time and expense of comprehensive restorative orthodontic and prosthodontic care may require an overlay partial denture. The overlay prosthesis can be quite versatile and can be an excellent compromise in the case where no other treatment option is available.

Levandoski's rationale and approach to the fabrication of occlusal overlay partial dentures involves some innovative advantages. The occlusal pad areas over the teeth are fabricated of an ultrathin retentive meshwork of a chrome-cobalt alloy. The meshwork has several unique strong points over the prior art of retentive beads or coatings applied to a solid occlusal overlay partial denture:

1. The meshwork very firmly engages the acrylic, which allows unprecedented retention and resistance to fracture.
2. The meshwork does not directly touch the teeth, which makes insertion adjustments very easy.

3. The meshwork is cheaper to fabricate.
4. The occlusal tooth surfaces are contacted by the overlay acrylic, which makes tooth wear less likely and ajustment very easy.
5. In the event that a tooth has to be restored under the denture, acrylic may be easily added to make up for any minor posttreatment discrepancies.
6. Repairs are very easy and do not require recoating or special framework preparation.
7. The buccal/lingual finish line at the height of the contour helps to strengthen the composite cap and provides a definitive finish line.
8. It is easier to finish light-cured composites applied to the occlusal cap area with the meshwork.

Some of the greatest advantages of overlay partial dentures are that they do not involve an irreversible procedure as would the full-mouth rehabilitative techniques of cast full crowns or onlays. The overlay partial denture prosthesis is almost invariably made for the lower arch. They are constructed on models mounted with a compound construction bite obtained as per the Levandoski transcranial vector analysis technique with the Levandoski articulator. It would be the same compound bite used to construct the mandibular stabilization prosthesis. After 6 to 9 months of wear of the stabilization prosthesis, a time during which the patient is asymptomatic, the clinician will be sure of the posterior vertical dimension and location of the mandible that is correct for that particular patient. It is wise to use a *removable* posterior "gap-filling" cast prosthesis for a 1- to 2-year period prior to restoring to permanent cast crown and/or onlay-type restorations just to make sure that the long-term compatibility of that particular mandibular position (vertical, lateral, and AP) and resultant condylar position at full occlusion have been secured.

The word *prosthesis* is pure Greek and originally meant "a putting to." The modern definition is "the replacement of an absent part by an artificial substitute." In the case of the type of prosthesis we are discussing here, the "absent part" happens to be the absence of sufficient posterior vertical dimension of occlusion, and it manifests itself once the condyles and mandible have been properly orthopedically and muscularly advanced to the correct physiological (down and forward) location, which results in the classic form of a posterior open bite (Christensen's old phenomenon). Once again, it is interesting to see what the prosthetic talent of Levandoski is capable of producing when his efforts are "put to" the problems of "filling in the gaps" of the posterior occlusion with the aforementioned overlay partial dentures. He has made important contributions here also.

The chief problem with the cast overlay partial has been with the hardness of the materials used for the occlusal surface. Overlay partials are not new to dentistry; their use goes back to the "bite-raising" techniques of the early TMJ investigators of 60 years ago. One approach to the problem of just how to construct these devices was to cast the entire partial denture out of metal. Economics requires that a nonprecious common partial denture framework of a lasting alloy of the chrome-cobalt type be used. Levandoski feels that the metal should be nickel free. A certain amount of wear and chemical reaction takes place in the mouth with respect to partial denture metal frameworks, and although it is slight, the possibility of nickel ion release cannot be ignored. This, Levandoski feels, is undesirable because (1) a considerable number of people are sensitive to nickel, (2) it has the potential of being immunosupresssive, and (3) it may cause metal allergy–type reactions as well as other heavy metal toxicity reactions. Additionally, with an overlay partial made entirely of metal, the minor occlusal adjustments required to mill the biting surfaces of the device into a comfortable and compatible chewing surface become quite difficult. This is especially true when one considers the most unusual occlusal surface pattern design Levandoski recommends for these types of prostheses.

Another more popular method of constructing overlay partials consists of casting a metal framework with the usual lingual bar and traditional Aker's or reverse-action clasps but then covering the occlusal surface of the appliance with "retention beads" of cast metal so as to facilitate the addition of acrylic. This acrylic is then shaped in the form of traditional occlusal dental anatomy to conform to the opposing maxillary posterior teeth. The problem with this technique is that although it results in an overlay partial with a highly desirable "softer" occlusal acrylic surface, the acrylic quite often breaks loose from the metal framework under heavy function. Levandoski has devised alterations in the technique of this type of construction that drastically reduce the incidence of breakage.

Instead of using cast retention beads to hold the acrylic to the metal framework, Levandoski constructs the appliance with a buccal and lingual finishing line of metal just at the buccal and lingual heights of the contour of the teeth. Then a cast metal meshwork, similar to that used on free-end tissue-born partial dentures, is used to cover the occlusal surfaces of the posterior teeth. There is a slight clearance of the material over the occlusal surfaces of the abutment teeth as a result of the use of 30-gauge relief wax over these teeth prior to making the refractory casts. The space between the occlusal surface and the metal mesh framework then allows the acrylic to flow under the framework for greatly enhanced mechanical retention and acrylic adaptation.

The master cast with framework is then articulated with the maxillary model by using the patient's stabilization prosthesis as the interocclusal record. Note that after 6 to 9 months of wear, the stabilization prosthesis contains all the information needed to fabricate an occlusal surface on a long-term prosthesis. In other words, the casts mounted with the

CASE HISTORY

PATIENT: Age 22 years, 10 months, male

MAIN PROBLEM:
1. Can't chew food properly, because of pain.
2. Pain and other TMJ symptoms.
3. Want lower jaw forward.
4. The frequent headaches.

DENTAL HISTORY:
1. Family dentist referred patient to orthodontist for orthodontic treatment.
2. Patient had orthodontic treatment at age 18. Orthodontist had two upper first bicuspids extracted and treated with fixed appliances (braces) for 2½ years. Patient wore a retainer for one year.
3. Pain started in the right TMJ after the braces were put on.
4. After braces removed, patient had abnormal bite, pain, and could not chew food normally.
5. Patient then saw Dr. Gelb in New York City for seven appointments. Dr. Gelb made a lower splint that relieved pain, allowed patient's mandible to bite forward, and patient could chew food without discomfort. No headaches with splint.
6. Patient had to travel 1000 miles each way to Dr. Gelb's office. Dr. Gelb referred to Dr. Witzig in Minneapolis, to finish the case, (300 miles each way from Madison, Wisconsin).

FINDINGS:
I. Orthodontic treatment finished in a Class II/Division 2 Malocclusion.
II. Severe insufficient Vertical Dimension without splint.
III. Incisal Interference without splint.
IV. Pain when splint out of mouth.
V. Upper central incisor teeth tipped lingually. (Retruded centrals.)
VI. Right TMJ has locked disc.

RADIOGRAPHIC FINDINGS:
1. Posterior-superior displaced condyles.

DIAGNOSIS: Internal derangement both TMJs with displaced condyles in both joints.

TREATMENT:
First Appliance
1. Sagittal (splint) appliance to . . .
   a. Move upper anterior teeth out of retrusion.
   b. Keep pain free.
   c. Allow to chew food.
   d. Allow mandible to bite normally.

Second Appliance
2. Biofinisher.
   a. Increase vertical dimension.

Third Appliance
3. Overlay prosthesis.
   a. Allows normal bite and occlusion.

RESULTS: 1. No Pain, No headaches with prosthesis.
            2. Can chew food properly with prosthesis.
            3. Patient can have overlay prosthesis changed to crowns, after
               wearing the overlay prosthesis for two years.
    One year overlay prosthesis:
            1. No headaches.
            2. No clicking or popping.

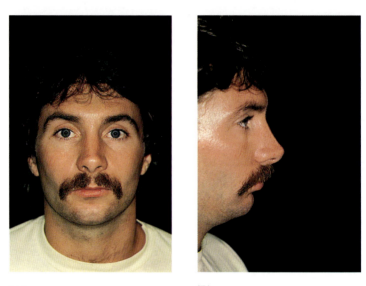

(A)   (B)

Figure 6–4   TMJ combination therapy: functional jaw orthopedics and
prosthodontics. **(A and B)** Pretreatment facial views of a 22-year-old male with
severe TMJ problems and a history of upper bicuspid extractions and fixed
appliance treatment (braces) for a Class II, Division 2 malocclusion. **(C and D)**
Pretreatment study casts of the completed orthodontic treatments for original
malocclusion. Note that the patient is still Class II, Division 2 with a deep bite
and retruded mandible. **(E)** Note the incredible curve of Spee of the
posttreatment maxillary dental arch! **(F and G)** Pre–TMJ treatment intraoral
views. **(H)** Construction bite for a Sagittal II (splint) appliance. Note how the
construction bite offers some modicum of increase in vertical and mandibular
advancement. **(I and J)** Acrylic bite blocks or "occlusal pads" of the appliance
provide a pain-relieving "splint effect." **(K)** Appliance in the mouth. **(L)**

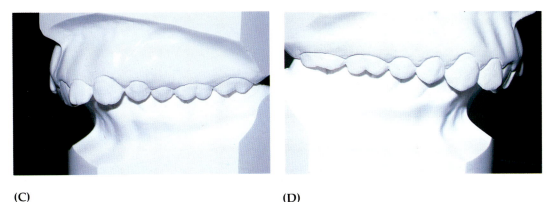

(C)

(D)

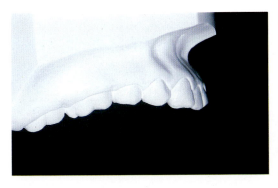

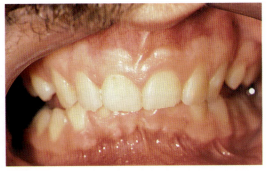

(E)

(F)

Biofinisher appliance. **(M)** Completion of the Biofinisher stage of treatment. At this point, with the posterior open bite only partially closed by Biofinisher technique the decision was made to complete the treatment of the remaining posterior open bite with a prosthetic overlay. **(N)** Condyles were finished in the Gelb 4/7 position. The ability of the prosthetic overlay partial to place the condyle in this position was verified by transcranial radiography (at full occlusion). **(O)** Overlay partial denture prothesis. **(P and Q)** Occlusion with an overlay partial in place: no TMJ clicking, no headaches. The patient relates that he can now bite where his jaw feels like it wants to go. **(R)** Note the greatly enlarged posterior joint spaces at full occlusion on an overlay prosthesis. **(S)** One year after TMJ treatment: no signs or symptoms. (Courtesy of Dr. John Witzig.)

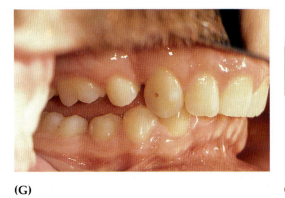

(G)

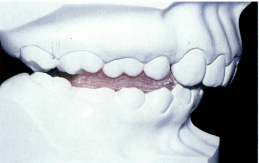

(H)

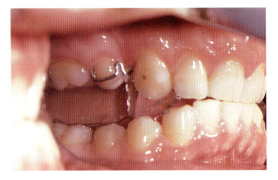

(I)

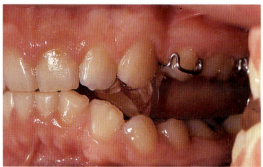

(J)

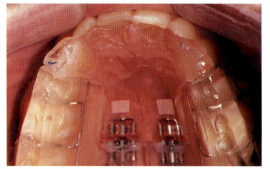

(K)

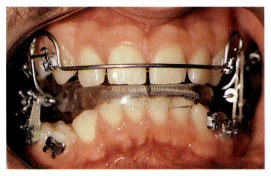

(L)

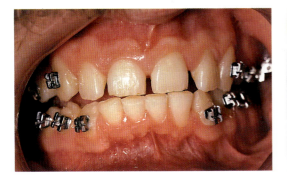

(M)

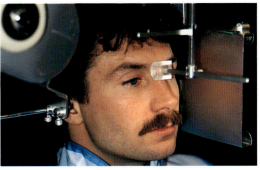

(N)

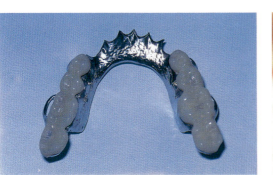

(O)

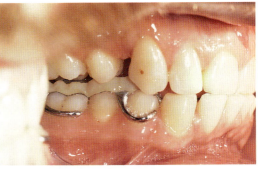

(P)

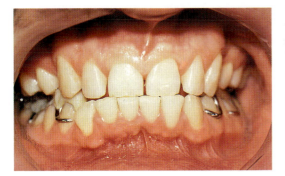

(Q)

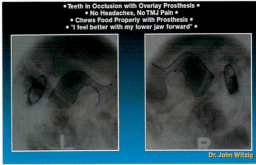

(R)

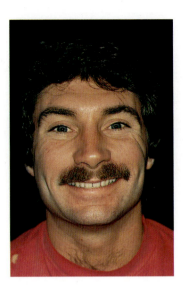

(S)

stabilization prosthesis now acting as an interocclusal transfer record will retain the precise AP positioning, posterior vertical dimension, and transverse (z axis) parameters that have helped get the patient into remission of signs and symptoms before mounting the casts on the Levandoski articulator. It is prudent to take a set of transcranial films with the patient in the intercuspal position of the splint. If the casts are to be mounted on the Levandoski articulator and it appears that the anterior vertical dimension should be increased or that the condyle must be advanced, then fine-tuning adjustments can be made. Greenstick compound can be placed on the occlusal surface of the stabilization prosthesis and the articulator closed. This corrected record is then placed in the patient's mouth, and another set of transcranial films are taken to confirm the correction. The patient is placed on a soft diet and advised to call the next day so that symptoms can be evaluated. If the patient feels comfortable with the correction, then that corrected position will be used to finish the occlusion in acrylic or light-cured composite on the pads of the framework.

The beauty of the technique of using the initial acrylic Levandoski supersplint as an occlusal registration for mounting construction casts is that even an old "barn door hinge–type" articulator will suffice for this particular phase of the treatment plan as long as no other changes in anterior or posterior vertical dimension are contemplated. This is because the supersplint had to be originally constructed on a Levandoski-type, fully adjustable articulator (Logic I) in conjunction with the transcranial vector analysis coordinates and cephalometric analysis. This gives the splint the capacity to properly position the condyles in the first place; hence it also acts as a perfect way to orient construction casts for the completion of the overlay partial because the x, y, and even z axis adjustments have already been programmed by the first articulator into the splint's occlusal acrylic surface. Functional milling and/or occlusal adjustments have further refined it. Therefore, any type of articulating device capable of merely holding the construction casts as per the dictates of the intervening splint, now acting as an occlusal registration device, will serve for the completion of construction of the overlay partial because x, y, and z coordinate corrections will anatomically be present. The question then arises, "But what about lateral excursive movements?" The answer is that in the way Levandoski prefers to construct these devices, there shouldn't be much of a lateral movement to the occlusion, at least not for a while.

Upon receiving the cast framework back from the laboratory, it is removed from the construction cast. Then the construction cast and a cast of the upper arch are mounted in any kind of articulator by using the former supersplint to orient the casts to each other. Light-cured or self-curing acrylic is then placed in somewhat thin layers over the posterior abutment teeth, and the cast framework is pressed firmly down onto the lower master construction cast so as to fully seat against the cast and squeeze out excessive acrylic from under it in the process. The acrylic is then quickly and easily pressure cured or light cured. This first layer is strong, hard acrylic such as Densply Triad and will serve as a substructure acrylic for the sake of strength. But Levandoski feels that such acrylics or composites are too hard for optimum compatibility with opposing occlusions of TMJ pain-dysfunction patients. He therefore uses a somewhat softer, more conventional acrylic such as Forestacryl in a second layer processed over the substructure layer for occlusal purposes. This second layer of softer acrylic is placed over the first layer of harder acrylic or composite that has already been cured, and the articulator is closed down into it so that the occlusal surfaces of the upper teeth form the acrylic to their surfaces. Once cured, the newly formed occlusal surface of the overlay partial is trimmed and polished to coincide as closely as possible to the anatomical surface of the original Levandoski-type supersplint, high buccal and lingual walls, cuspid rise, and all! The purpose in this is not only to continue to force the patient to function in the newly achieved advanced orthopedic position as was done originally with the splint but to also cut down on the amount of lateral excursive movements possible during functional occlusion as was also originally done with the splint.

Levandoski, as well as other advanced TMJ investigators, feels that lateral excursive movements during function are destabilizing factors and are universally hard on TMJs that have already suffered a considerable degree of degenerative osseous breakdown and/or ligament damage.

Joints with nonreducible articular discs, anteromedially displaced discs, or ligamentous perforations are in this category. When the disc is anteromedially displaced by a correspondingly superiorly and posteriorly displaced condyle, corrective advancement procedures that deliver the condyle out of its improper place in the bilaminar zone and reposition it in the vicinity of the Gelb 4/7 position may not always recapture the disc in severe functionally induced joint degeneration cases. Torn or elongated posterior attachments and other supportive ligaments within the joint may have suffered so much chronic abuse and damage as to preclude complete disc recapture. Yet substitute scar-type tissue will generally form upon which the condylar head may ride as long as the bilaminar zone remains unviolated and the joint remains decompressed at both function and rest. But this substitute tissue that develops in the joint under such postadvancement circumstances is still not articular discal tissue. And the elongated ligaments do not fully regain their original taut length. Tendon and ligament damage beyond a certain point is incapable of complete restoration to normal. Therefore, it is true that some advanced states of TMJ degenerative arthritis or functionally induced arthrosis may be considered lifelong conditions in that all of the individual joint components may never return to a fully normal status. They perpetually remain in this "guarded" condition and function reasonably normally, albeit tenuously, in pain-free operation. Therefore, some care must be exercised in certain types of cases as to the amount of physical loading and chronic functional "abuse" such joints should prudently be expected to endure. Retaining the protective "high buccal walls of the occlusal acrylic biting surface of the overlay partial denture is a move in the direction of trying to provide as much long-term protection to those fragile and physiologically threadbare joints as possible. Mastication is not a problem because the patient is quite used to functioning on such an occlusal scheme as represented by these types of devices. Patients do not need excessive functional lateral excursive movements to masticate well. They do need pain-free well-protected joints. Constructing the occlusal surface of the overlay partial to mimic the biting surface of the original splint provides much of that protection. So does a built-in cuspid rise wherever possible so that when such border movements are executed, for one reason or another, the posteriors are discluded as quickly as possible. This turns out to be far more compatible with the joint than is employing anterior incisal guidance involving centrals and laterals. The buccal and lingual walls of the posterior acrylic of the splint or overlay partial can only go so high. Once they cease to be effective, the cuspid rise should disclude the patient so that no lateral protrusive maneuver under occlusal pressure can be produced by the patient. Lateral protrusive bruxism is very destructive to impaired joints and is likely a major etiological agent in degenerative TMJ disease. Late canine rise to disclude the patient will protect the joints and avoid continued insult. The acrylic used for the occlusal surfaces of the final overlay partials may be much harder than that used for the biting surface of the original mandibular stabilization splint. This is because the joints have had about 6 to 9 months to "settle down" in properly positioned, pain-free, decompressed function and therefore have physiologically "bounced back" from their former pretreatment debilitated state. After such periods of intracapsular recuperation, they are better prepared to absorb the shock of a harder occlusal surface.

In light of this view, the original *all-acrylic* splints Levandoski constructed were made entirely of the softer-type acrylic. This allowed the patient to readily "mill in" the minor discrepancies of the occlusal surface through function. But the substructure of these original splints, being composed of the same softer-type acrylics, was subject to breakage. This led Levandoski to develop a modified technique of double layering where the main substructure of the splint is made out of an extrastrength acrylic that is very hard such as Forestacryl while the occlusal biting surface (the top 2 mm) is composed of a second layer of softer laboratory acrylic. This, as previously mentioned, makes for an occlusal surface that is easier not only for the clinician to adjust but also for the opposing teeth to functionally mill during chewing and for the joints to biomechanically accept. Caulk Ortho Resin is a type of softer acrylic favored for such double–acrylic-layering splint construction techniques. However, if the interocclusal distance, i.e., the amount of posterior open bite, is minimal and causes the resultant splint made for that patient to be relatively thin and therefore more subject to breakage, the entire splint may have to be made out of the stronger Forestacryl. The metal substructure of the permanent overlay partial denture obviates this consideration, and softer acrylic may be used for occlusal biting surfaces if desired. It may be easily "spotted" (added to) with cold-cure acrylic, and it is easily milled. However, it must be remembered that by the time more "permanent" prostheses such as these are constructed, the patient is usually under such good control that the use of the harder, more durable (and therefore more practical) acrylic poses no problem.

Yet if the clinician is concerned as to the acceptability of the harder acrylic to the patient, the double-layering technique may even be used with the cast framework of the overlay partial. The initial substructure acrylic may be made of the harder light-cured composite or conventionally cured acrylic, and an occlusal layer of softer acrylic may be processed on top of it. In either technique, of course, the final layer of acrylic is formed to the occlusal surfaces of the upper teeth by closing the articulator down onto the soft acrylic before it is cured. For the more severe cases, the double-layering technique represents a more cautious approach. In the event of occlusal wear of the softer surface layer of acrylic with time, the biting surfaces of the overlay partial may be easily "spotted" with additional acrylic and formed in the mouth when needed to compensate for wear. The end product of these techniques is a hybrid

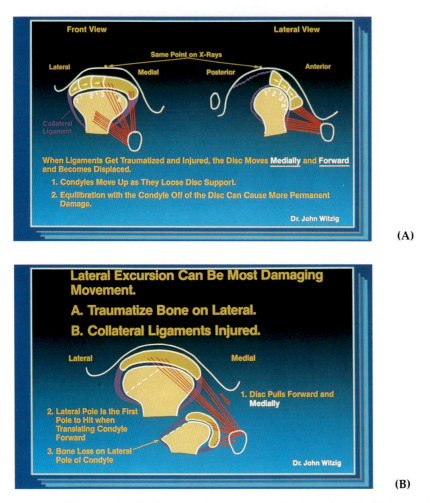

Figure 6–5 **(A)** Disc displacement anteriorly and medially leaves lateral pole of condyle unprotected. **(B)** This is why lateral excursive mandibular movements are very damaging.

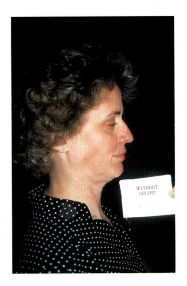

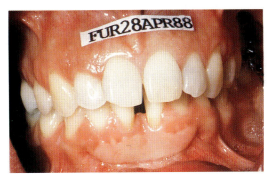

(B)

(A)

Figure 6–6   Generic manually produced "guesswork" splints vs. the science and mathematics of the Levandoski mandibular stabilization prosthesis. This middle-aged female suffered from a long history of TMJ problems of a functionally induced nature, some of which were masticatory problems, supraorbital and retro-orbital headaches (cephalalgia), neck aches (cervicalgia), torticolis (involuntary twitching and/or spasm of the neck musculature affecting head posture), earaches (otalgia), barohypoacusis, tinnitus, restriction of the range of movement of the mandible, and bilateral crepitus of the TMJs upon movement. **(A)** "Pretreatment" profile. Note that the term *pretreatment* indicates the condition of the patient prior to treatment by the Levandoski methods. She had a previous history of numerous other types of treatments from a number of other TMJ clinicians involving the use of a number of other types of splints. **(B)** "Pretreatment" intraoral view of occlusion. Note the deep bite and "tightness" of the anterior incisior coupling. This generates the NRDM/SPDC phenomenon in this patient, hence also her TMJ symptomatic picture. **(C)** Generic splint no. 1 in the patient's mouth. Note the status of the anterior acrylic area, a form of iatrogenic anterior incisal interference. **(D)** Splint no. 1. Note how the acrylic in the anterior area acts as a ramp to keep the mandible back during full occlusion on the splint. **(E)** Tracings of transcranial radiographs of the TMJs with the patient biting fully into splint no. 1. Note that the splint does nothing to decompress the superior and posterior joint spaces, which are suffering from severe condylar intrusion. It also did nothing to relieve the patient's signs and symptoms. **(F)** Profile with splint no. 1 inserted. **(G)** Splint no. 2. Note the even thicker anterior area of acrylic that opens the *anterior* vertical dimension of occlusion further still but at the same time does nothing for the *posterior* vertical or the condyle-fossa relationship. **(H)** Splint no. 2 in the mouth. **(I)** Transcranial radiographic tracings of TMJs with splint no. 2 in the patient's mouth at full occlusion. Note the failure of the splint to decompress the joints, NRDM/SPDC phenomenon being still in full force. **(J)** Profile with splint no. 2 in the patient's mouth at full occlusion. **(K)** Splint no. 3, this time an upper. Note how the acrylic in the anterior area adjacent to the lingual surfaces of the upper anterior teeth still acts as a ramp deflecting the mandibular denture (hence condyles) posteriorly, upon full intercuspation. **(L)** Splint no. 3 in the patient's mouth. **(M)** Transcranial radiographic tracings of TMJs with splint no. 3 in the patient's mouth at full occlusion. Note its failure to decompress the joints. It also failed to relieve the symptoms. **(N)** Profile with splint no. 3 in mouth at full occlusion. **(O)** Yet another splint (no. 4) made at another office. **(P)** Although no anterior ramp of acrylic exists here to act as a form of anterior incisal interference, the "construction-bite" occlusal record (produced manually) used for the orientation of the plaster casts for construction of this particular splint resulted in a device that drove the mandible back upon full intercuspal occlusion. Hence the NRDM/SPDC phenomenon is in full effect just the same. **(Q)** Transcranial radiographic tracings of TMJs with splint no. 4 in the patient's mouth at full occlusion. Note how it fails to decompress the joint, i.e., fails to force the condyle out of its superior posterior displaced position. It also failed to relieve the patient's symptoms. **(R)** Profile with splint no. 4 in the mouth at full occlusion. **(S)** Tracings of the transcranial radiographic record generated via a Levandoski (Logic I) articulator employing the corrections programmed into the three-way hinges from the transcranial vector analysis. Note how the compound occlusal record so generated (and hence the splint that will be generated as a result of it) forces the mandibular denture and, as a result, the condyles into a physiologically balanced stable relationship. Note the increased superior and posterior joint spaces in both joints. **(T)** Compound occlusal record on casts mounted on a Levandoski articulator. **(U)** Compound record in the patient's mouth. Subsequent transcranial radiographs confirm that this record forces the condyles to the Gelb 4/7 position at full intercuspal occlusion. A period of about 30 minutes is often required to allow distraught muscles time to relax enough to permit the full (but gentle) occlusion into the compound record that was initially generated on Levandoski articulator after transcranial vector analysis corrections have been performed. **(V)** Profile with a compound "occlusal correction" record in place at full intercuspation. **(W and X)** Orientation of the upper and lower dentitions to one another after coordinates from transcranial vector analysis corrections have been transferred to articulator hinges. With the transcranial vector analysis used to correct the occlusal table *posteriorly*, the Levandoski proportional analysis graph (keyed on effective maxillary and mandibular lengths) was used to correct the deficient vertical dimension *anteriorly*. It was opened 3.0 mm. **(Y and Z)** Facial views with a compound occlusal record–generated Levandoski mandibular stabilization prosthesis ("supersplint") inserted and the patient biting at full intercuspation. After a period of several months of splint wear note how the facial muscles assume a more relaxed nature resulting in improved facial appearance. With the splint inserted symptoms dramatically subsided. (Courtesy of Dr. Ronald Levandoski.)

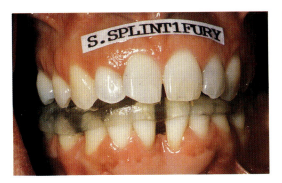

(C)

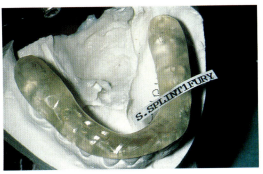

(D)

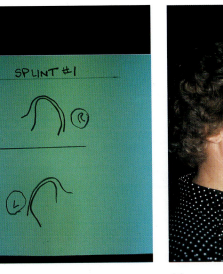

(E)

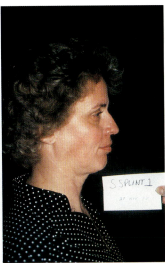

(F)

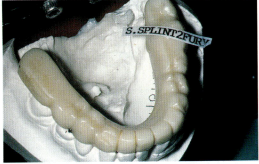

(G)

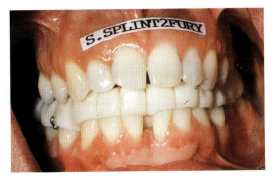

(H)

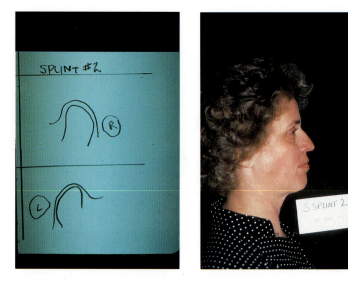

(I)

(J)

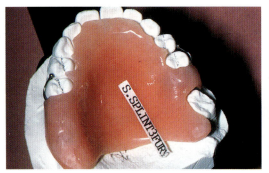

(K)

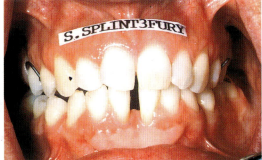

(L)

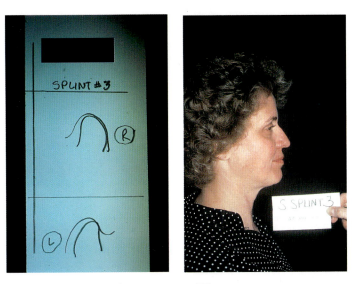

(M)

(N)

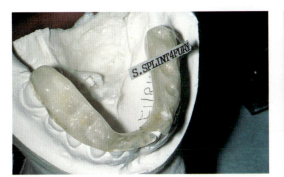

(O)

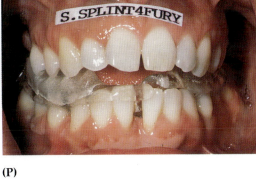

(P)

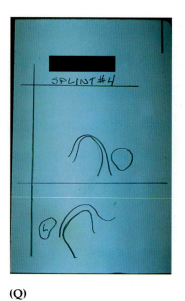

(Q)

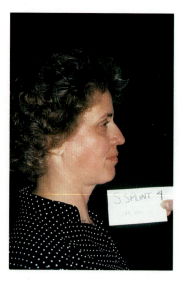

(R)

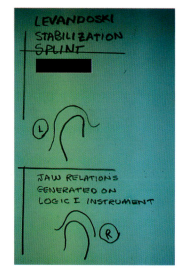

(S)

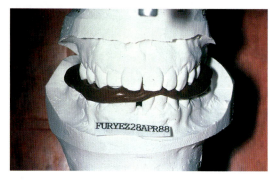

(T)

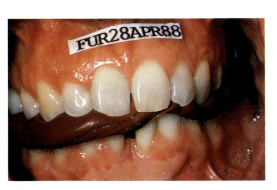

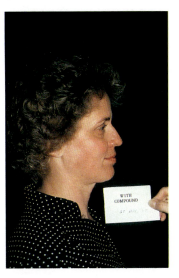

(U)

(V)

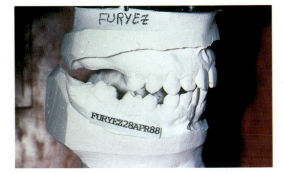

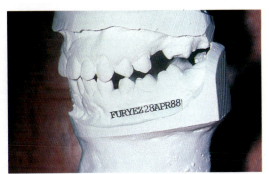

(W)

(X)

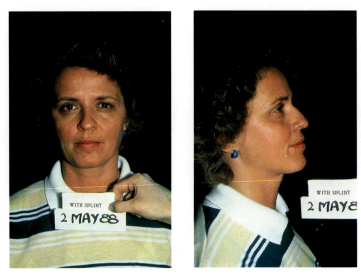

(Y)   (Z)

splint—appliance—prosthesis device that incorporates principles of all three: an intraoral acrylic TMJ splint, an orthodontic functional appliance, and a removable partial denture prosthesis. The double layering (2 laminae) of acrylic gives such devices even wider versatility and results in what might be termed as "bilaminar mandibular stabilization partial denture," with the play on words obviously intended.

A modification of the above methods of constructing the overlay partial denture that is popular with some clinicians involves the use of composite material for the occlusal portion of the prosthesis instead of the various types of acrylic. After the framework is cast in the "retention bead" style, a material known a Silicote is applied to the surface of the metal to receive the light-cured composite material. This material is mixed with a flame in a special blow torch designed for the purpose and then applied to the metal in a manner laboratory technicians refer to as "fire blasting." This results in a bonded, clear layer of burnt silica 2 μm thick over the metal surfaces to which it is applied. It is to this surface in turn that the light-cured composite is applied. The composite material offers better wear characteristics than the acrylics do. It has the additional advantage of spotting well when additional composite is needed. The initial layer of composite can be molded to the occlusal layer of the upper cast in the Levandoski fashion, or it may be constructed in the more conventional form of traditional occlusal dental anatomy. It is then light cured by the laboratory with special strobe lights in approximately 90 seconds. Of course, the more durable surface of the composite is harder and therefore is generally only indicated for a patient who has not suffered extensive long-term damage.

APPLICATION OF THE LEVANDOSKI METHODS TO THE PARTIAL DENTITION

When patients who have less than complete dentitions require treatments for functionally induced TMJ problems, the same principles of treatment previously discussed still apply, albeit with some slight modifications for those patients with free-end, extension base, partial denture needs.

If a patient is missing posterior teeth but is still capable of supporting fully tooth-borne partial dentures due to the presence of posterior

---

Figure 6–7 Splint failure due to the reverse Christensen effect. **(A–C)** Study casts of the occlusion of a 29-year-old female with a long history of functionally induced TMJ problems including severe cephalalgia, cervicalgia, TMJ arthralgia, crepitus, and a history of treatment with five different types of generic splints including a Herbst. The patient was referred for surgical treatment, which she refused. **(D and E)** Generic splint no. 1. Note how the splint opens the bite more in the anterior area than in the posterior area. Splint no. 1 had been ground to the point of perforating through the intraocclusal acrylic in the second molar area. **(F)** Generic splint no. 1 in the mouth. Note that although it is fitted to the upper dental arch, there is nothing to prevent lateral mandibular movement at full occlusion. **(G)** Profile with splint no. 1. **(H and I)** Generic splint no. 2 opens the anterior vertical even more while doing very little for the posterior vertical as evidenced by the proximity of the upper and lower posterior molars to each other. This is the complete opposite of the desired Christensen phenomenon, which would result in greater increase in posterior vertical (the creation of a posterior open bite) as the mandible-condyle unit is advanced out of its retruded pretreatment position. **(J)** Splint no. 2 in the patient's mouth. In spite of greater anterior vertical, it fails to decompress the condyles, prevent lateral excursive movements during occlusion, or relieve the patient's symptoms. **(K)** Profile with splint no. 2. **(L and M)** Herbst appliance used by another treating clinician. Levandoski feels these devices are contraindicated in TMJ pain-dysfunction patients because they prevent a natural return to centric relation, which, although not a functional position for TMJ conditions, oddly seems a requirement for Nature at such times as yawning. Levandoski believes that such patients should not have the restriction to such movements placed on them by such things as a Herbst appliance. It did nothing but worsen the patient's

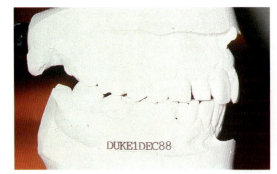

Figure 6–7(A)

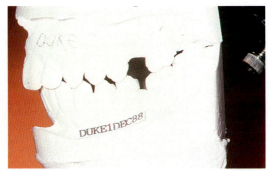

(B)

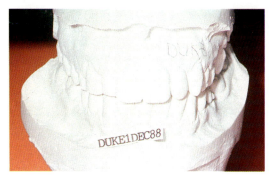

(C)

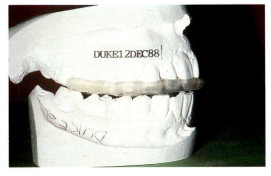

(D)

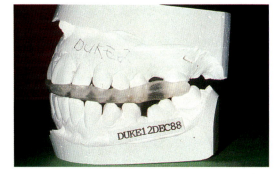

(E)

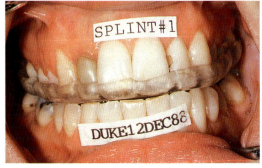

(F)

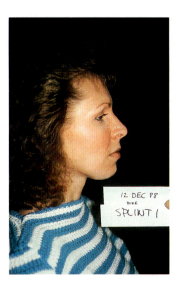

(G)

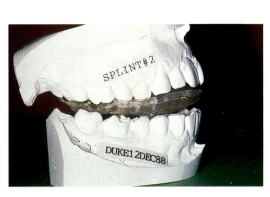

(H)

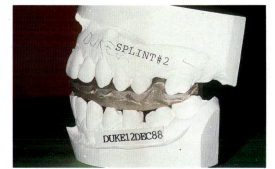

(I)

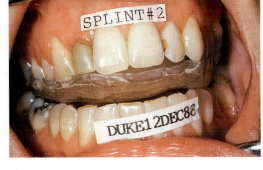

(J)

symptoms. **(N)** Herbst appliance in the patient's mouth. **(O)** Patient profile with the Herbst appliance in her mouth. **(P)** Transcranial radiographic tracings of the pretreatment condyle-fossa relationship (hatched lines) and corrected condyle-fossa relationship to the Gelb 4/7 position (solid line) as part of the Levandoski transcranial vector analysis. **(Q)** Compound occlusal record generated on a Levandoski (Logic I) articulator after corrections are made in the x, y-planes as per the numerical values of the vector analysis. **(R and S)** Relationship of the upper and lower dental arches to each other without a compound record in the way. Once corrections are made on articulator, the posterior vertical is corrected as per the dictates of the x, y-coordinates of the transcranial vector analysis. The anterior vertical is corrected (by adjusting the

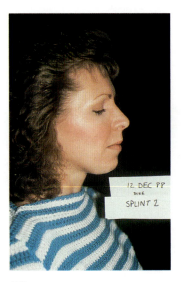

(K)

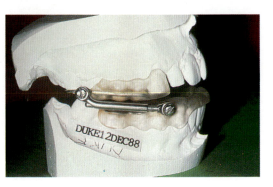

(L)

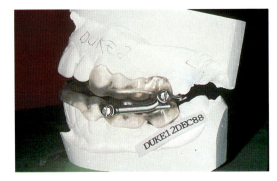

(M)

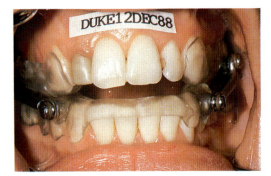

(N)

pin on the articulator) as per the cephalometric dictates of the Levandoski proportional analysis graph. Note how the posterior vertical is opened without simultaneously excessively opening the anterior vertical. This represents proper decompression of the joints and advancement down and forward of the mandible-condyle unit. This is a correct example of the Christensen phenomenon. **(T)** Levandoski mandibular stabilization prosthesis in the patient's mouth. Note that the high buccal walls of acrylic prevent lateral excursive movements during the final moments of full intercuspation. Small acrylic projections in the cuspid area provide a "canine rise" to protect the joints during wider-ranging lateral excursion. **(U)** Since the maxillary right cuspid shows excessive wear, the principle of group function is utilized to provide a "rise"

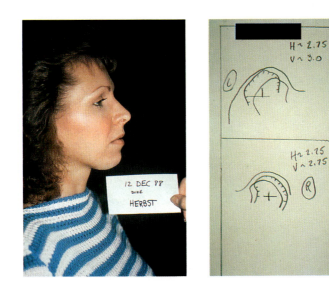

(O)   (P)

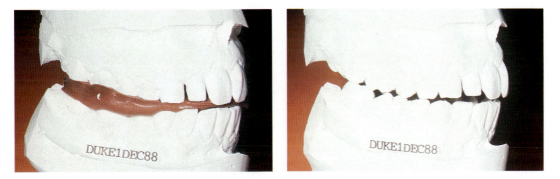

(Q)   (R)

during right lateral excursive movements. With use of this splint the patient's symptoms dramatically subsided. **(W and X)** Facial views with the Levandoski "supersplint" in place at full intercuspation. (Courtesy of Dr. Ronald Levandoski.)

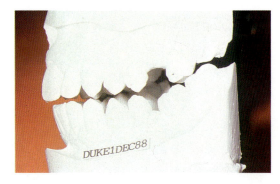

(S)

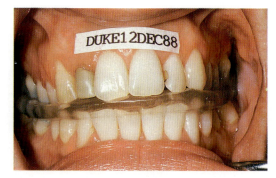

(T)

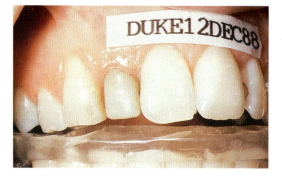

(U)

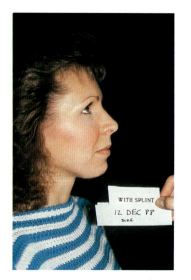

(V)

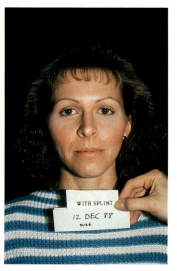

(W)

abutment teeth, the technique of construction of the Levandoski mandib-ular stabilization prosthesis or supersplint as well as that of the final cast overlay, metal-based partial denture is the same as described above. The only difference is that the splint and partial denture must fill in the eden-tulous areas between the abutment teeth. But for the patient who is miss-ing those all-important posterior abutment teeth, the clinician merely pro-duces a "construction-quality" set of master casts and directly proceeds to cast the metal partial denture framework. This then serves as the sub-structure for the splint/partial appliance to be constructed for that patient. Let us assume an example patient with a full natural upper dentition and a natural lower dentition consisting of only the remaining six lower ante-rior teeth. A cast metal framework is initially constructed as if a tradi-tional partial denture were going to be made complete with the appropri-ate types of clasps, lingual bar, or plate and meshwork extensions out over the edentulous areas. Acrylic is then processed as per methods de-scribed above, and the appliance serves as an initial stabilization prosthe-sis to get the joints (and musculature) under control for 6 to 9 months.

When it comes time to convert the splint to a partial denture, the master casts are mounted on the Levandoski articulator, with the stabili-zation prosthesis previously made for the patient with a traditional cast framework as the substructure used as the occlusal record. The stabiliza-tion prosthesis is again tried in the mouth, and transcranial films are taken. If condylar position corrections are required, the articulator is ad-justed, green stick compound is added to the stabilization prosthesis, and the articulator is closed. The corrected stabilization prosthesis is tried in the mouth, transcranial films are taken to confirm the correction, and the patient is allowed to wear the corrected stabilization prosthesis for a few days to confirm the corrections.

Once the master casts have been mounted and corrected, if need be, in the articulator as per the dictates of the Levandoski coordinates from the transcranial vector analysis, the acrylic is applied to the metal mesh-work extension and processed to form the acrylic-free end bases and acrylic portion of the substructure. Of course, the portion that rests on the edentulous areas in the patient's mouth is expected to fit as comfort-ably as any partial denture. The occlusal layer of the acrylic of choice is then processed onto the acrylic substructure by closing the articulator and its upper cast down into the acrylic before it is hardened so that the oc-clusion of the upper teeth forms the acrylic of the lower to a locking bite. It may at once be seen that this appliance serves as the initial splint and then in turn may be used as the final partial denture. Traditional pink denture-base acrylic may be used as the acrylic substructure from the be-ginning.

Actually, what this technique represents is nothing more than con-struction of a Kennedy class I free-end partial denture in the traditional fashion except that instead of teeth being processed onto the pink acrylic free-end bases, "bite-locking" occlusion-stabilizing acrylic is processed onto them in the Levandoski fashion. The occlusal registration used to produce the final occlusal surface of the partial denture against which the patient occludes is a simple product of mounting the master casts in a Levandoski articulator (Logic I) as per the patient's habitual occlusion and then modifying that relationship on the articulator to a correct (decompressed, advanced) maxillomandibular relationship as per the dictates of the Levandoski transcranial vector analysis and confirmatory follow-up transcranial radiographs.

Traditional wax bite blocks mounted on the cast framework may also be used at this point in the technique to transfer the corrected occlusal relationship back to the patient's mouth for the follow-up transcranial radiograph. Another method simply employs the processing of the pink acrylic free-end base substructure on the master cast and layering greenstick compound on the occlusal portion to register the corrected occlusal relationship once the appropriate x- and y-axis adjustments (z-axis adjustments are rare) have been made to the articulator and it has been closed down into the compound. Then the partial denture framework with the compound-corrected occlusion is transferred back to the mouth. A subsequent transcranial radiograph with the patient *gently* biting into the compound-covered partial soon divulges whether or not the corrections made on the articulator as per the first transcranial view are sufficient. Once satisfactory condyle-fossa alignment is achieved, the case may be processed. Softer acrylic used at the initiation of treatment may be replaced with harder, more durable material once the situation is determined to be under good control, a period of at least 6 months. The patients are, of course, instructed to wear their prostheses all the time and should *not* remove them during eating or even sleep as would be the case with conventional partial dentures. Prostheses so constructed again are a hybrid of the occlusal TMJ splint/functional appliance/partial denture. They are, at first, odd in appearance to the clinician unfamiliar with their use, but to the patients who wear them, they are a friend indeed.

APPLICATION OF THE LEVANDOSKI METHODS
TO THE ABSENT DENTITION

The main subject matter of this text and in fact the entire trilogy has been the diagnosis and treatment of malocclusion and functionally induced TMJ problems in patients with complete or nearly complete dentitions by means of FJO techniques. Yet the basic tenets that govern this approach are so profound, the principles of proper condylar position in the joint at function, proper muscular positioning of the mandible, and a proper occlusal relationship to reinforce all this are so fundamental to the basic design premise of the entire maxillofacial complex that such princi-

Figure 6–8 Combined orthodontic/prosthodontic/TMJ treatment. Combination treatment can produce dramatic results. **(A–D)** The comparison of facial appearance between an old upper full denture and a new one that is the product of the Levandoski approach is obvious in this young female TMJ pain-dysfunction patient. Her problems include chronic retro-orbital cephalalgia (headache), bilateral TMJ crepitus, missing posterior teeth, forward tipping of the remaining molars, inadequate anterior and posterior vertical dimension of occlusion, and a dissatisfaction with a recently made full upper denture that simply "looked like false teeth." Note the fuller, more natural appearance of the new denture made by using Levandoski techniques. **(E)** "Pretreatment" (i.e., pre–Levandoski treatment) occlusion. Note the deep overbite. **(F)** The old upper denture acted as a ramp deflecting the mandibular teeth, hence the whole mandibular-condyle unit, posteriorly and superiorly (due to a lack of posterior vertical). Note that areas in the denture are worn and even perforated by grinding from lower anteriors that slid up the lingual surfaces of the anterior denture teeth to strike the acrylic in the rugal area *(black arrow)*. **(G)** In this case the old upper denture acted as a base for adding acrylic that would force the mandible-condyle unit down and forward as per x, y-coordinate dictates of the transcranial vector analysis. Acrylic was added to the denture mounted against the lower model in the Levandoski articulator once corrections were made in the three-way articulator hinges as per the vector analysis. This also opened the bite anteriorly for orthodontic advancement of lingually tipped lower anteriors. **(H)** The lower anteriors were leveled, aligned, rotated, and advanced orthodontically. The mesially tipped lower molars were also uprighted all by means of the Brehm utility arch wire technique. **(I–L)** Before and after appearance of the lower teeth at completion of orthodontic treatment. Note how the posterior molars are uprighted and the lower anteriors are advanced (tipped) to a more correct angulation. This makes for a much more favorable path of origin and insertion for a future partial denture. (The design for the framework was drawn on post–orthodontic treatment casts). **(M)** The framework and upper occlusion rim are placed in the mouth. The occlusion rim is constructed in the usual "educated guesswork" fashion by using traditional parameters. A lead foil strip is placed over the anterior central incisor contact area. Transcranial and cephalometric radiographs are then taken with the patient biting into the occlusion rim. Levandoski transcranial vector analysis is then performed on the joint radiographs, and correction of the x, y-coordinates (if needed) that would be necessary to move condyle to the Gelb 4/7 position is noted. Levandoski proportional analysis is performed on the cephalogram to scientifically and mathematically determine the anterior vertical dimension corrections. Other traditional cephalometric analysis procedures are performed to see whether future anteriors (lead foil) will be protrusive enough to provide proper lip support, etc. The master casts are then mounted in a Logic I articulator using a Levandoski Vector I face-bow. **(N)** The necessary corrections are then made to the three-way hinges (as per the vector analysis) and the incisal guide pin (as per the proportional analysis). **(O and P)** Any posterior and/or anterior open bite that is then generated between the upper occlusion rim and the lower dentition as a result of these "joint- and face-protecting" corrections is then compensated for when the teeth are set. **(Q and R)** Completed new full upper denture and lower partial denture. Note the increased vertical. Subsequent transcranial

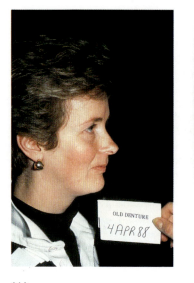

(A)

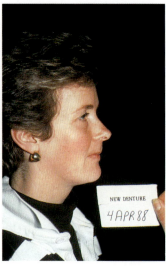

(B)

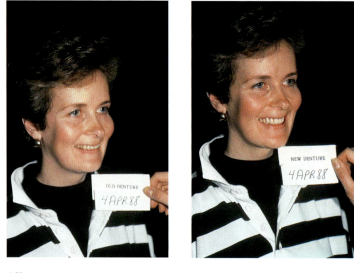

(C)   **(D)**

radiographs confirm the new occlusion positions of the condyle in the Gelb 4/7 position. **(S and T)** Note the improved facial appearance after the muscles accommodate to the new bite. The pains subsided. (Courtesy of Dr. Ronald Levandoski.)

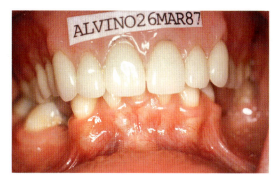

(E)

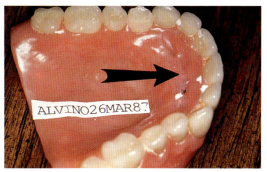

(F)

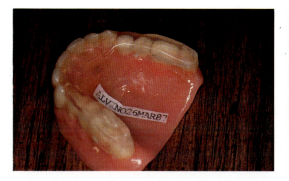

(G)

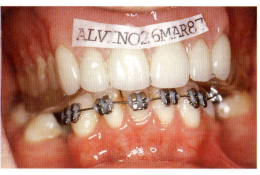

(H)

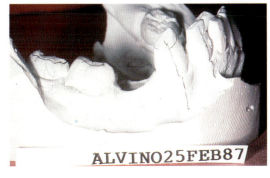

(I)

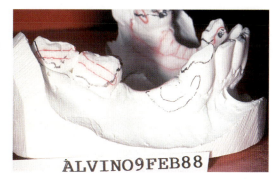

(J)

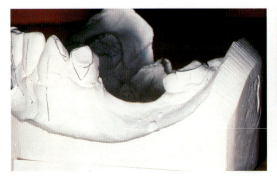

(K)

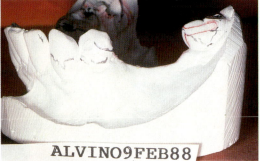

(L)

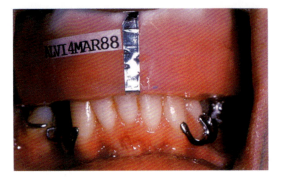

(M)

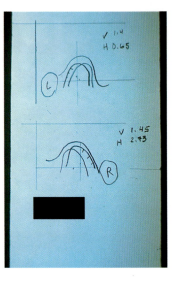

(N)

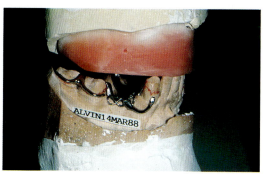

(O)

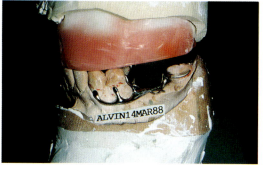

(P)

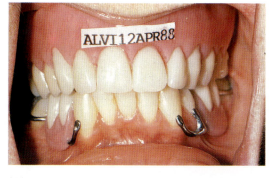

(Q)

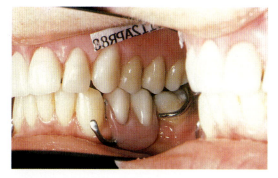

(R)

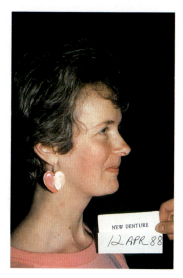

(S)

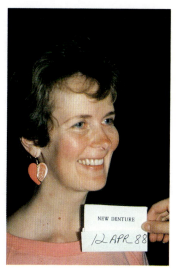

(T)

ples may even be relied upon in treating patients prosthodontically who have no natural dentition left at all. It is in this particular theater of operations that the full impact of the genius of Levandoski's prosthodontic skills may be appreciated. For it is in this field that he has made what surely must be his most revolutionary contributions to prosthodontic technique. And it all stems from his consummate knowledge of the TMJ.

As with the field of orthodontics, the field of prosthodontics has likewise been dominated by a number of notions that have long been held as solemn dogma for decade upon decade yet in modern times have been exposed as either ill founded or downright fallacious. The first and most important of these is the technique of registering an intramaxillary occlusal record during the wax occlusion rim stage of full-denture construction by means of the operator applying firm manual pressure on the patient's chin during closing. This was done in order to direct the mandible posteriorly while registering the interocclusal record so as to seat the condyle as far superiorly and posteriorly as possible in that mythical aphoristic Avalon of theoretical condylar full-occlusion positioning, centric relation! This principle of interocclusal registration has dominated prosthodontics for almost a century and, as previously noted in volume I, was selected not on the basis of any true knowledge of intracapsular kinematics but simply because it was supposedly reproducible (which it is not)! Although many modern-day clinicians are abandoning such registration techniques in favor of more "natural" methods, this author is unaware of any state board licensing examination involving the construction of full upper and lower denture prostheses that does not require that the interocclusal registration be performed in this manner. This, along with the propensity for full-denture patients to lose vertical dimension due to alve-

---

Figure 6–9 TMJ treatment and full-denture prostheses. **(A)** A 38-year-old female with a history of chronic disabling pain in both TMJs for 15 years. The patient had all teeth removed and full upper and lower dentures made 15 years previously. She also suffered from otalgia (ear aches) and tinnitus. She had several sets of economy dentures made that seemed to have made the pains worse. She was afraid of TMJ surgery. **(B)** Facial appearance with new dentures made by using Levandoski techniques, transcranial vector analysis, proportional analysis, and conventional cephalometric analysis. **(C and D)** Before and after quartering views. Note how well the muscle and facial tone improves after 10 days of "letting stubborn musculature get used" to new dentures. **(E)** original pretreatment dentures. **(F)** "Try-in" with lead foil to assist cephalometric evaluation of anterior tooth placement. Transcranial radiographs at this point confirm that the condyle location is correct (corrected in the occlusion rim stage on the Levandoski articulator by using vector analysis coordinates. **(G)** Final dentures are both esthetically pleasing and relieve the TMJ problems by positioning the condyles in the Gelb 4/7 position at full intercuspation. (Courtesy of Dr. Ronald Levandoski.)

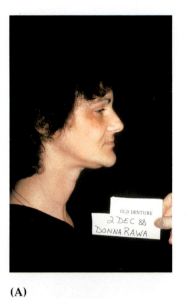

(A)

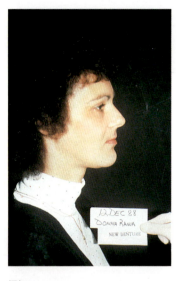

(B)

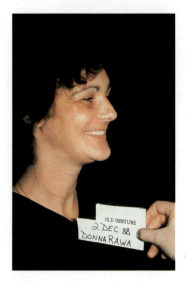

(C)

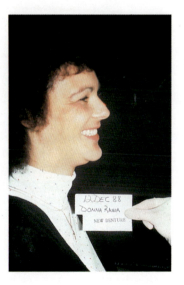

(D)

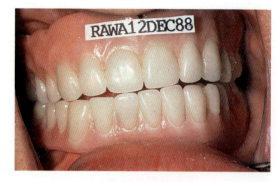

(E)

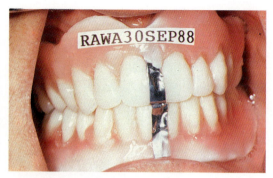

(F)

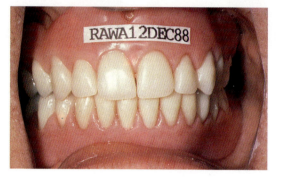

(G)

olar ridge resorption, may account for the fact that Levandoski has observed that there are very few patients with full dentures constructed in the conventional fashion who do not have posteriorly displaced condyles. Transcranial radiographs of the joints of denture patients should reveal that the upper and lower dentures at full occlusion should lock the condyle in the Gelb 4/7 position down and forward against the articular eminence, not up and back against the bilaminar zone. As also previously noted earlier in this text, very few patients may be found walking around with their thumbs on their chins.

Another theoretical notion to suffer the iconoclasm of Levandoski's revolutionary new ideas is that of the "Bennett movement." Although he accepts that a small amount of Bennett movement does in fact occur in a normal healthy joint, Levandoski strongly feels, as do others, that an extreme amount of Bennett shift is pathological and that it indicates excessive ligament distortion and an effort of muscles attempting to maneuver the condyle past a medially displaced disc. It has been proposed that the Bennett movement is an indicator of cusp form and posterior central grove width, i.e., the greater the Bennett movement, the correspondingly wider should be the central fossae of the artificial teeth used in the restoration of the occlusion. These occlusally flatter teeth are believed to better accommodate the Bennett shift. This is the equivalent to designing tooth forms that accommodate or reproduce pathology. No study has satisfactorily been able to equate tooth fossa width and cuspal height with, for instance, the temporal fossa slope or the Bennett shift seen in healthy functioning TMJs. In other words, the form (anatomy) of *individual* teeth in patients without TMJ disorders has no relationship to the form (anatomy) or range of motion of the TMJ! You cannot predict the slope of the temporal fossae from the angle of individual tooth cusps or the depth of their central fossae. What is important is (1) the position of teeth in three dimensions, (2) the influence of the teeth as a whole on the position of the maxilla and mandible in the intercuspal position, and (3) the lack of occlusal interferences that prevent the condyles from moving forward in all planes of motion. One can predict with great regularity where the condyles will be in a Class II, Division 2 malocclusion with excessive incisal misguidance! Dr. Levandoski states that he has never observed a patient with Class II, Division 2 malocclusion who did not have retruded condyles with compressed joint spaces. The ultimate solution to this dilemma is to utilize occlusal pads with high buccal/lingual walls to limit lateral protrusive movements. In Levandoski's mandibular stabilization prosthesis, there is late cuspid rise with complete freedom of the condyles to advance forward. The more degenerative and unstable the joints, the less lateral protrusive movement should be available to that patient and the later the cuspid rise.

One of the main goals of treatment with various stabilization prostheses (occlusal repositioning appliance, partial denture, full denture, bridgework, etc.) is not only to correctly position the mandible AP and vertically but also to induce the masticatory motion to adopt primarily a vertical motion, thus reducing the lateral excursive movements, which are considered damaging to already structurally compromised TMJs. This ties in with the time-proven medical orthopedic principle of splinting an incompetent joint to protect it from movement in the range of motion, which is contributing to the chronic dislocation and subsequent pathology. Dentists should begin to look at the TMJ in the light of common medical wisdom. The TMJ is somewhat unique, but it is still a set of bones and ligaments, and the general principles covering their physiology and pathology must not be ignored.

The extreme of this concept of accommodating the Bennett shift is represented by flat-plane teeth. Their non–occlusion-capturing, totally flat surfaces are the complete antithesis of the Levandoski approach of using closely interdigitating opposing occlusal surfaces to guide the mandible, and hence its condyles, to a predetermined structurally compatible

position. Flat-plane teeth are hard on TMJs that have already been structurally compromised and suffer from poor ligamentous support due to
functional abuse simply because such teeth fail to provide a stable occlusion that guides the mandible to its orthopedically correct full-occlusion
location. The muscles of mastication (which may need retraining from
their former Class II neuromuscular ways) are given no information as to
how to position the mandible with respect to AP or lateral dimensions.
Only information concerning the vertical dimension is provided. Patients
who suffer the dual miseries of having functionally induced TMJ problems and are also in need of full upper and lower dentures need an occlusion that guides them into a proper (condyle down and forward near
Gelb 4/7) condylar position. Their joints are debilitated, and they need an
occlusal home base. The steep cusp slopes of 33-degree posterior denture
teeth set with late cuspid rise and, of course, no anterior incisal misguidance can provide that home base, once verified as proper by transcranial
and cephalometric radiography. Flat-plane teeth cannot provide such AP
guidance. They also allow unfavorable loading of the joints during protrusive movements because they fail to exact the kind of posterior cuspal-
guiding plane support required during mandibular protrusion that is demanded by the Christensen phenomenon. It must be remembered that
during protrusive occlusal movements the posterior interocclusal vertical
dimension of occlusion opens faster than does the anterior vertical one.
This is intimately related to the angle of the slope of the articular eminence. As the mandibular denture advances during occlusal protrusive
movements, the flat-plane teeth fail to provide any occlusal stops that
would transfer force vectors through the teeth and denture base material
down onto the ridges. Instead, the force vectors are transmitted via the
condyle directly against what may be posterior attachment laminae (or
scar tissue if one is attempting to resolve a bilaminar perforation) in joints
with anteromedially displaced discs. Nothing posteriorly, i.e., no protective molar inclined planes, is present to support the condyle in a down-
and-forward direction. The entire mandible, and hence its condyles,
merely advance strictly horizontally (albeit actually quite a short distance)
until the condylar head makes full-force contact against the articular eminence and whatever tissues may remain between it and the eminence. If a
slight overbite exists in the anterior denture teeth, protrusion results in
loading at only three points, the anterior teeth and the anterosuperior
surface of the condylar head (capitulum) of each TMJ. The entire scenario
creates an unfavorable loading situation for the joint simply because the
flat-plane teeth do not support the condyle as it moves slightly forward
during protrusive movement but rather permit the condyle to slam
straight forward against already compromised intracapsular articular tissues the disc has anteromedially displaced (i.e., the condyle rides on a
posterior lamina) until the protrusion becomes extensive enough to force
the condyle in turn forward enough that the slope of the eminence be-

comes the only medium for indirectly bringing the condyle down as it comes forward. This, of course, is the case when the protrusive movement is executed in the full-occlusion position, a time when extreme loading forces are transmitted to the joint. This is the same principle behind the fact that certain flat-plane splints improperly made on hinge articulators can, under the right circumstances (or more correctly wrong circumstances), allow for the improper transmission of loading forces to the joint during slight protrusive movements during full occlusion, thus leaving the patient in even more distress during periods of bruxism when such full-force occlusion protrusive movements might be made. Flat-plane or near-flat-plane teeth in denture patients with TMJ problems wear the joints out by allowing excessive Bennett movement to occur. Thus they have no place in the Levandoski armamentarium of materials used to combat TMJ problems in the edentulous patient.

Determining the vertical dimension of occlusion for patients receiving full upper and lower artificial dentures has been a prosthodontic "no man's land" for generations of dentists. Numerous opinions abound as to how to determine the correct vertical, but most of them are centered around a plain old-fashioned educated guess. The concept of using cephalometrics to scientifically determine the range of correct anterior vertical for a given patient (or transcranial radiographs to determine correct posterior vertical and condylar position) was a notion all but totally foreign to the prosthodontic discipline, at least until now. Here is where the application of Levandoski's methods once again revolutionizes the discipline. Studying the step-by-step methods he uses to construct full upper and lower artificial dentures brings this to a clearer understanding.

THE LEVANDOSKI FACE-BOW

Some important considerations are necessary when designing a face-bow: (1) the design of the articulator, (2) the classification of the face-bow, and (3) the TMJ status of the patient. The Levandoski (Vector I) instrument was devised to complement the Levandoski three-dimensional articulator (Logic I) and also to address the need for a face-bow that could withstand the rigors of autoclaving sterilization procedures. Traditionally, a face-bow has been described as a caliper-like device used to orient the maxillary cast on an articulator. There are two basic types of face-bows: the so-called arbitrary and the hinge axis or kinematic. In actuality, what a face-bow does is orient the occlusal plane of the upper teeth (or occlusion rim) to the auditory meatus or some arbitrarily obtained landmark or to a manipulated nonphysiological hinge axis. Note that hinge axis measurements are of no value to the FJO aficionado because it is commonly agreed that pushing the mandible up and back is universally bad. Plus, it has been shown that the hinges' axis varies considerably. It is not sensible to arbitrarily force a joint to work constantly at the limit of its range of motion. This is very unstabilizing and would offend basic medical orthopedic values. Dentists are not immune to the laws of nature regarding the skeleton! In other words, just because I can rotate my neck 90 degrees to the left with some degree of reproducible regularity does not mean that I should wear a shirt that forces my head into this position and only fits when my head is 90 degrees to the left. Likewise, our occlusal treatments should not tend to elongate ligaments and destabilize the condyle-disc-fossa relationship. They should allow for freedom to move toward the limits imposed by ligaments.

The Vector I face-bow consists of an intrameatal caliper and a cuspid apex indicator. The intrameatal caliper is an interesting concept. It does not measure the intercondylar distance as has been claimed. It merely measures how far the ear rod can fit into the auditory meatus. This doesn't necessarily correlate with any measurement of the intercondylar width. The auditory meatus is a radiographic landmark used in cephalometrics — the porion. The location of this landmark as recorded by a face-bow can be useful in evaluating mounted casts.

After a preliminary set of upper and lower casts of the patient's maxillary and mandibular edentulous ridges is obtained by the usual alginate impression method (making sure they are properly extended and border molded into all vestibular areas), a set of acrylic custom trays is constructed. The master construction casts are produced from master impressions taken with these custom trays by using a totally passive impression material. The custom trays should be properly trimmed, fit as closely as possible to the patient's natural ridges, and be adequately extended into the vestibular areas. Only a relatively thin coat of passive (zinc oxide/eugenol wash–type) impression material need then be applied to the inside of the tray in a fashion similar to the way one would add moderate amounts of impression material to the tissue side of a denture that is to be relined. This prevents excessive impression material from being squeezed out the back of the tray as the impression is taken or otherwise distorting the tissues. This technique is also obviously predicated on the use of very accurate custom trays. The tray is seated front to back with one hand while the lips are retracted slightly with the other to allow air to escape from the vestibular areas. While gently seating the upper tray, Levandoski not only muscle trims the borders in the usual fashion but also has patients turn their heads from one side as far as they can go to the other. As with any procedure concerning the construction of artificial dentures, no step is more important than that upon which the operator is presently working. The preliminary alginate impressions *must* be properly extended so that all the important anatomical landmarks appear. Cook's plane across the hamular notch area of the maxilla, the retromolar pads of the mandibular area, and the labial, buccal, and lingual vestibular areas of both upper and lower arches should all be clearly visible and "bubble free." Only then may a highly accurate set of acrylic trays needed for such impression methods as these be produced for the registration of even more accurate master impressions. This in turn gives the most accurate upper and lower master casts for the construction of occlusion runs and eventually the final dentures.

Warmed and softened compound is adapted in a horseshoe-shaped fashion onto the occlusal table of the bite fork of the Levandoski face-bow transfer device. The softened compound is then carefully adapted to the maxillary edentulous alveolar ridge of the upper cast. Extensive coverage of the rugal area and palatal vault is not necessary, merely enough coverage of the bare ridge itself to permit stabilization of the bite fork once the compound cools and stiffens. Levandoski prefers this technique over inserting a heated bite fork into the base plate wax of occlusion rims. Once the rims have been properly contoured by the operator to act as a laboratory guide to tooth positioning and lip support, placing a heated bite fork into the labial surface of the wax of the upper rim and luting it to place with additional melted wax can destroy the contours of the wax labial surface of the occlusion rim so laboriously produced by the operator.

The compound-covered occlusal table of the bite fork is then stabilized against the edentulous maxillary ridge in the patient's mouth. It is held in place by the patient's thumb as the rest of the face-bow is subsequently attached and composed around it. Once the face-bow is properly registered, the entire apparatus is transferred to the Levandoski articulator where it serves as an orientation device for mounting the upper master cast.

With the face-bow properly attached to a fully "zeroed and leveled" articulator, the master cast is indexed for the mounting plaster, placed on the compound occlusal table of the bite fork, and mounted into place in the usual fashion with laboratory plaster (with the incisal guide pin preset to hold the upper and lower arms of the articulator parallel).

Next, the wax occlusion rims are placed in the mouth, and the vertical dimension of occlusion, AP alignment, and labial support are established in the usual fashion. This, quite frankly, means "eyeballing in" the occlusion rims by employing whatever methods the operator normally uses. Admittedly, this was the phase of artificial denture construction that relied most on the glorified educated guess. Very little science appeared here. But in these modern orthopedic times, the Levandoski techniques have changed all that.

When the operator is satisfied that his clinical experience and considered opinion have produced occlusion rims with as proper an anterior and posterior vertical dimension of occlusion, AP alignment, and lip support as is possible to produce by conventional techniques, the occlusal surface (or the rims) is notched bilaterally, and a 3-mm side strip of periapical x-ray lead is attached to the upper and lower occlusion rims at the midline and covered with a thin layer of base plate wax. The rims are

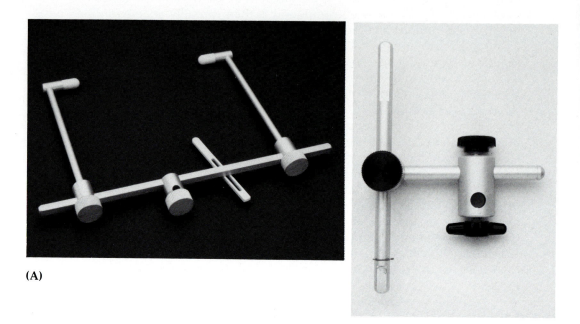

(A)

(B)

Figure 6–10 Levandoski Vector I face bow. **(A)** Horizontal plane caliper, or "face bow." The large middle lock nut is for attachment of **(B)** the vertical registration plate assembly that holds and orients **(C)** the bite registration plate (bitefork). **(D)** Adaptor plate. **(E)** Fully assembled face bow.
Operating Instructions
(F) In adult dentition, palpate the tip of the left maxillary canine and mark on the lateral nasal fold with a felt tip pen.
(G) If the patient has primary dentition, mixed dentition, or dentures mark half the height of the ala bulge.

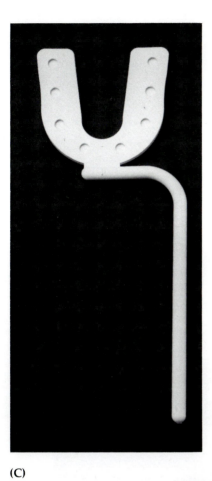

(C)

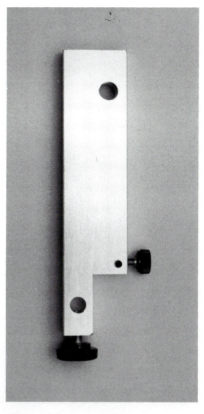

(D)

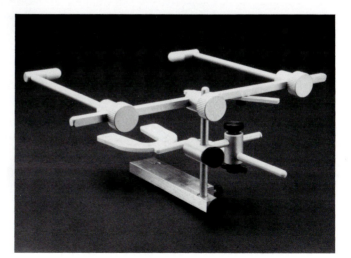

(E)

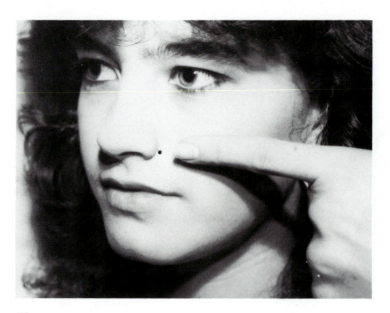

(F)

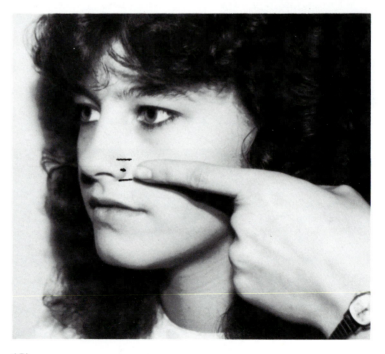

(G)

(H) Soak the maxillary cast in water. Cover the upper surface of the registration plate with a thin layer of melted impression compound, and gently press the wet maxillary cast, dentulous or edentulous, into the tempered compound. Make sure that the midline of the model aligns with the midline of the registration plate. The model is inserted to the same depth anteroposteriorly and transversely. Cook's plane is parallel to the registration plate (bitefork). Then attach the vertical rod to the horizonal plane caliper as follows: The vertical rod has a milled flat on both ends (see **B**). The longer flat inserts into the horizontal plane caliper, and must engage the vertical rod cap lock. The bottom of this milled flat must fully index against the cap lock rim **(H)**, with no gaps, as shown in **(I)**.

Instruct the patient to gently guide the ear inserts evenly into each auditory meatus. The doctor adjusts the intermeatal scale bar until the same number on the scale indexes at the medial edges of the threaded portion of **both** cap locks. The ear rods should be perpendicular to the intermeatal scale bar. When both right and left index numbers are the same, tighten both cap locks. Record the number shown on the scale.

Loosen the vertical lock nut, horizontal lock nut, and registration plate lock nut on the registration plate asembly (see **B**). Place the registration plate with compound occlusal imprint (from the model) in the mouth **(J)**. The patient now holds the registration plate against the maxillary teeth with his or her thumbs.

(K) While the patient holds the registration plate with thumbs, and horizontal plane caliper with fingers, insert the registration plate rod into the registration plate assembly. Fully insert the upper end vertical rod of the registration plate assembly into the horizontal plane caliper.

Adjust the anterior reference pointer to the anterior reference mark made on the patient's face with a pen.

(L,M) Tighten, in order, the vertical, horizontal, and bitefork lock nuts of the registration plate assembly. The bite registration process is complete.

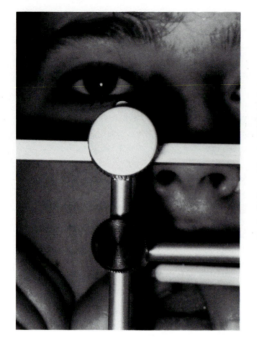

(H)

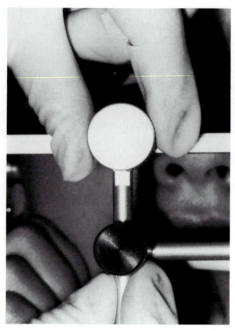

(I)

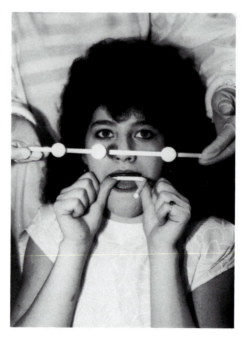

(J)

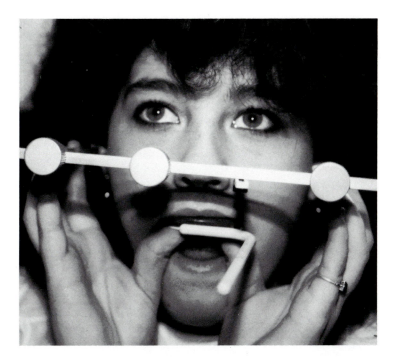

(K)

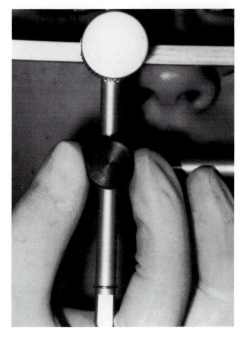

(L)

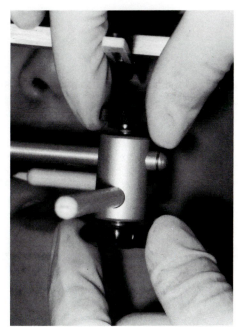

(M)

(N) To remove the registration plate assembly:
1. Be certain that the vertical, horizontal, and bitefork lock nuts are tight.
2. Loosen and retract the anterior pointer.
3. Have patient release the registration plate from teeth.
4. Loosen both ear rod cap locks; slide ear inserts out of auditory meatii.
5. Loosen the vertical rod cap lock and remove the horizontal plane caliper.
6. Gently remove the entire registration plate and assembly from the mouth.

Label the registration plate assembly with the patient's name, and set aside for mounting. Remove ear insert tips and anterior pointer from the horizontal plane caliper. After disinfecting the horizontal plane caliper, place fresh ear insert tips and a fresh anterior pointer on the horizontal plane caliper. The horizontal plane caliper is again ready for use with a new registration plate assembly.

Cast Mounting Procedure:

The Vector I allows the use of multiple registration plate assemblies with a single horizontal plane caliper. The registration plate assembly can be stored for subsequent model mounting or may be sent to the laboratory for mounting on Logic I or other compatible articulators. For lower beam adaptor plate attachment (see **D**) zero the Logic I articulators (as discussed in Chapter 5). Attach the adaptor plate to the lower beam with the ring nut.

(O,P) Zero the adaptor plate using the dial caliper as follows:
1. Tighten the ring nut.
2. Loosen the small Allen set screw with the hex key provided.
3. Loosen the zeroing screw on side adaptor plate.
4. Use the dial caliper to zero the right side of the adaptor plate to the right side of the lower beam by measuring and adjusting the zeroing screw until the distance from the right side of the beam to the right side of the adaptor plate is the same at the front and the back (see **O,P**).
5. Tighten the small Allen lock screw.

(Q) Make peripheral index cuts in the bases of both upper and lower models.

Mounting the Maxillary Cast:

Attach an upper cast mounting plate with plaster retention insert to the upper beam.

(R) Position the lower end of the vertical rod of the registration plate assembly **(B)** into the vertical rod recess of the adaptor plate, and tighten the recess locking screw at front of the adaptor plate.

(S) Place the model on impression compound index of bite registration plate, and open the upper beam of the articulator (beams paralleled at start).

(T) Apply plaster to upper mounting plate. Throughly fill the undercut of the mounting plate insert. Apply plaster to maxillary cast and peripheral index cuts of cast. Gently close the upper beam of the articulator, mold plaster into the peripheral index cuts, and allow the plaster to set. Open the upper beam of the articulator with the attached maxillary cast, and remove the adaptor plate and registration plate assembly from the lower beam adaptor plate so that the lower mmodel may now be mounted.

Mounting the Mandibular Cast:

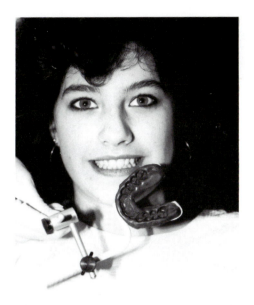

(N)

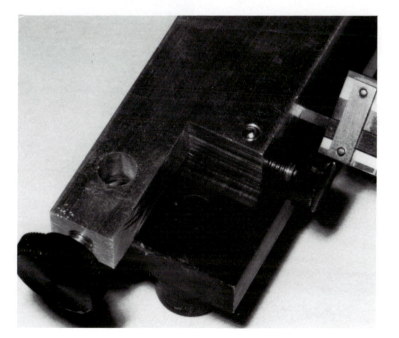

(O)

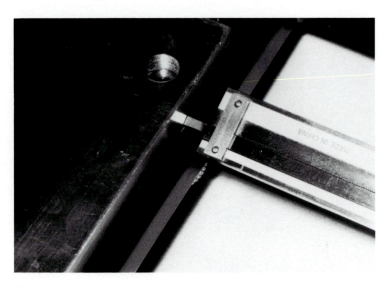

(P)

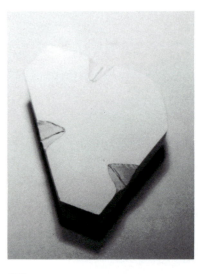

(Q)

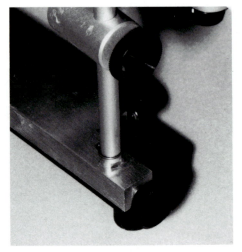

(R)

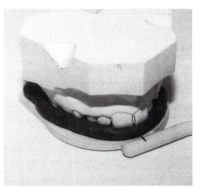

(S)

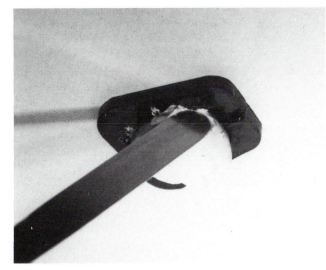

(T)

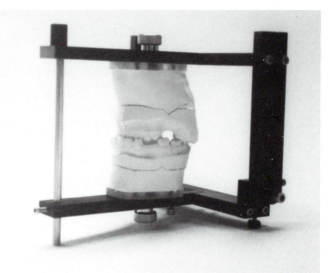

(U) Invert the articulator. Place the mandibular cast in the maximum intercuspal position. Do not use a wax occlusion record! Place sticky wax on casts to hold them together. If the intercuspal position of the casts is unclear, the doctor must check the occlusion in the mouth and mark the casts with lines delineating the true intercuspal position. If the case is either fully or partially edentulous, use occlusion rims, adjusted and occluded in the mouth, to facilitate mounting. These same occlusion rims must be in the patient's mouth when taking TMJ x-rays for Logic I articulator adjustments. Check to make sure that the lower beam, with lower mounting plate, mounting plate insert, and optional plaster shim, can be closed with at least 8 mm clearance to the mandibular cast when that cast is in maximum intercuspation with the upper model. Place mounting plaster on the mounting plate, being sure to fill the undercut of the mounting plate insert. Place mounting plaster on the lower model. Gently close the lower beam into the plaster, and mold the excess into the peripheral index cuts in the mandibular model. Allow the plaster to set, then upright the articulator. Perform visual check: Does everything look right?

placed back in the mouth, the patient is asked to close on occlusion-recording medium, and the rims are luted together by traditional methods. Levandoski is fond of using common plaster with an accelerator or boxing wax to make such occlusal records because of its physical characteristics, ease of manipulation, and economy. The patient is instructed to keep the jaws firmly imbedded in the occlusion rims, and transcranial and cephalometric radiographs are taken. The upper and lower wax occlusion rims, which are securely luted together, are removed in one piece from the patient's mouth, a procedure at times requiring no small amount of alacrity. But, as Levandoski himself wryly quips, "They'll come out in one piece, in spite of how much the patients fuss and fume!" If one will forgive a brief moment of metaphysical levity, this is obviously an instance in which the end justifies the means.

The rims are then transferred to the articulator where the upper cast has already been mounted against the upper beam of the articulator by using the face-bow, and by turning the articulator upside down, the lower master cast is carefully fitted into the lower occlusion rim and secured in conventional fashion, again with common laboratory plaster.

Transcranial vector analysis is then performed on the radiographs of the joints. Remember, these transcranial radiographs represent the condylar position reflecting condylar alignments generated by the "guesstimate-produced" occlusion rims in their present orientation. Many astute clinicians are humbled when they see irrefutable evidence that their "golden hands" approach to occlusal records is totally unreliable in placing the condyles where they belong! The horizontal and vertical vectors for condylar correction are programmed into the articulator. Almost always the patient will exhibit a posterior open bite. These corrections take care of the posterior vertical dimension portion of the intermaxillary relationship. For the proper relationships in the anterior portion, Levandoski abandons the "educated-guess technique" for that of the mathematical exactness of cephalometrics.

It must be remembered that all cephalometric radiographs, including the ones we are discussing here that are involved in this particular technique, may not be truly representative of the patient's actual maxillomandibular skeletal relationships. This, of course, is due to one simple, basic fact. The roentgenocephalogram in norma lateralis is produced with the patient biting in full habitual occlusion. This means that if that occlusion happens to be one of the types that drives the mandible back, the "normal" maxillomandibular relationship that Nature intends may be usurped by a counterfeit maxillomandibular relationship that the occlusion intends. If an orthodontic treatment plan, a TMJ splint, or any reconstruction of the occlusion is built around a cephalometric evaluation of a pathological mandibular position, then at least we are perpetuating pathology and, at worse, we are hurting the patient. Is the true A-B difference as great as the cephalogram depicts? Is the ANB angle as bad as its value indicates? Is the pogonion as retruded as it appears? Or do we have a normal "Class I" mandible simply being driven back to a large A-B difference, a large ANB angle, and a retruded pogonion location making it appear "smaller" because something in the occlusion forces the mandible back as a whole. The coordination of cephalometric analysis with that of transcranial analysis holds the answers to such questions. Taken to its logical conclusion, this line of reasoning leads to the relatively new concept of the "corrected Ceph."

In light of the discussion above, it may now be seen that the significance of certain cephalometric measurements and relationships may be mitigated by the correctness (or incorrectness) of the condyle-fossa relationship. Any cephalogram produced from a patient with a functionally induced TMJ problem, i.e., retruded condyles at full occlusion, has an automatic bias coerced into some of its cephalometric relationships. Levandoski was sensitive to this occlusion-induced distortion of skeletal relationships. Thus after taking a cue from Cecil Steiner and James McNamara (who moved tracings of mandibles also), Levandoski developed a simple method for producing a corrected cephalometric tracing that proves very useful in the construction of full upper and lower artificial dentures. The method is the essence of both genius and simplicity and puts true science in the place of the guesswork phase of full-denture construction.

With the completed transcranial vector analysis coordinates of the case close at hand, a conventional tracing of the cephalogram in norma lateralis is drawn on the tracing paper, preferably in a dark ink or heavy pencil line. The center of the condyle (C-point, Bimler) is arbitrarily registered. Next, a second tracing *of the mandible only* is produced on a second tracing sheet with the registration of the C-point in the exact same location in a different-color pencil. Horizontal and vertical base reference lines are also drawn at identical locations along the side and top or bottom edge of both tracings. The second tracing of the mandible only now lays on top of the first tracing of the entire maxillofacial complex of our edentulous patient. Now it must be remembered that this initial cephalogram represents the maxillomandibular relationship dictated by the "eyeballed" occlusion rims in the patient's mouth at the time of exposure. If the condylar position needs correction, as would be indicated by the findings of the transcranial vector analysis (also a product of the relationship of the occlusion rims), these corrections may be transferred to the cephalometric tracing. While keeping the horizontal and vertical base reference lines at the edges of the tracings parallel, the topmost of the two tracings (the mandible only) is moved down and forward against the background of the full tracing beneath it. It is moved by the exact amount represented by the x and y coordinates of the transcranial analysis. This places the mandible in the correct AP orthopedic relationship and also automatically sets up the correct posterior orthopedic vertical. The anterior vertical dimension of occlusion still remains unresolved—but not for long. By inserting a compass point (or even a straight pin) through the top tracing of the mandible only at the C point (Bimler), which is now "advanced," against the background tracing of the entire skull and penetrating it right through to the film itself, the top tracing of the mandible may be rotated about this pinpoint hinge to find the satisfactory anterior vertical. The pin forces the top tracing of the mandibular condyle to stay in its corrected location with respect to the outline of the fossa of the first tracing beneath it. The initial ANS-Me lower face height measurement is made on the original tracing of the noncorrected cephalogram and noted. The previously discussed graph of the Levandoski proportional analysis, which relates ANS-Me lower face height as a function of the McNamara effective maxillary and mandibular lengths, is then consulted. The patient's own effective maxillary and mandibular lengths are also taken directly from the first tracing (condylion–A point, condylion-pogonion). The effective mandibular length is not affected by how far posteriorly the mandible is forced by the occlusion. The effective maxillary length may be "corrected" to a more accurate value in retrusive mandibular situations by subtracting the x coordinate (horizontal displacement value) of the transcranial vector analysis from the value for the effective maxillary length taken from the tracing. This correction factor is not great, however, because it usually falls in the range of 1 to 3 mm, which accounts for only about 1% to 3% of the overall effective length.

Thus, by employing the values of the proportional analysis graph and remembering Levandoski's admonition to add several more millimeters to the ANS-Me lower face height graph reading obtained in adults, the top tracing of the mandible may be rotated "open" to the value so indicated. Then the superimposition of the top tracing of the mandible only against the background tracing of the entire maxillofacial complex beneath it results in a corrected cephalometric tracing representing what the true skeletal relationships of the mandible to the maxilla would have or should have been had not the misdirecting dental occlusion gotten in the way. The difference between the corrected ANS-Me lower face height and the occlusion rim–determined noncorrected ANS-Me lower face height is simply determined by subtracting the latter from the former. For the sake of discussion, let us assume that the pretreatment (occlusion rim–determined) anterior vertical had to be increased by 6.0 mm. A dial caliper is opened to an arbitrary 50 mm. The beaks of the caliper are placed against the plaster art bases of the upper and lower master casts in the Levandoski articulator. Now it must be remembered that when these casts were mounted, the arms of the articulator were set parallel to each other and held that way by the "zeroed-in" styluses at the back of the articulator and the incisal guide pin in the front. That parallelism is, of course, now lost because of the corrections imported to them as a product of the transcranial vector analysis. But that only corrects the posterior portion of the maxillomandibular relationship. It also only affects the back part of the articulator. The anterior portion, represented by the yet unadjusted incisal guide pin, is still the same as when the casts were mounted as per the dictates of the luted occlusion rims. We have determined that that anterior relationship is 6.0 mm less cephalometrically than we desire as per the proportional analysis graph and the corrected cephalometric tracing techniques just described. We also have our mounted models in our articulator with marks on the most anterior portion of the casts an arbitrary 50 mm apart. The setscrew holding the incisal guide pin is loosened, and the articulator is opened until the marks on the upper and lower casts are now 56 mm apart. The incisal guide pin is then locked at that position by tightening the setscrew. Thus the desired maxillomandibular orthopedic relationship for that individual patient is secured. The occlusion rims are then re-waxed to this new corrected position.

An interesting adjunct to this technique developed by Levandoski that proves handy is that when the original occlusion rims have been carved to just about the ideal "eyeballed" dimensions of labial protrusion (lip support) and before they are luted together in the registration of the interocclusal record, a thin strip of common lead foil from a common intraoral bite-wing film is placed over the wax rim in the anterior incisor area. The strip should cover a portion of the labial, incisal, and even a small part of the lingual aspects of the wax occlusion rim. This then produces a visible image on the cephalogram that indicates the amount of labial protrusion that upcoming upper and lower anterior incisors will provide. Employment of the Bowbeer cephalometric analysis with its concern for proper lip support and incisor location is then greatly facilitated. Levandoski notes in this regard that it is often difficult to get patients to accept the fully allotted portion of anterior incisor protrusion and lip support that such analysis methods indicate. People who wear full dentures seem to have a propensity for expecting to look a bit "sunken in" around the lips and corners of the mouth, and they also do not expect to have a lot of their artificial dentures show when smiling, laughing, or even talking. This could easily be a product of social conditioning and having seen so many patients with underdeveloped artificial dentitions. Beauty may truly lie in the eye of the beholder, but full-denture construction now lies fully in the mathematics of cephalometrics.

Another surprise to come out of this method of denture construction is that not only do patients have dentures that preclude TMJ problems of a functional nature but the need for surgical tuberosity reduction is almost entirely eliminated. Such tissue reduction procedures are usually reflective of the fact that the posterior vertical dimension is too small, not that the maxillary tuberosities are too large. When problems are corrected on a Levandoski articulator by the methods described above, one will observe that the distance between the maxillary tuberosity and the mandibular retromolar pad is increased by more than enough to accommodate a layer of upper and lower denture base material. The maxillary tuberosity does not collide with the mandibular retromolar pad in a normal, healthy, well-balanced individual with a full dentition. Why should it do so once that dentition has been lost and alveolar resorption resulting from socket healing has taken place? Analysis of such a case by the Levandoski methods will usually reveal that a set of artificial dentures needs to be constructed that will force the mandible *down and forward* to a correct Gelb-4/7–type position at full occlusion; once they do so, there will quite often be plenty of room not only for the maxillary tuberosity but also for the denture base material that must cover it. Likewise with the mandibular retromolar pad. All this, of course, is predicated upon a locking type of occlusion that gives the mandible and its supportive musculature a home base to seek out during function. Not only should that home base position the mandible at a proper vertical dimension of occlusion, but it should also produce a proper condyle-disc-fossa relationship. That is where the selection of artificial denture teeth becomes important.

The most important denture teeth as far as Levandoski is concerned are the 33-degree posteriors. He prefers the steep occlusal inclined cuspal planes of these teeth because they offer the best chance of locking the mandible and its condyle in the best possible predetermined "home" position. Thus these teeth are expected to operate in a similar fashion to the occlusion-locking, Levandoski-type overlay partials and acrylic splints. In view of the fact that the occlusal relationship is determined scientifically and that (1) the condylar position, (2) the mandibular AP position, and (3) both the anterior and posterior vertical dimensions of occlusion in such artificial dentures so constructed in effect are a reflection of what Nature originally intended (on average), it is no surprise that the patients do quite well with this arrangement. As with all cases of TMJ treatment with appliances (and in the edentulous patient the dentures themselves become the appliances), *a certain initial period of adjustment* may be required to allow the patients to become accustomed to the new occlusal relationship. But being that the new occlusal relationship is a very close imitation to Nature's original design intent, that period of adjustment does not take long. It is also a period of time surprisingly free from necessitated adjustments of the denture base material due to sore spots. Although adjustments may be necessary, their numbers are greatly reduced when the dentures are produced by using these methods.

Other Levandoski favorites as far as tooth selection is concerned are the Bioform 23E and the Bioblend 21X upper anterior tooth forms in a basic 8.25 × 11.0-mm tooth. The 230LLS and the 233L are often used posteriors, with the 230LLS being handy from the standpoint that it requires less grinding at its base when occlusal height problems arise. For lower anteriors, tooth-type "H" seems the variety most often selected.

Upon careful reflection, it may readily be seen that the contributions of the former construction worker and radio disc jockey turned prosthodontist supreme, Dr. Ronald Levandoski, act as a figurative clasp that holds the graceful necklace of the modern theories of TMJ therapeutics together. Many important links of that necklace were fashioned by many great doctors from several continents and across many decades. But the fact that Levandoski can apply the fundamental tenets of the FJO philosophy of condylar positioning, mandibular positioning, and muscle reconditioning to something as seemingly distant and unrelated to orthodontics as full artificial denture construction imparts a final benediction to the FJO family of techniques that proves they are applicable to all types of dental patients regardless of the complete or incomplete status of their dental structure. His bold fervor for such concepts puts him in the same league as the numerous other great TMJ clinicians who have aligned themselves with this movement. And like all pioneers in any field, he too has had to suffer a certain modicum of rejection and derision of his theories from those ironically most qualified and responsible for recognizing their true value, his own colleagues. But again, like all the others, his insights into the true nature of the functionally induced TMJ problem is fired by the courage of his convictions. He and the other great intrepid leaders of this new movement in maxillofacial orthopedics are uncommon men fighting for a common cause. The application of the Levandoski methods will no doubt stand the test of time because they have already stood the test of Nature.

"Felix, qui protuit recrum
cognoscere causas."
"Happy is he who is able
to learn the causes of things."

Virgil

References

1. Bonwill WGA: Scientific articulation of human teeth as founded on geometrical mathematical and mechanical laws, *Dent Items Interest* 1899; 21:617–636, 873–880.
2. Gysi A: Problems of articulation. *Dent Cosmos* 1910; 52:148.
3. Snow GB: Articulation. *Dent Cosmos* 1900; 42:51–55.
4. Christensen C: A rational articulator. *Ash's Q Circ* 1901; 409–420.
5. Posselt U: *"Physiology of Occlusion and Rehabilitation.* Oxford, Blackwell Scientific Publications, Inc, 1971.
6. Christensen C: The problem of the bite. *Dent Cosmos* 1905; 47:1184–1195.
7. Bennett MG: A contribution to the study of the movements of the mandible. *J Prosthet Dent* 1958; 8:41–54.

CHAPTER 7
Practical Application

There is no way to illustrate the application of the principles of functional jaw orthopedics (FJO) in a manner that would be all-inclusive to every situation, for such situations are as varied as the patients who present for treatment on a daily basis. Yet we have attempted to convey the basic principles of this discipline in a fashion universal enough that its basic techniques may be applied to the greatest number of patients who suffer from functionally induced temporomandibular joint (TMJ) problems. The extremely rare case requiring unusual or extremely sophisticated treatment methods is obviously out of the realm of this discussion. Yet it is firmly believed by many authorities that the principles of diagnosis and treatment represented by the level of knowledge discussed in this trilogy of texts are so profound that if it is not sufficient to deliver the patient to a reasonably pain-free posttreatment state, the patient is suffering from more than a mere functionally induced TMJ arthrosis and therefore the timely persuit of other forms of diagnosis and general medical evaluation are indicated. If putting the compressed condyle in a more physiologically correct down and forward position does not produce results, something else is going on.

As far as choosing representative cases to illustrate the application of FJO principles of diagnosis and treatment to the problems of TMJ pain and dysfunction, several things must be confronted. First, it must somewhat paradoxically be stated that no two TMJ cases are alike. Yet in many ways they are all alike. This is what gives the basic diagnostic and treatment methods discussed here their universality. One person's TMJs are made of pretty much the same stuff as the next persons and will usually respond in pretty much the same way to both functional abuse as well as functional corrections. It must be remembered that Nature is the treating clinician's most important partner and, if given the chance, can deal with things on a far deeper level than we can ever begin to understand.

Second, it must be realized that in using examples of before and after illustrations of TMJ cases one of several things might be observed. In some cases the amount of condylar advancement needed to resolve the patient's pain and dysfunction problems might be very slight. A 1.0-mm increase in the superior and posterior joint space may be all that is needed. If so, the changes in the anterior profile and cephalometric measurements may be difficult to detect because they will not be great on a relative basis. Sometimes the amount of advancement of the mandible may be so slight as to even be difficult to detect in the joint area itself. In a structure as small and highly stressed as the human TMJ, 1.0 mm is the same as a mile!

Yet in other cases both the amount of condylar repositioning in the joint as well as the changes in anterior profile and cephalometric measurements are both great enough to be easily detected by what ever measuring and analysis system one would choose. It must also be remembered that the complications of before and after cephalometric comparisons of treated TMJ cases in children and adolescents are compounded by changes in base reference lines and landmark location due to growth and development.

Therefore it may be debated by some that cephalometric analysis is not critical to diagnosis and treatment of TMJ problems if one is planning on finishing the case prosthodontically. However, the value of the cephalometric component of the diagnostic and treatment planning process has been well established, especially if the clinician plans on treating the patient orthodontically. Yet of one thing there can be no doubt. Some form of image of the joint is mandatory to modern TMJ therapeutics. And in view of the importance of a physiologically stable TMJ in the overall operation of the maxillofacial complex, any major orthodontic, occlusal rehabilitative, or prosthodontic treatment plan that does not include considerations of some form of examination and/or image of the joint places the treating clinician responsible for that treatment plan in an extremely vulnerable and compromised situation. The lamp has been lit. And from what we see now, there's no going back!

Note: The following series (Figs 7–2 through 7–10) of before and after transcranial radiographs illustrate how repositioning compressed condyles down and forward (in the vicinity of the Gelb 4/7 position) relieves functionally induced TMJ pain and dysfunction problems. Each case listed below shows a pretreatment transcranial radiograph of both the right and left joints in the full biting position, relaxed (rest) position, and fully opened position. In each of these cases the patients' problems of TMJ pain and dysfunction (which means the usual raft of symptoms of headache, facial muscle soreness, neck ache, clickings, etc.) were successfully ameliorated in a new occlusion that repositioned the condyles in a physiologically correct and stable Gelb 4/7 position.

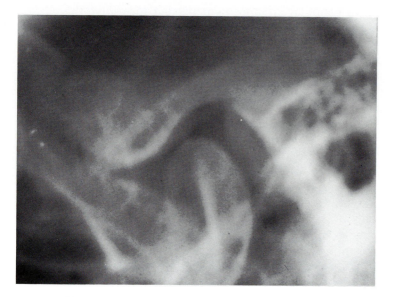

Figure 7–1   TMJ ideal. The goal of every TMJ treatment plan is to relieve the patient's TMJ pain and dysfunction problems and secure the condyles into a physiologically proper and stable position in the joint, a position referred to at times as the Gelb 4/7 position. Shown here is a transcranial radiograph of a TMJ after disc recapture by treatments that resulted in an occlusion that instead of pushing the condyle up and back brought it down and forward into the physiologically correct and stable Gelb 4/7 position. (Courtesy of Dr. Steven G. Messing).

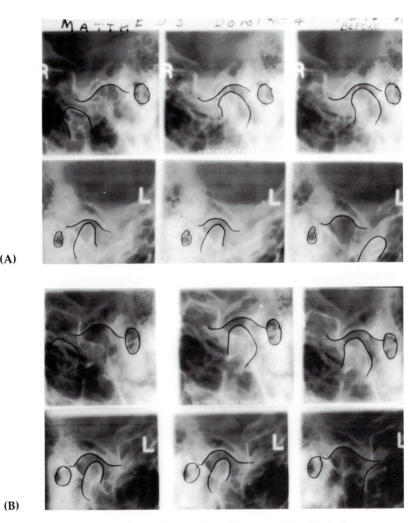

Figure 7–2 A 39-year-old female. Problem: headaches, fibromyositis. Clinical findings: interincisal opening of 43.5 mm, closing click in the left joint. **(A)** Pretreatment; **(B)** posttreatment. (Courtesy of Dr. Harold Gelb).

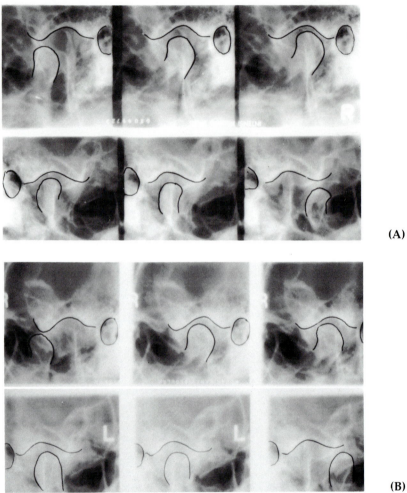

(A)

(B)

Figure 7–3   A 30-year-old female. Problem: myalgia, back pains. Clinical findings: interincisal opening of 49 mm, closing click in the left joint. **(A)** Pretreatment; **(B)** posttreatment. (Courtesy of Dr. Harold Gelb).

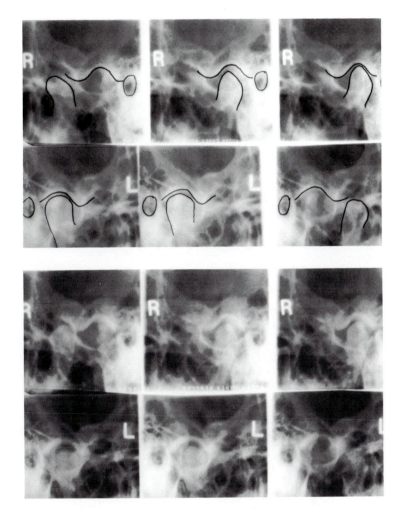

(A)

(B)

Figure 7–4 A 30-year-old female. Problem: ear pains, reciprocal clicking, fibromyalgia, internal disc derangement. Clinical findings: interincisal opening of 50 mm, opening and closing click in the right joint. **(A)** Pretreatment; **(B)** posttreatment. (Courtesy of Dr. Harold Gelb).

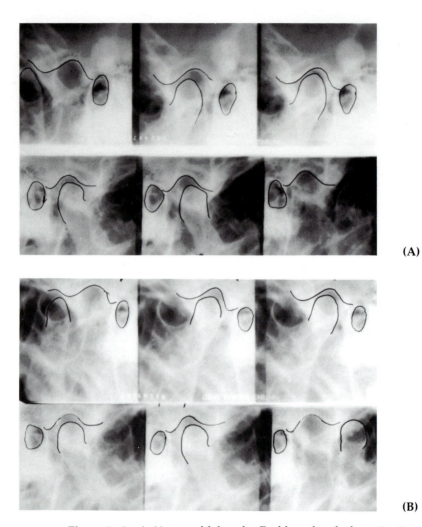

(A)

(B)

Figure 7–5 A 44-year-old female. Problem: headaches, tinnitus. Clinical findings: interincisal opening of 48.5 mm, clicking upon full opening. **(A)** Pretreatment; **(B)** posttreatment. (Courtesy of Dr. Harold Gelb).

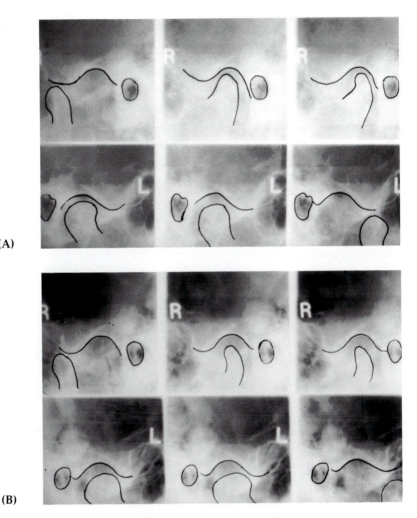

Figure 7–6   A 46-year-old male. Problem: headaches, ear aches (dominant on the left side). Clinical findings: interincisal opening of 41.5 mm, bilateral reciprocal clicking. **(A)** Pretreatment; **(B)** posttreatment. (Courtesy of Dr. Harold Gelb).

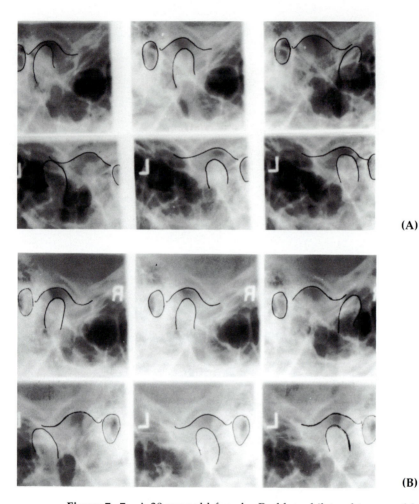

(A)

(B)

Figure 7-7   A 30-year-old female. Problem: bilateral temporal headaches, neck aches, shoulder aches, tinnitus. Clinical findings: interincisal opening of 51.5 mm, TMJ tenderness. **(A)** Pretreatment; **(B)** posttreatment. (Courtesy of Dr. Harold Gelb).

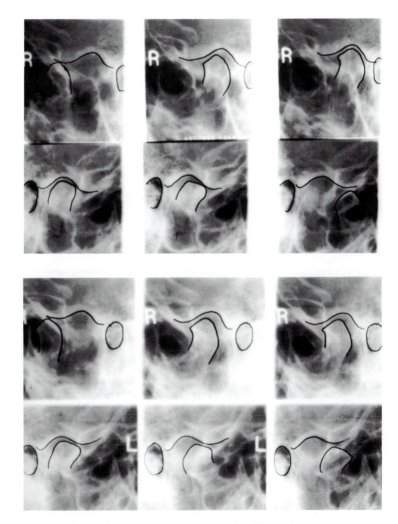

(A)

(B)

Figure 7–8 A 46-year-old female. Problem: vertigo, cervicalgia. Clinical findings: interincisal opening of 42 mm. **(A)** Pretreatment; **(B)** posttreatment. (Courtesy of Dr. Harold Gelb).

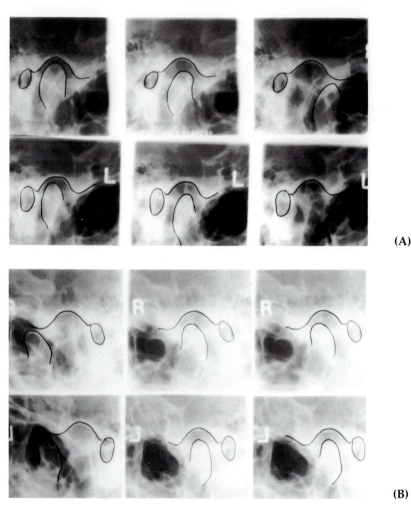

(A)

(B)

Figure 7–9   A 34-year-old female. Problem: fibromyalgia, internal disc derangement, bilateral reciprocal clicking. Clinical findings: interincisal opening of 39 mm. **(A)** Pretreatment; **(B)** posttreatment. (Courtesy of Dr. Harold Gelb).

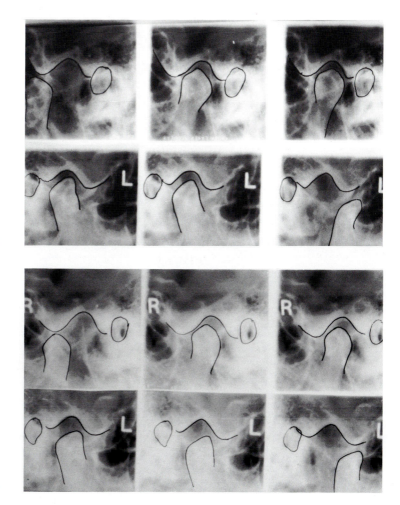

Figure 7–10 A 40-year-old female. Problem: headaches. Clinical findings: interincisal opening of 47 mm. **(A)** Pretreatment; **(B)** posttreatment. (Courtesy of Dr. Harold Gelb).

CASE HISTORY

<u>PATIENT</u>: Age: 14 years, 1 month

MAIN PROBLEM:
1. Pain in right ear.
2. Problem in opening mandible.
3. After sleeping, difficulty in opening mouth.

MEDICAL-DENTAL HISTORY:
1. Saw medical doctor first when it was possible to open mandible just a little bit.
2. Then saw a dentist who has a strong reputation for TMJ treatment.
    a. He constructed a full coverage bulky splint, which relieved the pain.
    b. Patient wore splint for one year.
    c. Then tried without splint, pain immediately returned.
    d. Patient and parents were told by dentist she would either have to have surgery or wear splint for remainder of her life.
3. Parents transferred patient to Dr. Witzig.

FINDINGS:
1. With splint: No pain
                  No joint noises.
2. Without splint: Joint and muscle pain
                     Clicking
3. Class II/Division II Malocclusion
4. Deep overbite
5. Incisal misguidance

RADIOGRAPHIC FINDINGS:
1. Left TMJ—posterior-superior condyle displacement.
2. Right TMJ—posterior-superior condyle displacement.

DIAGNOSIS: Internal derangement with posterior-superior displaced condyles.

TREATMENT:
First appliance—sagittal splint (Sagittal II appliance) for (7 months).
    1. Pain relief
    2. Allow joints to heal
    3. Move upper anterior teeth out of retrusion
Second appliance—Orthopedic Corrector I (7 months)
    1. Correct deep overbite permanently.
    2. Correct Class II to Class I.

RESULTS:
18 months after all appliances removed:
    1. No pain.
    2. No headaches.
    3. Class II to Class I corrected permanently.
    4. Deep overbite corrected permanently.
Six years after all appliances removed:
    1. 48.9 mm opening
       13.2 mm right
       13.9 mm left
    2. No clicking, no pain, no headaches.

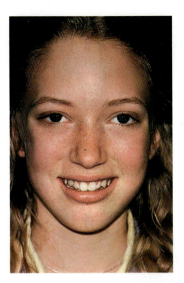
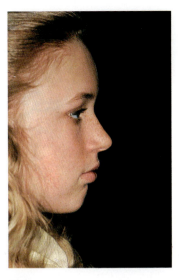

(A)   **(B)**

Figure 7–11   (A and B) Pretreatment facial views of a 14-year-old girl with severe TMJ problems. **(C)** Tomogram of the right condyle. **(D)** Tomogram of the left condyle. Note that both condyles are severely superiorly and posteriorly displaced. **(E–G)** Pretreatment study casts of malocclusion. **(H)** First appliance, the Sagittal II (splint) appliance, to advance the upper anteriors out of the way and to provide "splint effect" pain relief to the TMJ. **(I)** Appliance inserted. **(J)** After 7 months with the Sagittal II (splint) appliance an Orthopedic Corrector I (OCI) was constructed. **(K and L)** Facial views after completion of the OCI phase of treatment that advanced the mandible and increased the vertical dimension of occlusion. **(M and N)** Occlusion after completion of the OCI phase of treatment (7 months). Note the Class II to Class I correction and increased vertical dimension. **(O)** Post–TMJ treatment transcranial radiographs of the joints. Note the advanced condyles. **(P)** 6½ years after completion of FJO TMJ treatments. The changes are permanent. **(Q)** Facial appearance 6½ years after withdrawl of functional appliances. No headaches, no clicking, and no other signs or symptoms of TMJ pain or dysfunction were present. (Courtesy of Dr. John Witzig.)

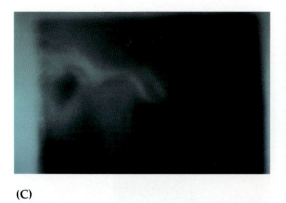

(C)

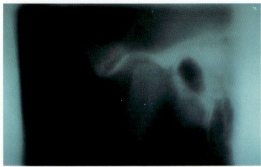

(D)

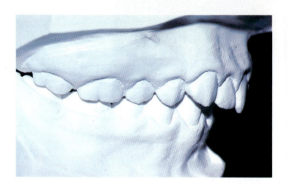

(E)

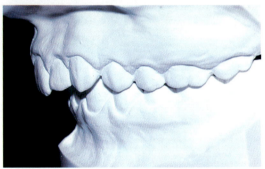

(F)

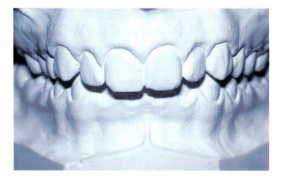

(G)

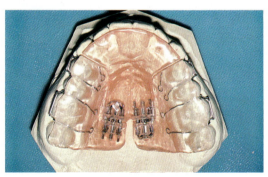

(H)

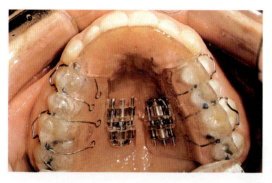

(I)

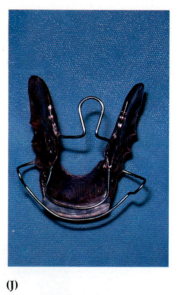

(J)

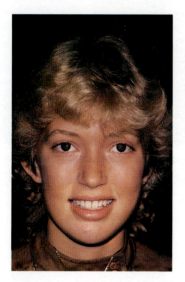

(K)

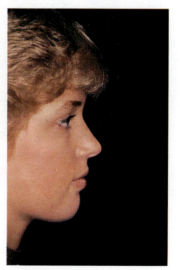

(L)

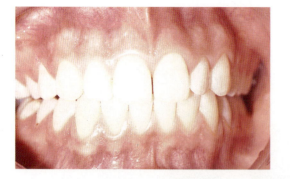

(M)

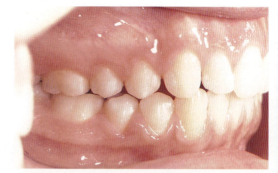

(N)

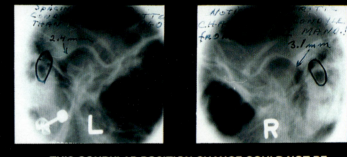

(O)

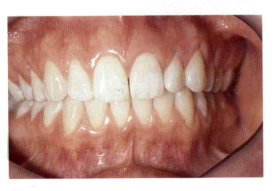

(P)

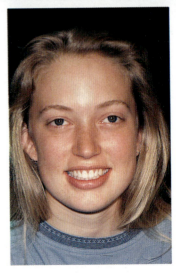

(Q)

CASE HISTORY

PATIENT: Age: 34 years old, female

MAIN PROBLEM:
1. Headaches every day.
2. Ringing in the ears.
3. Dizzy spells daily.
4. Patient was referred to an oral surgeon for TMJ pain by family dentist.

FINDINGS:
1. Left side—locking of disc.
    —crepitus.
    —severe TMJ pain.
2. Right side—locking of disc.
    —pain in TMJ.
3. Mandible will sometimes lock in closed position.
4. Class II/Division II malocclusion with deep overbite.
5. Lower first molars missing on both sides.
6. Severe vertical deficiency.
7. Upper central incisors tipped back lingually.
8. Incisal interference.

RADIOGRAPHIC FINDINGS:
1. Left—Posterior-superior displaced condyle.
2. Right—Flattening of condyle head.
    —Posterior-superior displaced condyle.

DIAGNOSIS: Internal derangement of both TMJs with locking. Severe degenerative arthritis both sides. Crepitus (bone against bone) in left TMJ with probable perforation.

TREATMENT:
1. First appliance: Upper Sagittal II (splint)
   (7 months)   appliance.
   a. Relieve pain.
   b. Upper central incisors move out labially.
2. Second appliance: Upper Straight Wire brackets for
   (7 months)   straightening teeth.
                       Lower Gelb splint for proper vertical dimension and bite.
   Upper retainer was made for patient to wear during sleep.
   Patient will have lower inadequate bridges replaced. Until this is completed, patient will wear lower Gelb splint.

RESULTS:
1. Changed patient's life from constant headaches to free of pain.
2. Condyles finished in a pain-free condition. The new occlusion has the condyles down and forward from their pretreatment displacement of up and back.
3. No TMJ pain now.

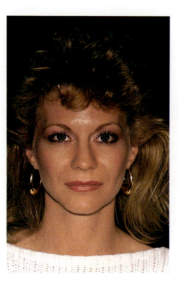

(A)   **(B)**

Figure 7–12   Adult TMJ problems in a 34-year-old female. **(A)** Pretreatment facial view. **(B)** Pretreatment occlusion. **(C)** Pretreatment transcranial radiographs of the right and left TMJs. Note the severity of the superior and posterior condylar displacement. **(D)** Pretreatment study casts showing the severity of the overbite. **(E and F)** Teeth marked "G" are gold crown abutments or pontics of old bridgework. Note the deep curve of Spee, which acts to both drive mandible back upon full occlusion and interfere (in the second molar area) with mandibular advancement techniques. **(G)** Sagittal II (splint) appliance to advance the upper teeth and provide a "splint effect" of pain relief to the TMJs. **(H)** Appliance at completion of the active-plate phase of treatment. Note the open screws on the appliance. The first phase of treatment with the Sagittal appliance lasted 7 months (active treatment and retention with the appliance acting as its own retainer.) **(I)** Brackets were placed to level, align, and rotate the teeth in final arch-perfecting steps for the maxillary dental arch. After the fixed appliance brackets were removed, a Gelb splint was used to treat the posterior open bite. It also acts to position the mandible down and forward so that the condyle is held in a stable and physiologically correct location (Gelb 4/7) during function. It will serve until bridges can be remade to the correct mandibular/condylar position. **(J and K)** Posttreatment correctness of (advanced) condylar position verified via transcranial radiography. Note the before and after changes in the size of the joint spaces. **(L and M)** Facial views 4 months posttreatment. No signs or symptoms of TMJ pain or dysfunction were present. (Courtesy of Dr. John Witzig.)

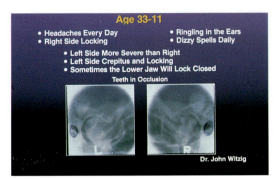

(C)

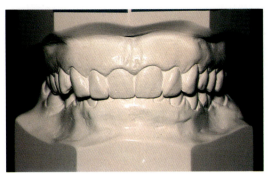

(D)

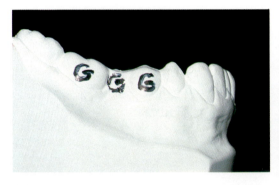

(E)

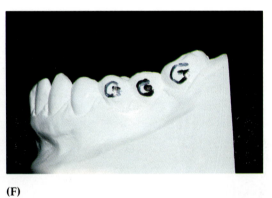

(F)

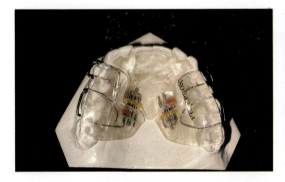

(G)

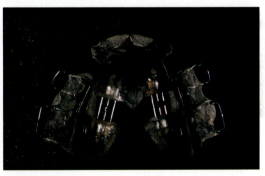

(H)

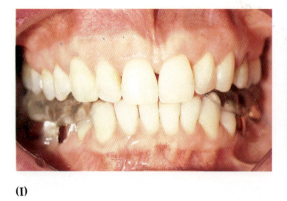

(I)

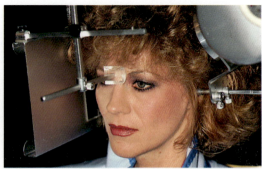

(J)

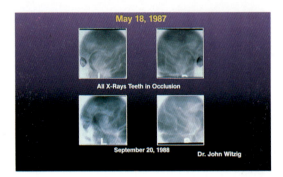

(K)

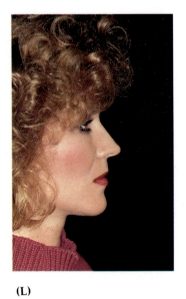

(L)

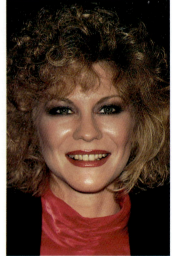

(M)

CASE HISTORY

PATIENT: Age: 12 years, 2 months

MAIN COMPLAINT:
1. Pain in front of ears, kept awake at night. Would take aspirin to get to sleep.
2. Headaches.
3. Wants teeth straightened.

FINDINGS:
1. Clicking both TMJs.
2. TMJs painful to palpation.
3. Painful to open normally.
4. Dental malocclusion with deep overbite, crowded cuspids, and retruded upper anterior teeth.
5. Incisal interference.

RADIOGRAPHIC FINDINGS:
1. Posterior-superior displaced condyles.

DIAGNOSIS: Internal derangement, both left and right TMJs.

TREATMENT:
1. Upper Sagittal (splint) appliance—13 months.
   Lower transverse appliance—wore same time as upper.
2. Upper straight wire appliance—6 months.
   Lower Sagittal appliance.
3. Upper retainer—4 months.
   1. Finish of treatment:
      a. No headaches.
      b. No pain by ears.
      c. Condyles are now down and forward in the temporal fossa.
      d. Teeth are straight.
      e. No clicking in TMJs.
   2. One year after retention.
      a. No headaches
      b. Opening of 44½ mm.
   3. Four years after
      a. No headaches

Figure 7–13 Combined orthodontic and TMJ treatment. **(A and B)** Pretreatment facial views of a 12-year-old girl with orthodontic malocclusion and TMJ pain and dysfunction. **(C–F)** Pretreatment occlusion. **(G–I)** Pretreatment study casts of occlusion. Even though the molars are near Class I dentally, notice the deep anterior overbite and steep "Division 2" angulation of the upper anteriors. This incisal interference with what would be a more orthopedically correct (advanced) mandibular arc of closure to final occlusion initiates the NRDM/SPDC phenomenon that forces the mandible-condyle unit too far back. **(J and K)** Progression radiography of the TMJs during treatment. **(L)** Panograph showing that arch crowding may be corrected via second molar replacement and Sagittal I distalizing techniques, but only after the anteriors are first moved far enough forward by using second molar anchorage. Then the remaining crowding (if still present) may be relieved via lateral development and/or distalization techniques (directional decrowding). **(M)** Patient wearing the Sagittal (splint) appliance. **(N)** Upper Sagittal appliance. **(O)** A lower transverse appliance (Schwarz appliance) was used because the lower arch needed development laterally to match the uppers. It was worn at the same time as the upper appliance (splint). Upper appliance worn actively for 4 months (screws turned twice a week to advance the uppers) and then passively as its own retainer for 11 months during which time the mandible autoadvanced! **(P and Q)** Upper arch after the Sagittal appliance has moved the teeth forward. **(R)** Straight-wire fixed appliance to level, align, and rotate the teeth and perfect the upper dental arch. **(S)** Posttreatment radiograph showing the third molars moved into position to replace the second ones. **(T)** Final occlusion 1 year postretention. **(U)** One year postretention (upper retainer used for 4 months after the brackets were removed). There were no signs or symptoms of TMJ pain or dysfunction. **(V and W)** Pretreatment cephalometric analysis (Functional Orthopedic) and printout. **(X and Y)** Posttreatment cephalometric analysis (Functional Orthopedic) and printout. (Courtesy of Dr. John Witzig.)

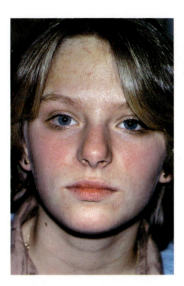

Figure 7–13(A)

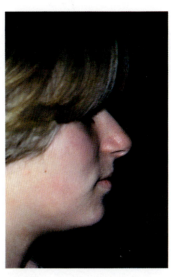

(B)

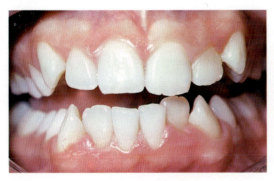

(C)

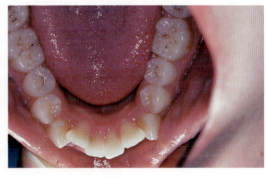

(D)

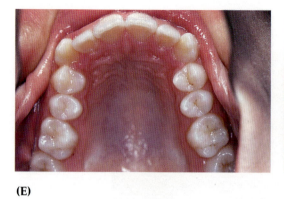

(E)

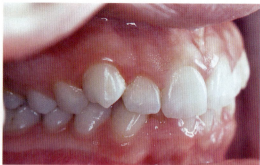

(F)

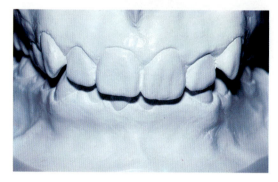

(G)

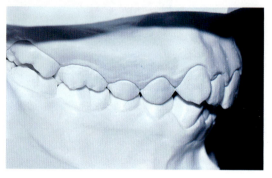

(H)

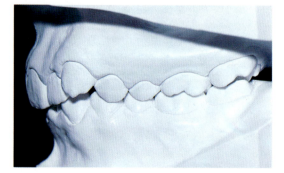

(I)

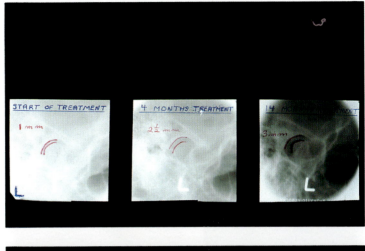

(J)

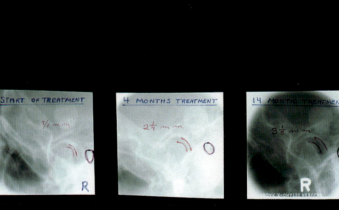

(K)

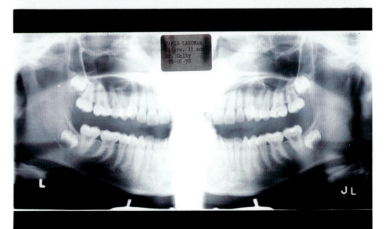

(L)

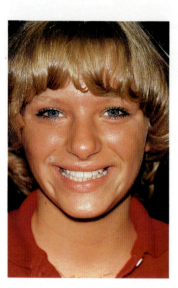

(M)

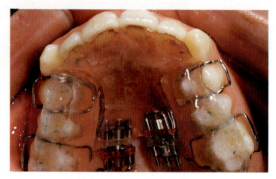

(N)

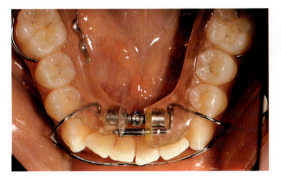

(O)

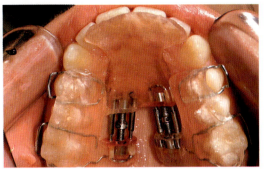

(P)

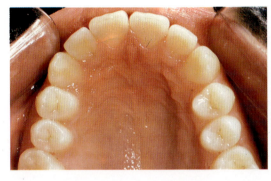

(Q)

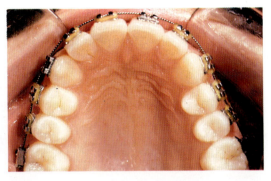

(R)

(S)

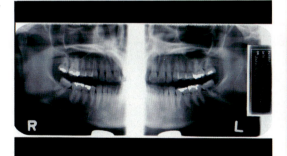

(T)

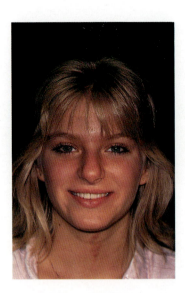

(U)

FUNCTIONAL ORTHOPEDIC ANALYSIS

MEASUREMENT	NORM	ACTUAL	COMMENT
A. RELATING THE MAXILLA TO THE CRANIAL BASE			
A Pt to N Perp	-2.0mm to 2.0mm	1.3mm	
B. RELATING THE MANDIBLE TO THE MAXILLA			
Eff. MAXILLA Lgth	***	88.7mm	
Eff. MANDIBLE Lgth	110.3mm to115.3mm	110.2mm	SHORT MANDIBLE
Diff=MAX-MAND Lgth	***	22.8mm	
Lower Facial Ht[Vert Dim]	62.3mm to 66.3mm	60.3mm	SHORT VERTICAL DIMENSION
C. RELATING THE UPPER INCISOR TO THE MAXILLA			
Up1 to A Perp	4.0mm to 6.0mm	3.9mm	
D. RELATING THE LOWER INCISOR TO THE MANDIBLE			
Low1 to A-Pg Line	1.0mm to 3.0mm	2.3mm	
E. MANDIBULAR POSITION			
Pg to N Perp	-5.4mm to -1.6mm	-3.7mm	
F. OTHER USEFUL CEPHALOMETRIC MEASUREMENTS			
SNA	80.0° to 84.0°	81.7°	
SNB	78.0° to 82.0°	77.5°	RETROGNATHIC MANDIBLE
ANB	0.0° to 4.0°	4.2°	SKELETAL CLASS II
Interincisal Angle	120.0° to140.0°	133.1°	
Mandibular Plane Angle	20.0° to 30.0°	19.9°	LOW VERTICAL DIMENSION
Facial Axis (Ricketts)	86.5° to 93.5°	88.1°	
WITS	-2.0mm to 2.0mm	3.2mm	SKELETAL II

ORTHO-DIAGNOST

(V)

FUNCTIONAL ORTHOPEDIC ANALYSIS.

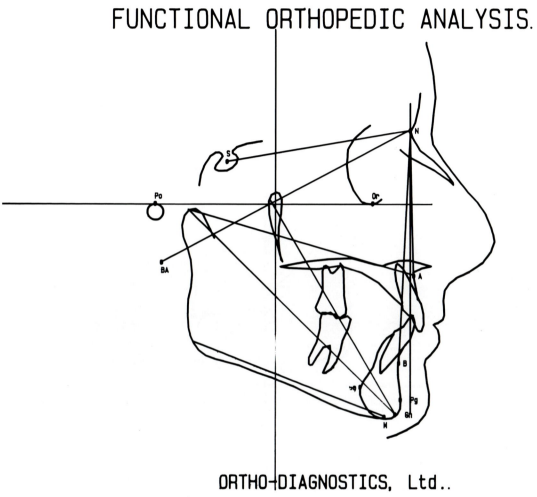

ORTHO-DIAGNOSTICS, Ltd..

(W)

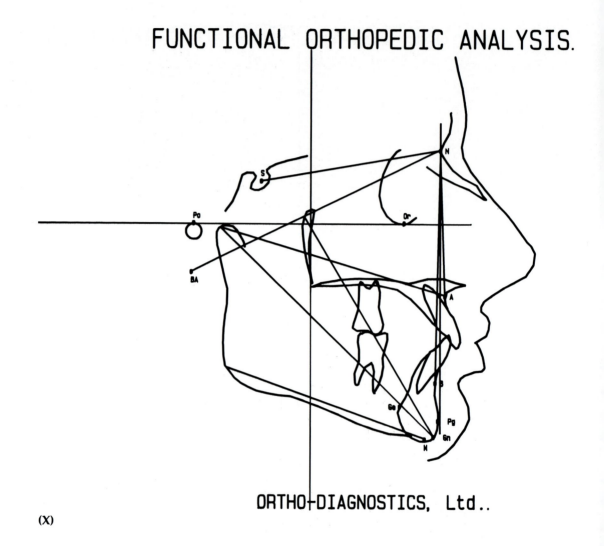

FUNCTIONAL ORTHOPEDIC ANALYSIS.

ORTHO-DIAGNOSTICS, Ltd..

(X)

FUNCTIONAL ORTHOPEDIC ANALYSIS

MEASUREMENT	NORM	ACTUAL	COMMENT
A. RELATING THE MAXILLA TO THE CRANIAL BASE			
A Pt to N Perp	-1.0mm to 3.0mm	1.8mm	
B. RELATING THE MANDIBLE TO THE MAXILLA			
Eff. MAXILLA Lgth	***	88.7mm	
Eff. MANDIBLE Lgth	110.2mm to115.2mm	113.1mm	
Diff=MAX-MAND Lgth	***	26.2mm	
Lower Facial Ht[Vert Dim]	62.2mm to 66.3mm	61.2mm	SHORT VERTICAL DIMENSION
C. RELATING THE UPPER INCISOR TO THE MAXILLA			
Up1 to A Perp	4.0mm to 6.0mm	5.9mm	
D. RELATING THE LOWER INCISOR TO THE MANDIBLE			
Low1 to A-Pg Line	1.0mm to 3.0mm	3.1mm	
E. MANDIBULAR POSITION			
Pg to N Perp	-3.9mm to 0.9mm	-0.8mm	
F. OTHER USEFUL CEPHALOMETRIC MEASUREMENTS			
SNA	80.0° to 84.0°	82.0°	
SNB	78.0° to 82.0°	78.9°	
ANB	0.0° to 4.0°	3.1°	SKELETAL CLASS I
Interincisal Angle	120.0° to140.0°	125.5°	
Mandibular Plane Angle	20.0° to 30.0°	18.6°	LOW VERTICAL DIMENSION
Facial Axis (Ricketts)	86.5° to 93.5°	85.9°	CLOSED BITE TENDENCIES
WITS	-2.0mm to 2.0mm	0.6mm	SKELETAL CLASS I

(Y)

CASE HISTORY

PATIENT: Age: 19 years, 11 months.

MAIN COMPLAINT: Left TMJ is cracking, sore, and aching. Headaches.

FINDINGS:
1. Clicking in both TMJs.
2. Class II/Division 1 malocclusion, with crowding and anterior open bite. First bicuspids and all anterior, upper and lower, are in open bite.
3. Maximum openings = 39½ mm.

RADIOGRAPHIC FINDINGS:
1. Posterior—superior displaced condyles, both TMJs.
2. Bone loss on both condyles.
3. Arthritic changes, both TMJs.

DIAGNOSIS: Internal derangement both left and right TMJs, with degenerative arthritis.

TREATMENT:
1. Upper second molar removal, third molar replacement.
2. Seven months—upper transverse splint.
3. Lower second molar removal, third molar replacement.
4. Nine months—Orthopedic Corrector II appliance to change Class II to Class I occlusion and bring condyles down and forward. Averaged 13 hours of wear daily.

RESULTS:
1. Headaches stopped.
2. No pain in either TMJ. Left TMJ "clicks" occasionally.
3. Opening of 50 mm.
4. Patient has been seen posttreatment once a year for 4 consecutive years. No recurring headaches and no TMJ pain.
5. Condyles are no longer posteriorly-superiorly displaced.

Figure 7–14 Anterior open-bite/TMJ case. Sometimes it is not anterior incisal interference that initiates the NRDM/SPDC phenomenon, but rather posterior bicuspid and/or molar interference that prevents the mandible from biting as far forward as the condyle-disc units would like. Posterior maxillary crossbites are hard on TMJs. So is maxillary posterior arch narrowing. Also it must be remembered that when the condyles start "melting down" due to functional abuse-inititated regressive remodeling the anterior bite tends to open. **(A and B)** Pretreatment facial views of a 20-year-old female with severe TMJ problems. **(C)** Pretreatment anterior open-bite malocclusion. **(D)** Pretreatment transcranial radiograph. Note the extremely tight joint spaces and condylar resorption and deformity (a narrow upper arch forces the lower arch, hence the condyle, back too far upon full occlusion). **(E)** Panograph showing all third molars present. Removal of all second molars prior to lateral development allows for better stability and less chance of recrowding. Since the upper thirds can easily replace the seconds at this age (although it would be almost too late for the lowers to do so) and since lateral development of the maxillary arch will be the initial phase of treatment in this case, all four second molars were removed. **(F)** Upper Transverse appliance with occlusal pads of acrylic to give a "splint effect" and relieve TMJ abuses. Activation of screws gradually widens the arch so that it will be compatible with a wider lower arch once the lower arch is advanced. **(G) (H)** Since not only mandibular retrusion but also an anterior open bite exists in this patient, an Orthopedic Corrector II (OCII) is the next appliance used. After 7 months (active and passive) of treatment with the Transverse (splint) appliance the OCII is used to steadily advance the mandible and close down the anterior open bite (which becomes progressively more difficult as the patient passes from childhood to adolescence on through to young adulthood. **(I,J)** Facial view and transcranial radiographs 1 month after completion of the OCII phase of treatment and closing down of the anterior open bite. **(K and L)** Appearance of the patient and occlusion 1 year after completion of treatment. **(M–O)** Posttreatment study casts. **(P)** Posttreatment panograph 2 years after appliances. Note how the third molars replaced the second ones nicely, even on the lower arch, quite a task for the lowers considering the patient's age! **(Q and R)** Pretreatment cephalometric analysis (Sassouni Plus) **(S and T)** Posttreatment cephalometric analysis (Sassouni Plus) (Courtesy of Dr. John Witzig.)

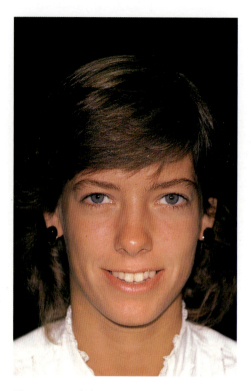 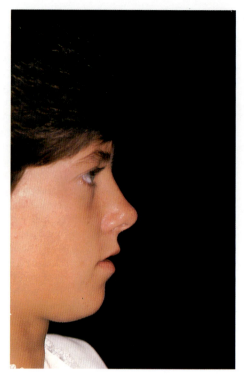

Figure 7–14(A)   **(B)**

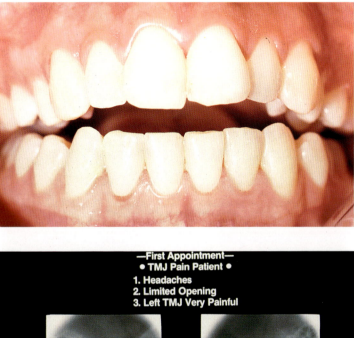

(C)

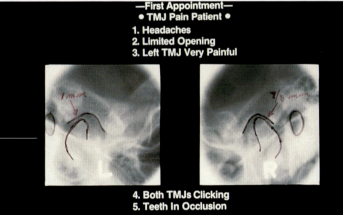

(D)

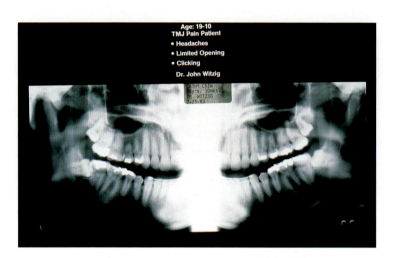

(E)

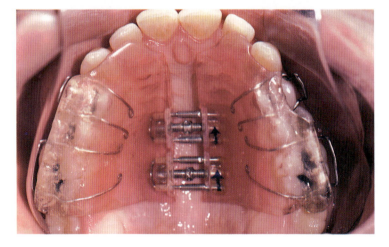

(F)

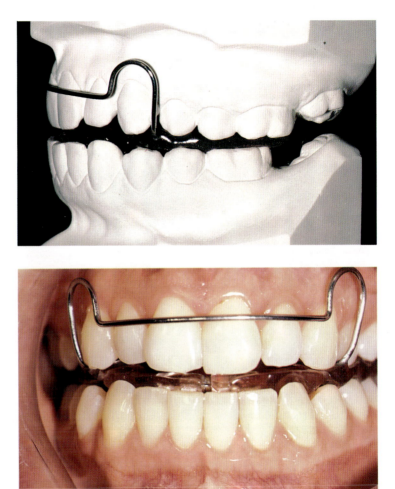

(G)

(H)

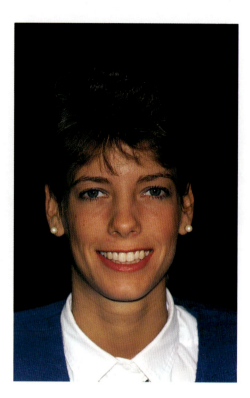

(I)

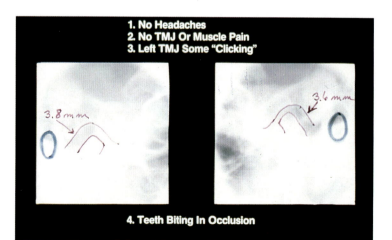

(J)

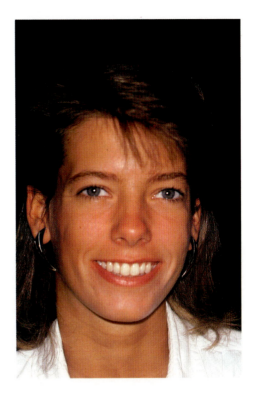

(K)

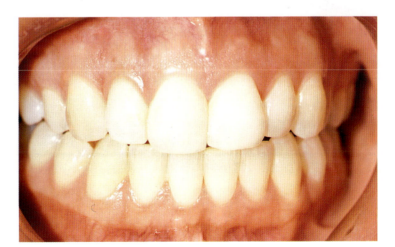

(L)

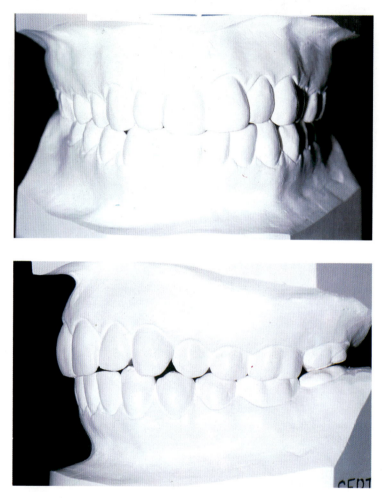

(M)

(N)

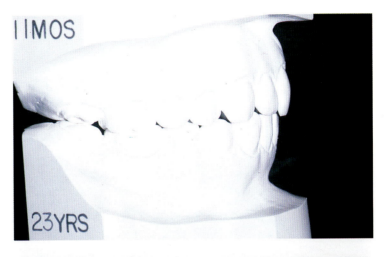

(O)

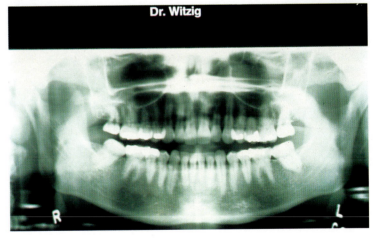

(P)

SASSOUNI PLUS.

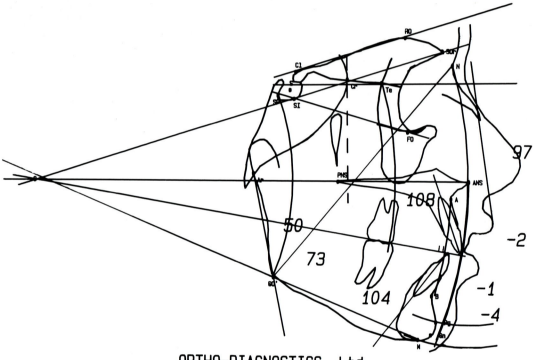

ORTHO-DIAGNOSTICS, Ltd..

(Q)

SASSOUNI PLUS

SKELETAL AP . . . . Class I with Class II Tendency

SKELETAL VERTICAL . . Normal with Open Bite Tendency

UPPER INCISOR . . . . . Retrusive

LOWER INCISOR . . . . . Protrusive

GROWTH DIRECTION . . . Clockwise tendency

MAXILLA LENGTH . . . . Long Posteriorly

MAXILLA POSITION . . . Normal

UPPER 6 POSITION . . . Anterior

MANDIBLE LENGTH . . . . Short Anteriorly Posteriorly

MANDIBLE POSITION . Undefined

UPPER LIP ANGLE . . . . Flat

MEASUREMENTS

SKELETAL AP
   B point is posterior to the A arc by 1.3 mm.
   ANS is anterior to the anterior arc by 0.4 mm.
   Pg is posterior to the anterior arc by 3.8 mm.
SKELETAL vERTICAL
   Vertical Dimension is long relative to age adjusted 'normal' by 4.0 mm.
UPPER INCISOR
   The tip of the maxillary central incisor is posterior
to the ANS arc by 1.5 mm.
LOWER INCISOR
   The tip of the mandibular central incisor has anterior
relation to the mandibular plane of 9.9 degrees.
GROWTH DIRECTION

MAXILLA LENGTH
   The maxilla is long by 4.9 mm.
MAXILLA POSITION
   PNS is posterior to the Cr 'vertical' by 4.5 mm.
UPPER 6 POSITION
   The upper first permanent molar is anterior
to the mid-facial arc by 1.6 mm.
MANDIBLE LENGTH
   The mandible is short relative to the cranial base by 7.7 mm.
MANDIBLE POSITION
   Actual Gonion is anterior to normal gonion by 4.2 mm.
UPPER LIP ANGLE
   The upper lip angle has posterior relation to the optic plane of 7.7 deg.
UPPER INCISOR ANGLE: 108.5 degrees
WITS: 1.9 mm

(R)

SASSOUNI PLUS.

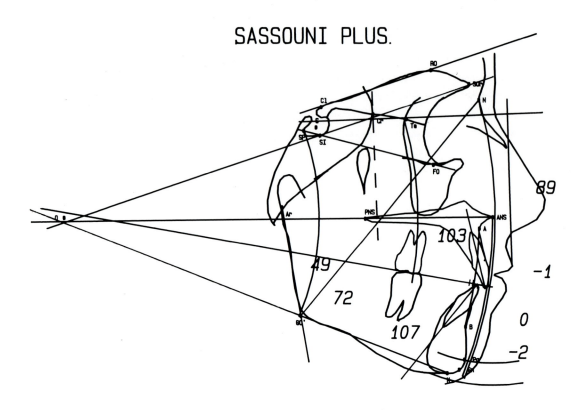

ORTHO-DIAGNOSTICS, Ltd..

(S)

SASSOUNI PLUS

SKELETAL AP . . . . Class I

SKELETAL VERTICAL . . Normal

UPPER INCISOR . . . . . Retrusive

LOWER INCISOR . . . . . Protrusive

GROWTH DIRECTION . . . Clockwise tendency

MAXILLA LENGTH . . . . Long Posteriorly

MAXILLA POSITION . . . Posterior

UPPER 6 POSITION . . . Anterior

MANDIBLE LENGTH . . . . Short Anteriorly Posteriorly

MANDIBLE POSITION . Undefined

UPPER LIP ANGLE . . . . Retruded

MEASUREMENTS

SKELETAL AP
   B point is anterior to the A arc by 0.1 mm.
   ANS is posterior to the anterior arc by 1.2 mm.
   Pg is posterior to the anterior arc by 2.1 mm.
SKELETAL VERTICAL
   Vertical Dimension is long relative to age adjusted 'normal' by 1.8 mm.
UPPER INCISOR
   The tip of the maxillary central incisor is posterior
to the ANS arc by 1.1 mm.
LOWER INCISOR
   The tip of the mandibular central incisor has anterior
relation to the mandibular plane of 12.1 degrees.
GROWTH DIRECTION

MAXILLA LENGTH
   The maxilla is long by 4.1 mm.
MAXILLA POSITION
   PNS is posterior to the Cr 'vertical' by 5.3 mm.
UPPER 6 POSITION
   The upper first permanent molar is anterior
to the mid-facial arc by 2.6 mm.
MANDIBLE LENGTH
   The mandible is short relative to the cranial base by 8.0 mm.
MANDIBLE POSITION
   Actual Gonion is anterior to normal gonion by 4.5 mm.
UPPER LIP ANGLE
   The upper lip angle has posterior relation to the optic plane of 15.6 deg.
UPPER INCISOR ANGLE: 102.8 degrees
WITS: -1.5 mm

ORTHO - DIAGNOSTICS, LTD.

(T)

"Books are good enough in their own way,
But they are a mighty bloodless substitute for life."

Robert Louis Stevenson, 1850–1894

CHAPTER 8
Why Stop?

There are few things of this temporal world that satisfy like the individual's own participation in the triumph of right principles. It truly takes a great deal of courage for us to stand firm for the sake of the well-being of the patient against the conflicts to health represented by the onslaughts of disease and degeneration. Yet in these controversial times relative to orthodontic therapeutics, it may take even greater courage to stand firm for the sake of our convictions against the conflicts represented by dissension toward new ideas that might occur among ourselves. Such is the plight of the modern-day practitioner who now has the privilege of availing himself of a broader and more extended range of orthodontic and maxillofacial orthopedic treatment modalities than was ever possible at any previous time in the profession's history. We stand at the dawn of a new era of development in which high technology will steadily expand the horizons of our knowledge and abilities ever farther. With such advancements will no doubt come even more sweeping new ideas to challenge the limits of our progress as did those represented by some of the aspects of the philosophical approach of functional jaw orthopedics (FJO). Some of these new ideas will merely augment those more basic tenets already in existence. Others will completely replace former ones altogether. However, in many instances this will not occur rapidly but rather by degrees, and not without a certain amount of professional growing pains. It is difficult to leave the comforts of therapeutic familiarity and strike out toward new and more advanced forms of treatment. Yet fortune is ally to the brave; therefore it is a journey each health care professional must endeavor to take because only we have the power and the resources to do so. The patients cannot do it for themselves. They rely on us.

With the internal turmoil brought about by rapidly changing circumstances, we must not lose sight of the fine example of those who have gone before us in this field. Their professionalism and dedication to the advancement of the science always acted as a standard by which they judged the value of their efforts. Theirs was a high-trust, low-fear environment that served to help not only their patients but also each other. With the more technically advanced environments of our modern times, it may be quietly wondered by some if maybe a little of this standard has been sadly lost, like so many other of the more human things of the past. When confronted with similar circumstances in our own professional careers, we should endeavor to evaluate both our activities and our services relative to three main areas of concern: the patient, the practitioner, and the profession!

Relative to the patient, we should evaluate a particular technique or procedure not only for what it does to a specific component of that patient but also as to how it affects the total patient, and we should ensure that it be consistent with the overriding concepts of total patient care. Earlier on in the development of the discipline, orthodontics seemed to focus its concentration on the arrangement of teeth alone and seemed less concerned with deeper structures further distally in the maxillofacial complex. The attractive smile anteriorly served as one of its paramount ends. Simplistically, it started at the front and worked its way back in the shaping of the mouth. However, in these modern days in which the clinician has the ability to unleash the tremendous powers of structurally oriented maxillofacial orthopedic appliances, the approach should be most properly changed to one of starting at the back, at the very foundations of the maxillofacial complex itself, i.e., the temporomandibular joint, and therapeutically working forward. We should conceptually build from there, and once the foundations have been secured fast, we may go on to create the anterior relationships in their full balance and beauty accordingly. The therapeutic government of the temporomandibular joint, this most basic and fundamental of structural entities, now lies fully within the realm of the discipline of orthodontics, which is exactly as it should be. We've finally come all the way.

Relative to the practitioner, we should evaluate the amenities and benefits that our treatment modalities generate, not only for our patients, but also for ourselves. Our patients are very important, to be sure, and their safe keeping is the lofty end to which we subjugate the efforts of our talents, but we as practitioners are important too. In spite of the cold intervening finger of technology, ours is still a science of humans treating humans. The newer methods and approaches to treating malocclusions described in this series of texts bring with them the blessings of not only making things easier and better for the patient but also easier and better for the doctor! Not only are the levels of intensity of personal efforts often reduced for the individual practitioner in much of the technique of FJO methodology, but the technique also brings with it the satisfaction in many cases of far superior results to those obtained with other methods. As a result, discerning clinicians experience higher levels of satisfaction with their daily efforts and a greatly diminished degree of frustration that, due to the inherently compulsive nature of most practitioners, can erode over a period of time even the most stalwart of characters. A professional career in a field as dynamic as dentistry should be one of a path of ascent and exhilaration, not a gauntlet of rigor and degeneration. The high level of professional skills represented by the modern-day practitioner was obtained at a price dearly paid in human terms. The successful clinician should be rewarded for his efforts by something more than just a fee.

Relative to the profession, we should judge our activities by their ability to either deter or enhance that single most shining attribute of our profession—knowledge. Knowledge provides the academic backbone that allows the profession to stand firm and is the foundation upon which is built the body of the services it delivers. It is knowledge that provides the energy and driving force that allow the practitioner to succeed in his battle against disease and deformity. It has always been likened to a light that dispels the darkness of ignorance and confusion. As a guiding beacon, it serves not only to lead us to higher levels of consciousness, but actually becomes a power, maybe the only true and most absolute form of power there is! Yet there is another facet to consider here. It is that knowledge for its own sake, knowledge that is confined, knowledge without direction is all but power*less*. When the guiding and facilitating power of knowledge comes into its full force is when it takes on the characteristics of disseminated knowledge. It is only then that the most good may be derived from its existence. Then it no longer portrays itself as a master but rather assumes the role of a servant. By virtue of the very nature of its philosophical approach and enhanced by the ingenuity of its techniques, the knowledge represented by the discipline of FJO is truly a power ready for dissemination to the general body of dental professionals. With this power, of course, comes the obligation and responsibility to manage it wisely. It is the duty of the individual practitioner to assume this responsibility forthrightly and ensure that the powers such knowledge represents are used properly and correctly in the treatment of the patient. Given access to such powers, the professional integrity of the main body of practitioners may be relied upon to guide the practical application of such entities and ensure that seldom if ever will it be abused to an untoward result. The wide distribution of this type of knowledge to the profession at large serves a noble end. For not only are a greater number of health care professionals going to be engaged in its use, but more importantly, as a result an even greater number of patients will become the direct recipients of its benefits. This in turn will free the orthodontic specialists and individuals who limit their practices exclusively to this particular discipline to aggressively advance the cause of the treatment of the more difficult malocclusions to even greater heights. Unburdened by the large number of what may be referred to by modern standards as "garden variety" cases, the specialists may devote more of their advanced training and skills toward the refinement of existing procedures or even the exploration of new and uncharted areas of the science, a movement that is sorely needed. Just how the demographics of orthodontic health care delivery will change in the near future is open to some degree of speculation, but one thing is becoming evident. To the mutual benefit of the patients, the practitioners, and the profession as a whole, it appears that the days of the practice of orthodontics being limited to an inner circle of a gifted few are over!

As stated at the onset, this series of texts was never intended to be a compendium of all forms of orthodontic technique. We have devoted our discussion to only those fundamental appliances and techniques pertinent to basic maxillofacial orthopedics. By necessity we have delved into the intricacies of various techniques, but have also stressed the basic concepts of treatment so that the knowledge of *how* we do it may also be accompanied by the knowledge of *why* we do it. It is also hoped that the information contained in these pages will act as a catalyst and a guide to stimulation of further study in the areas supportive to this field. Although some of the material discussed may at first seem difficult to those unfamiliar with a given technique or concept, with time and practical application the warm comforts of familiarity will soon develop and allow the mind to probe even deeper into the meaning of what is transpiring. For although initial technical knowledge is necessary to begin the use of such methodologies, such primary knowledge can only act as a medium for approaching a different kind of knowledge on a far deeper level, a level that allows one to not merely know but, more importantly, to understand. It is this understanding that liberates the practitioner to maximize the benefits to be derived from making individual judgments on each case and that allows that case to be brought to its finest level of completion.

The basic goal of this trilogy is to serve as a introductory medium to those totally unfamiliar with the FJO philosophy of treating malocclusions. The material may at times sound simplistic and may appear to skirt a variety of issues pertinent to modern-day treatment of maxillofacial dysplasias and temporomandibular joint conditions. But this is by design, not by accident. It is hoped that the general knowledge contained in these chapters will act as a foundation, a germ from which further pursuits in extending the range of one's technical expertise may blossom. The amount of information contained herein may give one to believe that the subject matter travels far beyond the realm of the mere introductory level, especially when it is practically applied in the treatment of patients suffering from the types of malocclusions discussed. However, by virtue of the organized and methodical approach used in describing FJO treatment techniques, the clinician will find that the insights derived from this somewhat agrestic little series of texts will truly enable one to correctly and successfully treat an incredible number of cases that present on a daily basis. Within a period of time and after a certain amount of clinical experience is gained in these methods, the temptation may become strong in the individual to tout the new found powers as a sort of intellectual lavaliere, if not externally, then at least internally. But no matter how extensive our knowledge becomes, it is infinitesimal when compared with what must yet be learned. The word *doctor* means "teacher." We all learn from others who have gone before us and in turn contribute each in our own way to those who will follow. But one thing will be certain, the more we broaden the borders of our horizon of technical expertise, the more there will be for us to expand ourselves into. Scientific knowledge is multiplying at an ever-increasing rate. In our efforts to merely keep current with the latest developments in the dental arts, we must not lose sight of the original purpose of the professional knowledge that we hope to continually advance. Ironically, in an age of extremely impersonal technological sophistication, the ultimate end of these efforts is still a very human one: the betterment of the plight of our fellow humans, the charges for whom we have been delegated the responsibility of rendering health care. This is why it has been emphatically stated that one of the cardinal traits of the FJO system has been its overwhelmingly human appeal to both patient and practitioner alike. These texts have been written in a style purposefully designed to stress this attribute. The health care professions are, frankly, a stress-filled business. If a number of techniques are available, all of which accomplish the same end, there is nothing wrong with choosing that particular treatment method that works most expeditiously in a given practitioner's own hands. By the standards of our age, if something attains a goal more simply and easily, it is by its very nature automatically better. Although a commonly observed phenomenon, the inadvertent construction of a scholastic presidio of technique, which may serve to quell the apprehensive ego of the practitioner but of itself only forces the patient to adapt to its demands instead of vice versa, only serves to add to the gap in empathy between the practitioner and patient and retard the progress on this most important human level. What is far better is to strive to understand fundamental treatment principles so as to allow a liberated mind to aggressively create new and "better" techniques to serve the patient's needs, making the treatment fit the patient, not making the patient fit the treatment.

"Have you the lion's part written?
Pray you if it be, give it me,
for I am slow of study."
A Midsummer Night's Dream, *Act I, scene 2*
William Shakespeare

A FINAL CHARGE

As may be seen from a brief review of the material discussed in these pages, there is currently available an enormous amount of information and technical knowledge that is expanding at almost an exponential rate in all the subordinate fields of dental health care. Over a period of time these innovations and advancements gradually find their way into the common workings of daily office procedures. The practitioner who strives after new knowledge and endeavors to perpetually renew and expand his area of expertise is to be commended. One of the hallmarks of this profession is that its members undertake these measures of self-improvement entirely on their own initiative. Once having left the academic environment of the college or university in which they were trained, they continue supplementing their educational process by means of not only the accumulation of practical experience but also through collaboration with their professional colleagues, institutional or privately produced continuing education courses, professional journals, independent lectures, and alas, even from books! Those who assist and encourage their comrades in this continuous process of learning ennoble not only themselves but the entire profession as well. There are a number of clinical educators who provide excellent educational opportunities for working practitioners by means of offering entire series of courses devoted to the use and management of both fixed and removable orthodontic and orthopedic appliances. Although each individual clinical instructor is methodologically different in his own way and delves into varying aspects of this discipline according to his own particular tastes, each is nevertheless dedicated to the same cause. They sincerely promote the philosophies and techniques of orthodontics to the highest and most practicable levels for the sake of both the doctor and ultimately the patient, the latter being the prime purpose for which the profession exists. It would greatly behoove individuals pursuing knowledge and advancement in the field of orthodontics to hear as many of these fine instructors as time and circumstances permit. This offers the student-doctors the benefit of the vast clinical experience these clinical instructors possess and exposes them to the outlook of some of the various great minds in the field. After studying their points of view and sifting the information they offer in turn through the sieve of their own intelligence and judgment, the student-doctor listeners may draw out what they deem most appropriate to their own particular needs and situations. As their talents and skills progress, their judgment on these matters will become steadily more adroit, and they will be able to select and apply to their daily practices ever-increasing amounts of the vast body of practical information such instructors have to offer. However, due to the professional demands of a busy practice and the problems associated with managing the business aspects of that practice, there often arises the problem for the practitioner of fitting such periods of advanced study into an already substantially burdened schedule. A professional career in the health sciences serves the role of a "jealous mistress" in the lives of each of its participants, a mistress with which they must constantly wrestle over the attentions that are to be divided between professional advancement and their personal lives. It is for these reasons that individuals will select a pace for their own progress in the continuous learning process that is compatible with their own personal circumstances. But the pace selected by each individual is not important. What is important is that one way or another the effort be maintained.

It is universally accepted that with time and experience one's level of understanding will deepen. In the clinical applications of FJO principles or any other area of the healing arts, as this understanding becomes progressively more profound, one tends to conclude that the power to effect cures and manipulate Nature for the sake of the betterment of our fellow humans is *not* the result of any innate human-generated ability of the practitioner to heal but rather is due to a vital force that is ever present and has its source in Nature itself. We, as practitioners, are merely temporary stewards of this power, and although we may revel in the satisfaction of watching our treatments transform a disfiguring and potentially harmful malocclusion into a well-balanced, well-functioning thing of beauty, we must remember that the grand design for such has always been potentially present within the patient from the very start, even down to the level of being totally programmed and perpetually contained within the nucleus of each and every cell. Our appreciation and respect for such powers in Nature grows progressively with the depth of our understanding of the incredible levels of profundity of its truths. Its deepest of mysteries will long remain inaccessible to us on a level approaching that of the sacred. The serene dignity of these truths by their very essence gently commands to those who act as its attendants that a tribute of scholastic vigilance on their part be faithfully maintained.

And if there be a final thought in parting to be offered by this treatise, it would humbly present itself in the form of a charge to the reader to consider the proposition that since fate has delegated us as practitioners to stand as guardians over the physical well-being of our own kind, then not only is the proper scholastic maintenance and nurturing of this stewardship a professional right, but it is also a solemn obligation. Therefore, in light of this charge, it may be stated with all probity that the point at which we have now arrived in this discussion of orthodontic therapeutic technique is in fact not the end, but truly only just the beginning!

"For I have learned
To look on Nature, not as in the hour
Of thoughtless youth; but hearing oftentimes
The still, sad music of humanity,
Nor harsh, nor grating, though of ample power
To chasten and subdue. And I have felt
A presence that disturbs me with the joy
Of elevated thoughts; a sense sublime
Of something far more deeply interfused,
Whose dwelling is the light of setting suns,
And the round ocean and the living air,
And the blue sky, and in the mind of man."

"Lines Composed a Few Miles
Above Titern Abbey"
July 13, 1798
William Wordsworth, 1770–1850
English Poet Laureate

INDEX